ATLAS OF DISEASES OF THE

KIDNEY

ATLAS OF DISEASES OF THE

KIDNEY

VOLUME ONE

Volume Editors

Tomas Berl, MD

Head, Division of Renal Diseases and Hypertension

University of Colorado School of Medicine

Denver, Colorado

Joseph V. Bonventre, MD, PhD

Massachusetts General Hospital

Charlestown, Massachusetts

Series Editor

Robert W. Schrier, MD

Professor and Chairman

Department of Medicine

University of Colorado School of Medicine

Denver, Colorado

With 32 Contributors

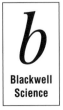

Blackwell Science

Developed by Current Medicine Inc., Philadelphia

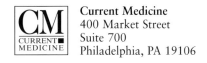

Current Medicine
400 Market Street
Suite 700
Philadelphia, PA 19106

Director of Product Development	*Lori J. Bainbridge*
Developmental Editor	*Paul Arthur*
Assistant Editor	*Debbie Singer*
Art Director	*Paul Fennessy*
Design and Layout	*Rick Ward, Erika Mangan, Christopher Allan*
Illustration Director	*Ann Saydlowski*
Illustrators	*Beth Starkey, Wendy Jackelow, Lisa Messina, Paul Schiffmacher, Lisa Weischedel, Debra Wertz*
Cover Design	*Rick Ward*
Cover Illustration	*Beth Starkey*
Production	*Lori Holland, Amy Watts*
Indexing	*Linda Van Pelt*

Atlas of diseases of the kidney/editor, Robert W. Schrier.
   p. cm.
   Includes bibliographical references and index.
   Contents: v.1. Disorders of water, electrolytes, and acid base/[edited by]
Tomas Berl; Acute renal failure/[edited by] Joseph V. Bonventre
   ISBN 0-632-04385-7
   1. Kidney Diseases atlases. I. Schrier, Robert W.
   [DNLM: 1. Kidney Diseases atlases. WJ 17A8812 1998]
RC903.A846   1998
616.6'1'00222—dc21
DNLM/DLC
for Library of Congress   98-5985
                                                       CIP

Library of Congress Cataloging-in-Publication Data
ISBN 0-632-04385-7

Printed in the United States of America by Quebcor.
5 4 3 2 1

Series Preface

The *Atlas of Diseases of the Kidney* series offers unique educational images including colored photographs, schematics, tables, and algorithms. The nine section editors have selected contributing authors who are not only experts in their field but are also superb educators. The resultant five volumes contain 67 chapters with more than 2500 images and provide the best teaching materials available in the field. In Volume I, disorders of water and sodium balance; potassium, magnesium, phosphate, and calcium metabolism; and acid-base balance are eloquently covered in Tomas Berl's section. Joseph Bonventre edited the section on acute renal failure including ischemic and nephrotoxic insults. His contributors assembled lucid and state-of-the-art educational materials related to the cellular and molecular mechanisms of renal injury and repair. Diagnostic evaluation, renal histology, nutrition and support therapies including intermittent hemodialysis, peritoneal dialysis, and continuous renal replacement therapies are illustrated.

The exciting advances in immunopathology and the latest treatments of the glomerulonephritides and vasculitides are the focus of the first half of Volume II, coedited and written by Richard Glassock and Arthur Cohen. Jean Pierre Grünfeld is the editor for section covering the numerous causes of tubulointerstitial disease. These include urinary tract infections, reflux, obstruction, cystic diseases, metabolic disorders, and the array of renal tubular disorders.

The kidney and hypertension are interrelated in cause and effect: renal parenchymal disease causes hypertension, and hypertension contributes to the progression of renal disease. Adrenal, renal vascular, and diabetes are other topics discussed in Volume III, ably edited by Christopher Wilcox. The final chapters in this volume deal with urgent and emergent hypertension as well as the treatment of hypertension.

Saulo Klahr edited Volume IV, which deals with the spectrum of systemic diseases and the kidney. Malignancies, paraproteinemias, HIV, hepatitis, cryoglobulinemia, sickle cell disease, sarcoidosis, and tropical diseases are just a few of the systemic diseases that affect the kidney and are addressed in this volume. Images of kidney diseases and hypertension are also included.

William Henrich edited the section of Volume V on dialysis as treatment of end stage renal disease. Principles of hemodialysis and peritoneal dialysis are followed by excellent images related to dialysate composition, access, recirculation, and prescription. The numerous complications of dialysis are also covered. The final section of Volume V on transplantation as a treatment of end-stage renal diseases is edited by William Bennett. As the first vital major organ to be successfully transplanted, many advances in histocompatibility, immunosuppressive therapy, and surgical technique of renal transplantation are well presented. Posttransplant and treatment, rejections, infections, complications, and recurrent disease are also covered in this section as is transplantation in children and kidney-pancreas transplants.

These section editors and authors deserve the major credit for this exciting Atlas of Diseases of the Kidney, which was initiated by Abe Krieger, president of Current Medicine. Thanks also to the developmental editor, Paul Arthur, the excellent illustrators at Current Medicine, as well as the support from Shirley Artese in my office.

Robert W. Schrier, MD

Contributors

HORACIO J. ADROGUÉ, MD
Professor
Department of Medicine
Baylor College of Medicine
Chief, Renal Section
Department of Veterans Affairs Medical Center
Houston, Texas

ROBERT J. ANDERSON, MD
Professor
Department of Medicine
University of Colorado
Denver, Colorado

ROBERT BACALLAO, MD
Associate Professor of Medicine
Department of Medicine
Indiana University
Clarian Health, Richard Roudebusch VAH
Indianapolis, Indiana

KEVIN T. BUSH, PhD
Postdoctoral Fellow
Department of Medicine
Harvard Medical School
Postdoctoral Fellow
Renal Division
Brigham and Women's Hospital
Boston, Massachusetts

MARC E. DE BROE, MD, PhD
Professor in Medicine
Department of Medicine/Nephrology
University Hospital Antwerp
Edegem, Antwerp
Belgium

WILFRED DRUML, MD
Professor
Department of Nephrology
Vienna General Hospital
Vienna, Austria

BRIAN G. DWINNEL, MD
Assistant Professor
University of Colorado Health Science Center
Denver, Colorado

DAVID H. ELLISON, MD
Associate Professor
Department of Internal Medicine
University of Colorado
Chief, Renal Section
VA Medical Center
Denver, Colorado

MICHAEL S. GOLIGORSKY, MD, PhD
Professor of Medicine and Physiology
Department of Medicine
State University of New York at Stony Brook
Stony Brook, New York

KATRINA J. KELLY, MD
Assistant Professor
Department of Internal Medicine
University of Cincinnati College of Medicine
Cincinnati, Ohio

RAJIV KUMAR, MBBS
Professor of Medicine
Department of Internal Medicine
Mayo Medical School
Chair, Division of Nephrology
Mayo Clinic
Rochester, Minnesota

SUMIT KUMAR, MB
Assistant Professor
Department of Medicine/Nephrology
Indiana University School of Medicine
Indianapolis, Indiana

MOSHE LEVI, MD
Professor
Department of Internal Medicine
University of Texas Southwestern Medical Center
Chief, Nephrology Section
VA North Texas Care System
Department of Nephrology
Renal Clinic
Dallas, Texas

FERNANDO LIAÑO, MD, PhD
Associate Professor
Department of Medicine
Universidad de Alcala
Alcala, Spain
Servicio de Nephrology
Hospital Ramon y Cajal
Madrid, Spain

WILFRED LIEBERTHAL, MD
Professor of Medicine
Department of Medicine
Boston University
Boston, Massachusetts

STUART L. LINAS, MD
Professor
Department of Medicine
University of Colorado
Chief of Nephrology
Denver Health Medical Center
Denver, Colorado

NICOLAOS E. MADIAS, MD
Professor of Medicine
Tufts University School of Medicine
Chief, Division of Nephrology
New England Medical Center
Boston, Massachusetts

JAMES T. MCCARTHY, MD
Professor of Medicine
Department of Internal Medicine
Mayo Medical School
Vice Chair, Division of Nephrology
Mayo Clinic
Rochester, Minnesota

RAVINDRA L. MEHTA, MD, MBBS
Associate Professor of Medicine
Department of Medicine
University of California San Diego School of Medicine
Associate Director of Dialysis
Division of Nephrology
University of California San Diego Medical Center
San Diego, California

STEVEN B. MILLER, MD
Associate Professor
Department of Internal Medicine/Nephrology
Washington University
Director
BJC/WUSM Renal Network
Barnes-Jewish Hospital
St. Louis, Missouri

BRUCE A. MOLITORIS, MD
Professor of Medicine
Indiana University
Director, Division of Nephrology
Clarian Health
Indianapolis, Indiana

CYNTHIA C. NAST, MD
Associate Professor
Department of Pathology
University of California, Los Angeles
Attending Pathologist
Cedars-Sinai Medical Center
Los Angeles, California

SANJAY K. NIGAM, MD
Associate Professor
Department of Medicine
Harvard Medical School
Associate Physician
Renal Division
Brigham and Women's Hospital
Boston, Massachusetts

FREDRICK V. OSORIO, MD
Nephrologist
East Valley Nephrology Associates
Mesa, Arizona

BABU J. PADANILAM, PhD
Research Assistant Professor
Department of Internal Medicine/Renal
Washington University
St. Louis, Missouri

JULIO PASCUAL, MD, PhD
Servicio de Nefrología
Hospital Ramon y Cajal
Madrid, Spain

MORDECAI POPOVTZER, MD
Professor of Medicine
Department of Nephrology and Hypertension
Chief, Nephrology and Hypertension Services
Director, Hadassah Jerusalem Osteoporosis Center
Hadassah University Hospital
Jerusalem, Israel

LORRAINE C. RACUSEN, MD
Assistant Professor
Department of Pathology
Johns Hopkins
Baltimore, Maryland

HIROYUKI SAKURAI, MD
Postdoctoral Fellow
Department of Medicine
Harvard Medical School
Postdoctoral Fellow
Renal Division
Brigham and Women's Hospital
Boston, Massachusetts

RICK G. SCHNELLMAN, PhD
Professor
Department of Pharmacology and Toxicology
University of Arkansas for Medical Sciences
Little Rock, Arkansas

KIM SOLEZ, MD
Professor of Pathology
Department of Laboratory Medicine and Pathology
University of Alberta
Edmonton, Alberta, Canada

TATSUO TSUKAMOTO, MD, PhD
Postdoctoral Fellow
Department of Medicine
Harvard Medical School
Renal Division
Brigham and Women's Hospital
Boston, Massachusetts

Contents

Disorders of Water, Electrolytes, and Acid-Base

Introduction
Tomas Berl

Over a century ago, Claude Bernard aptly noted that the medium in which we live is neither air nor water but rather the plasma that bathes all tissues. The maintenance of what he called the "interior environment" has been entrusted to the kidneys, which Homer Smith designated as the "master chemists" of this environment. The manner in which the kidneys fulfill the role to regulate the constancy and distribution of water and a number of electrolytes in body fluids is the subject of this section.

It is evident that the mechanisms whereby the volume and composition of extracellular fluid is maintained constant involves the regulated excretion of solute and water by the kidneys in quantities that match ingestion and metabolic production. The understanding of the processes that underlie the control of the renal excretion of solutes and water has evolved over the last three decades. Thus, one of the concepts that is graphically exposed in this volume reintroduces the reader to principles that have become integrated into general medical practice. However, the last 10 years have witnessed a virtual explosion in the unraveling of the structural complexity of the nephron and in the recognition of their functional heterogeneity. These years have also witnessed the isolation, characterization, and cloning of a large number of specific transporters and channel proteins. Studies on the regulation of these proteins have taken our understanding of the mechanisms that control the movement of solutes and water across diverse epithelia to the cellular and molecular level. Therefore, every chapter in this section contains descriptions of the cellular processes involved in the transport of the substance under discussion. The description of the transporters has also enhanced our knowledge of the manner in which diuretics operate to inhibit sodium excretion. Likewise, they have shed new light on the mechanism of a number of pathophysiologic conditions that are caused by inherited mutations leading to disorders of potassium, sodium, acid-base, and water balance. The nature of these disturbances is revealed in various chapters of this volume. They most likely provide only a first glimpse into what is likely to be a field of inquiry that will witness an explosion of new knowledge as we unravel the molecular basis of human disease.

The chapters of this section therefore bridge concepts in classic renal pathophysiology with today's understanding of cell transport and cell biology and place them in the context of clinically relevant disturbances of water and electrolyte metabolism. These graphically oriented chapters with descriptive text lucidly lay out to the reader the current knowledge of these disorders.

Diseases of Water Metabolism

Sumit Kumar
Tomas Berl

The maintenance of the tonicity of body fluids within a very narrow physiologic range is made possible by homeostatic mechanisms that control the intake and excretion of water. Critical to this process are the osmoreceptors in the hypothalamus that control the secretion of antidiuretic hormone (ADH) in response to changes in tonicity. In turn, ADH governs the excretion of water by its end-organ effect on the various segments of the renal collecting system. The unique anatomic and physiologic arrangement of the nephrons brings about either urinary concentration or dilution, depending on prevailing physiologic needs. In the first section of this chapter, the physiology of urine formation and water balance is described.

The kidney plays a pivotal role in the maintenance of normal water homeostasis, as it conserves water in states of water deprivation, and excretes water in states of water excess. When water homeostasis is deranged, alterations in serum sodium ensue. Disorders of urine dilution cause hyponatremia. The pathogenesis, causes, and management strategies are described in the second part of this chapter.

When any of the components of the urinary concentration mechanism is disrupted, hypernatremia may ensue, which is universally characterized by a hyperosmolar state. In the third section of this chapter, the pathogenesis, causes, and clinical settings for hypernatremia and management strategies are described.

CHAPTER

1

Physiology of the Renal Diluting and Concentrating Mechanisms

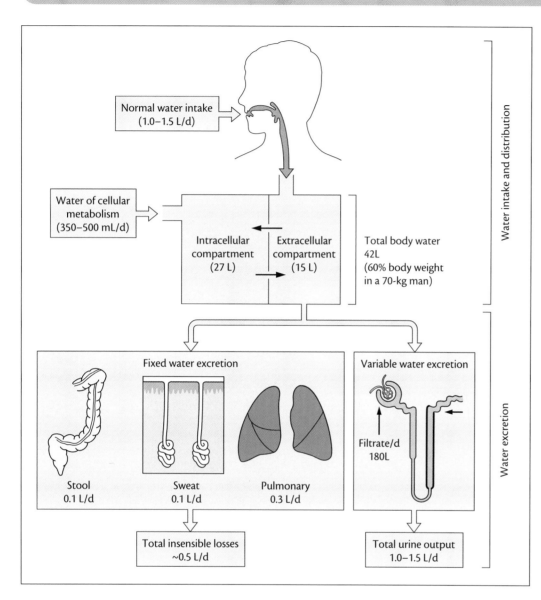

FIGURE 1-1

Principles of normal water balance. In most steady-state situations, human water intake matches water losses through all sources. Water intake is determined by thirst (*see* Fig. 1-12) and by cultural and social behaviors. Water intake is finely balanced by the need to maintain physiologic serum osmolality between 285 to 290 mOsm/kg. Both water that is drunk and that is generated through metabolism are distributed in the extracellular and intracellular compartments that are in constant equilibrium. Total body water equals approximately 60% of total body weight in young men, about 50% in young women, and less in older persons. Infants' total body water is between 65% and 75%. In a 70-kg man, in temperate conditions, total body water equals 42 L, 65% of which (22 L) is in the intracellular compartment and 35% (19 L) in the extracellular compartment.

Assuming normal glomerular filtration rate to be about 125 mL/min, the total volume of blood filtered by the kidney is about 180 L/24 hr. Only about 1 to 1.5 L is excreted as urine, however, on account of the complex interplay of the urine concentrating and diluting mechanism and the effect of antidiuretic hormone to different segments of the nephron, as depicted in the following figures.

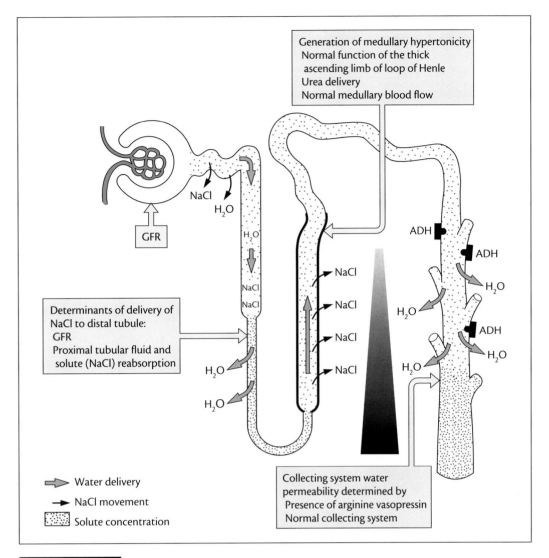

Water delivery

NaCl movement

Solute concentration

FIGURE 1-2

Determinants of the renal concentrating mechanism. Human kidneys have two populations of nephrons, superficial and juxtamedullary. This anatomic arrangement has important bearing on the formation of urine by the countercurrent mechanism. The unique anatomy of the nephron [1] lays the groundwork for a complex yet logical physiologic arrangement that facilitates the urine concentration and dilution mechanism, leading to the formation of either concentrated or dilute urine, as appropriate to the person's needs and dictated by the plasma osmolality. After two thirds of the filtered load (180 L/d) is isotonically reabsorbed in the proximal convoluted tubule, water is handled by three interrelated processes: 1) the delivery of fluid to the diluting segments; 2) the separation of solute and water (H_2O) in the diluting segment; and 3) variable reabsorption of water in the collecting duct. These processes participate in the renal concentrating mechanism [2].

1. *Delivery of sodium chloride (NaCl) to the diluting segments of the nephron* (thick ascending limb of the loop of Henle and the distal convoluted tubule) is determined by glomerular filtration rate (GFR) and proximal tubule function.
2. *Generation of medullary interstitial hypertonicity*, is determined by normal functioning of the thick ascending limb of the loop of Henle, urea delivery from the medullary collecting duct, and medullary blood flow.
3. *Collecting duct permeability* is determined by the presence of antidiuretic hormone (ADH) and normal anatomy of the collecting system, leading to the formation of a concentrated urine.

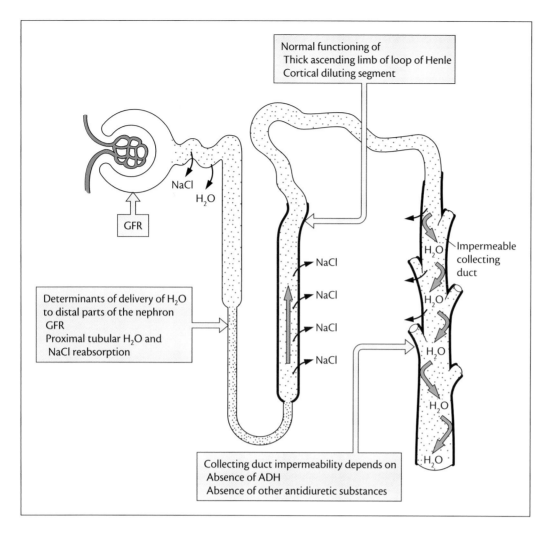

Normal functioning of
Thick ascending limb of loop of Henle
Cortical diluting segment

GFR

NaCl

H_2O

Determinants of delivery of H_2O
to distal parts of the nephron
GFR
Proximal tubular H_2O and
NaCl reabsorption

NaCl

NaCl

NaCl

NaCl

H_2O
H_2O
H_2O
H_2O
H_2O

Impermeable
collecting
duct

Collecting duct impermeability depends on
Absence of ADH
Absence of other antidiuretic substances

FIGURE 1-3

Determinants of the urinary dilution mechanism include 1) delivery of water to the thick ascending limb of the loop of Henle, distal convoluted tubule, and collecting system of the nephron; 2) generation of maximally hypotonic fluid in the diluting segments (*ie*, normal thick ascending limb of the loop of Henle and cortical diluting segment); 3) maintenance of water impermeability of the collecting system as determined by the absence of antidiuretic hormone (ADH) or its action and other antidiuretic substances. GFR—glomerular filtration rate; NaCl—sodium chloride; H_2O—water.

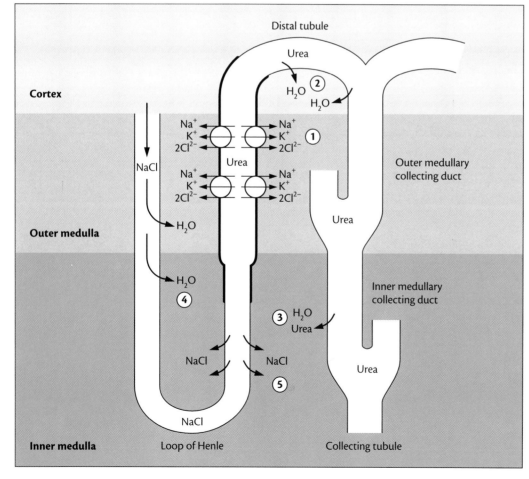

Cortex

Outer medulla

Inner medulla

Distal tubule

Urea

H_2O ②
H_2O

Na^+
K^+
$2Cl^{2-}$

Na^+
K^+
$2Cl^{2-}$ ①

NaCl   Urea

Na^+
K^+
$2Cl^{2-}$

Na^+
K^+
$2Cl^{2-}$

→ H_2O

→ H_2O
④

③ H_2O
Urea

NaCl   NaCl
⑤

NaCl

Loop of Henle

Outer medullary
collecting duct

Urea

Inner medullary
collecting duct

Urea

Collecting tubule

FIGURE 1-4

Mechanism of urine concentration: overview of the passive model. Several models of urine concentration have been put forth by investigators. The passive model of urine concentration described by Kokko and Rector [3] is based on permeability characteristics of different parts of the nephron to solute and water and on the fact that the active transport is limited to the thick ascending limb. 1) Through the Na^+, K^+, 2 Cl cotransporter, the thick ascending limb actively transports sodium chloride (NaCl), increasing the interstitial tonicity, resulting in tubular fluid dilution with no net movement of water and urea on account of their low permeability. 2) The hypotonic fluid under antidiuretic hormone action undergoes osmotic equilibration with the interstitium in the late distal tubule and cortical and outer medullary collecting duct, resulting in water removal. Urea concentration in the tubular fluid rises on account of low urea permeability. 3) At the inner medullary collecting duct, which is highly permeable to urea and water, especially in response to antidiuretic hormone, the urea enters the interstitium down its concentration gradient, preserving interstitial hypertonicity and generating high urea concentration in the interstitium.

(Legend continued on next page)

FIGURE 1-4 (continued)

4) The hypertonic interstitium causes abstraction of water from the descending thin limb of loop of Henle, which is relatively impermeable to NaCl and urea, making the tubular fluid hypertonic with high NaCl concentration as it arrives at the bend of the loop of Henle. 5) In the thin ascending limb of the loop of Henle, NaCl moves passively down its concentration gradient into the interstitium, making tubular fluid less concentrated with little or no movement of water. H_2O—water.

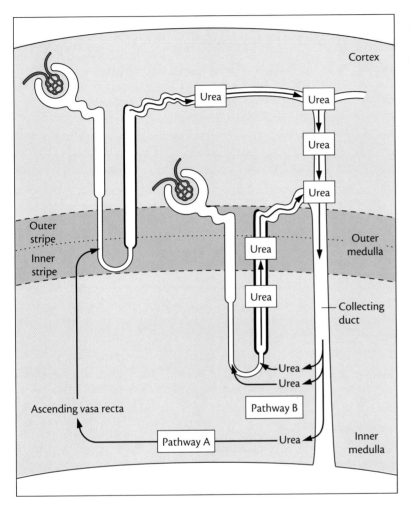

FIGURE 1-5

Pathways for urea recycling. Urea plays an important role in the generation of medullary interstitial hypertonicity. A recycling mechanism operates to minimize urea loss. The urea that is reabsorbed into the inner medullary stripe from the terminal inner medullary collecting duct (*step 3* in Fig. 1-4) is carried out of this region by the ascending vasa recta, which deposits urea into the adjacent descending thin limbs of a short loop of Henle, thus recycling the urea to the inner medullary collecting tubule (*pathway A*).

Some of the urea enters the descending limb of the loop of Henle and the thin ascending limb of the loop of Henle. It is then carried through to the thick ascending limb of the loop of Henle, the distal collecting tubule, and the collecting duct, before it reaches the inner medullary collecting duct (*pathway B*). This process is facilitated by the close anatomic relationship that the hairpin loop of Henle and the vasa recta share [4].

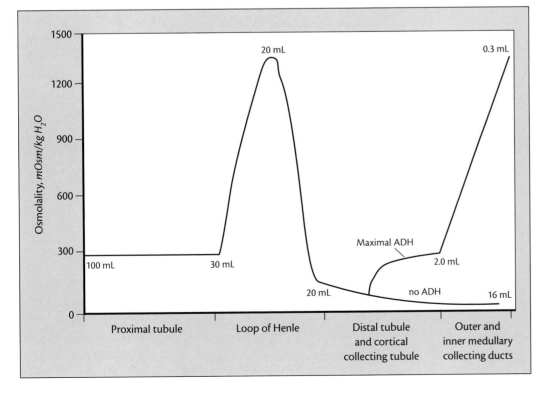

FIGURE 1-6

Changes in the volume and osmolality of tubular fluid along the nephron in diuresis and antidiuresis. The osmolality of the tubular fluid undergoes several changes as it passes through different segments of the tubules. Tubular fluid undergoes marked reduction in its volume in the proximal tubule; however, this occurs iso-osmotically with the glomerular filtrate. In the loop of Henle, because of the aforementioned countercurrent mechanism, the osmolality of the tubular fluid rises sharply but falls again to as low as 100 mOsm/kg as it reaches the thick ascending limb and the distal convoluted tubule. Thereafter, in the late distal tubule and the collecting duct, the osmolality depends on the presence or absence of antidiuretic hormone (ADH). In the absence of ADH, very little water is reabsorbed and dilute urine results. On the other hand, in the presence of ADH, the collecting duct, and in some species, the distal convoluted tubule, become highly permeable to water, causing reabsorption of water into the interstitium, resulting in concentrated urine [5].

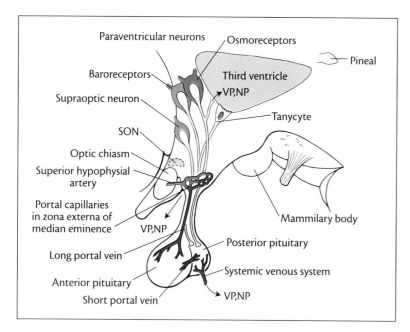

FIGURE 1-7

Pathways of antidiuretic hormone release. Antidiuretic hormone is responsible for augmenting the water permeability of the cortical and medullary collecting tubules, thus promoting water reabsorption via osmotic equilibration with the isotonic and hypertonic interstitium, respecively. The hormone is formed in the supraoptic and paraventricular nuclei, under the stimulus of osmoreceptors and baroreceptors (*see* Fig. 1-11), transported along their axons and secreted at three sites: the posterior pituitary gland, the portal capillaries of the median eminence, and the cerebrospinal fluid of the third ventricle. It is from the posterior pituitary that the antidiuretic hormone is released into the systemic circulation [6]. SON—supraoptic nucleus; VP—vasopressin; NP—neurophysin.

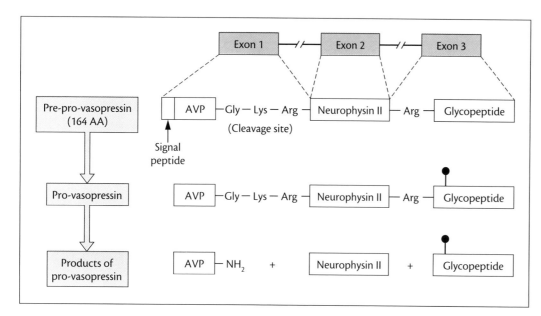

FIGURE 1-8

Structure of the human arginine vasopressin (AVP/antidiuretic hormone) gene and the prohormone. Antidiuretic hormone (ADH) is a cyclic hexapeptide (mol. wt. 1099) with a tail of three amino acids. The biologically inactive macromolecule, pre-pro-vasopressin is cleaved into the smaller, biologically active protein. The protein of vasopressin is translated through a series of signal transduction pathways and intracellular cleaving. Vasopressin, along with its binding protein, neurophysin II, and the glycoprotein, are secreted in the form of neurosecretory granules down the axons and stored in nerve terminals of the posterior lobe of the pituitary [7]. ADH has a short half-life of about 15 to 20 minutes and is rapidly metabolized in the liver and kidneys. Gly—glycine; Lys—lysine; Arg—arginine.

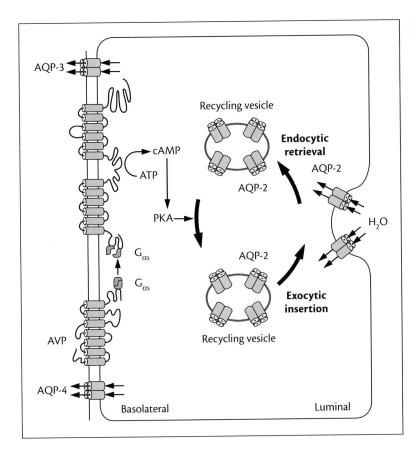

FIGURE 1-9

Intracellular action of antidiuretic hormone. The multiple actions of vasopressin can be accounted for by its interaction with the V2 receptor found in the kidney. After stimulation, vasopressin binds to the V2 receptor on the basolateral membrane of the collecting duct cell. This interaction of vasopressin with the V2 receptor leads to increased adenylate cyclase activity via the stimulatory G protein (Gs), which catalyzes the formation of cyclic adenosine 3', 5'-monophosphate (cAMP) from adenosine triphosphate (ATP). In turn, cAMP activates a serine threonine kinase, protein kinase A (PKA). Cytoplasmic vesicles carrying the water channel proteins migrate through the cell in response to this phosphorylation process and fuse with the apical membrane in response to increasing vasopressin binding, thus increasing water permeability of the collecting duct cells. These water channels are recyled by endocytosis once the vasopressin is removed. The water channel responsible for the high water permeability of the luminal membrane in response to vasopressin has recently been cloned and designated as aquaporin-2 (AQP-2) [8]. The other members of the aquaporin family, AQP-3 and AQP-4 are located on the basolateral membranes and are probably involved in water exit from the cell. The molecular biology of these channels and of receptors responsible for vasopressin action have contributed to the understanding of the syndromes of genetically transmitted and acquired forms of vasopressin resistance. AVP—arginine vasopressin.

AQUAPORINS AND THEIR CHARACTERISTICS

	AQP-1	AQP-2	AQP-3	AQP-4
Size (amino acids)	269	271	285	301
Permeability to small solutes	No	No	Urea glycerol	No
Regulation by antidiurectic hormone	No	Yes	No	No
Site	Proximal tubules; descending thin limb	Collecting duct; principal cells	Medullary collecting duct; colon	Hypothalamic—supraoptic, paraventricular nuclei; ependymal, granular, and Purkinje cells
Cellular localization	Apical and basolateral membrane	Apical membrane and intracellular vesicles	Basolateral membrane	Basolateral membrane of the prinicpal cells
Mutant phenotype	Normal	Nephrogenic diabetes insipidus	Unknown	Unknown

FIGURE 1-10

Aquaporins and their characteristics. An ever growing family of aquaporin (AQP) channels are being described. So far, about seven different channels have been cloned and characterized; however, only four have been found to have any definite physiologic role.

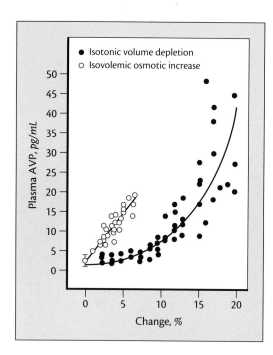

FIGURE 1-11

Osmotic and nonosmotic regulation of antidiuretic hormone (ADH) secretion. ADH is secreted in response to changes in osmolality and in circulating arterial volume. The "osmoreceptor" cells are located in the anterior hypothalamus close to the supraoptic nuclei. Aquaporin-4 (AQP-4), a candidate osmoreceptor, is a member of the water channel family that was recently cloned and characterized and is found in abundance in these neurons. The osmoreceptors are sensitive to changes in plasma osmolality of as little as 1%. In humans, the osmotic threshold for ADH release is 280 to 290 mOsm/kg. This system is so efficient that the plasma osmolality usually does not vary by more than 1% to 2% despite wide fluctuations in water intake [9]. There are several other nonosmotic stimuli for ADH secretion. In conditions of decreased arterial circulating volume (*eg*, heart failure, cirrhosis, vomiting), decrease in inhibitory parasympathetic afferents in the carotid sinus baroreceptors affects ADH secretion. Other nonosmotic stimuli include nausea, which can lead to a 500-fold rise in circulating ADH levels, postoperative pain, and pregnancy. Much higher ADH levels can be achieved with hypovolemia than with hyperosmolarity, although a large fall in blood volume is required before this response is initiated. In the maintenance of tonicity the interplay of these homeostatic mechanisms also involves the thirst mechanism, that under normal conditions, causes either intake or exclusion of water in an effort to restore serum osmolality to normal.

Control of Water Balance and Serum Sodium Concentration

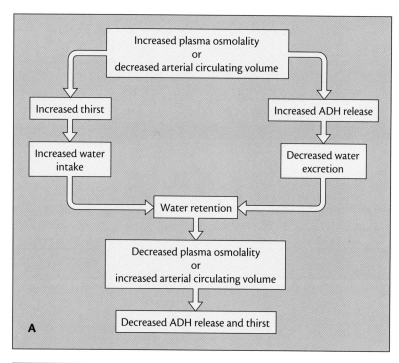

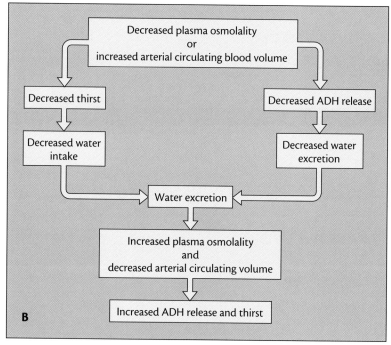

FIGURE 1-12

Pathways of water balance (conservation, **A**, and excretion, **B**). In humans and other terrestrial animals, the thirst mechanism plays an important role in water (H_2O) balance. Hypertonicity is the most potent stimulus for thirst: only 2% to 3 % changes in plasma osmolality produce a strong desire to drink water. This absolute level of osmolality at which the sensation of thirst arises in healthy persons, called the *osmotic threshold for thirst*, usually averages about 290 to 295 mOsm/kg H_2O (approximately 10 mOsm/kg H_2O above that of antidiuretic hormone [ADH] release). The so-called thirst center is located close to the osmoreceptors but is

anatomically distinct. Between the limits imposed by the osmotic thresholds for thirst and ADH release, plasma osmolality may be regulated still more precisely by small osmoregulated adjustments in urine flow and water intake. The exact level at which balance occurs depends on various factors such as insensible losses through skin and lungs, and the gains incurred from eating, normal drinking, and fat metabolism. In general, overall intake and output come into balance at a plasma osmolality of 288 mOsm/kg, roughly halfway between the thresholds for ADH release and thirst [10].

FIGURE 1-13

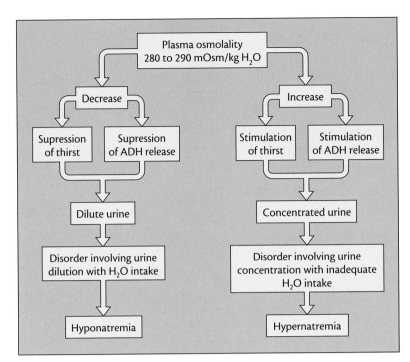

Pathogenesis of dysnatremias. The countercurrent mechanism of the kidneys in concert with the hypothalamic osmoreceptors via antidiuretic hormone (ADH) secretion maintain a very finely tuned balance of water (H_2O). A defect in the urine-diluting capacity with continued H_2O intake results in hyponatremia. Conversely, a defect in urine concentration with inadequate H_2O intake culminates in hypernatremia. Hyponatremia reflects a disturbance in homeostatic mechanisms characterized by excess total body H_2O relative to total body sodium, and hypernatremia reflects a deficiency of total body H_2O relative to total body sodium [11]. (*From* Halterman and Berl [12]; with permission.)

Approach to the Hyponatremic Patient

EFFECTS OF OSMOTICALLY ACTIVE SUBSTANCES ON SERUM SODIUM

Substances the increase osmolality *without* changing serum sodium	Substances that increase osmolality and *decrease* serum sodium (translocational hyponatremia)
Urea	Glucose
Ethanol	Mannitol
Ethylene glycol	Glycine
Isopropyl alcohol	Maltose
Methanol	

FIGURE 1-14

Evaluation of a hyponatremic patient: effects of osmotically active substances on serum sodium. In the evaluation of a hyponatremic patient, a determination should be made about whether hyponatremia is truly hypo-osmotic and not a consequence of *translocational* or *pseudohyponatremia*, since, in most but not all situations, hyponatremia reflects hypo-osmolality.

The nature of the solute plays an important role in determining whether or not there is an increase in measured osmolality or an actual increase in effective osmolality. Solutes that are permeable across cell membranes (eg, urea, methanol, ethanol, and ethylene glycol) do not cause water movement and cause hypertonicity without causing cell dehydration. Typical examples are an uremic patient with a high blood urea nitrogen value and an ethanol-intoxicated person. On the other hand, in a patient with diabetic ketoacidosis who is insulinopenic the glucose is not permeant across cell membranes and, by its presence in the extracellular fluid, causes water to move from the cells to extracellular space, thus leading to cell dehydration and lowering serum sodium. This can be viewed as translocational at the cellular level, as the serum sodium level does not reflect changes in total body water but rather movement of water from intracellular to extracellular space. Glycine is used as an irrigant solution during transurethral resection of the prostate and in endometrial surgery. Pseudohyponatremia occurs when the solid phase of plasma (usually 6% to 8%) is much increased by large increments of either lipids or proteins (eg, in hypertriglyceridemia or paraproteinemias).

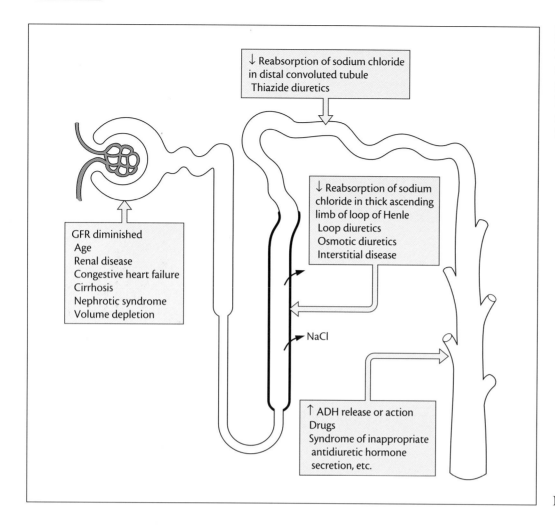

FIGURE 1-15

Pathogenesis of hyponatremia. The normal components of the renal diluting mechanism are depicted in Figure 1-3. Hyponatremia results from disorders of this diluting capacity of the kidney in the following situations:

1. *Intrarenal factors* such as a diminished glomerular filtration rate (GFR), or an increase in proximal tubule fluid and sodium reabsorption, or both, which decrease distal delivery to the diluting segments of the nephron, as in volume depletion, congestive heart failure, cirrhosis, or nephrotic syndrome.
2. *A defect in sodium chloride transport* out of the water-impermeable segments of the nephrons (*ie*, in the thick ascending limb of the loop of Henle). This may occur in patients with interstitial renal disease and administration of thiazide or loop diuretics.
3. *Continued secretion of antidiuretic hormone (ADH)* despite the presence of serum hypo-osmolality mostly stimulated by nonosmotic mechanisms [12].

NaCl—sodium chloride.

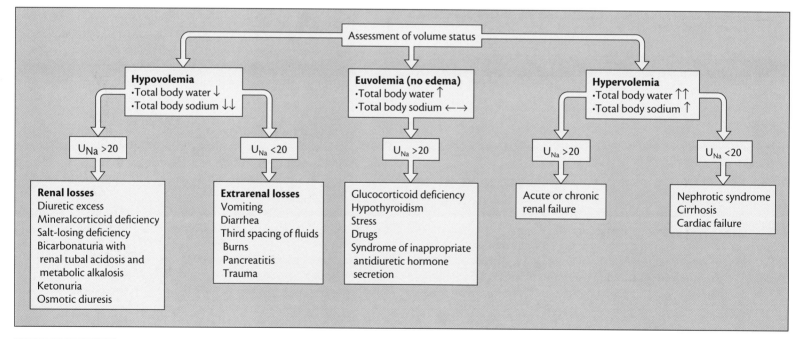

FIGURE 1-16

Diagnostic algorithm for hyponatremia. The next step in the evaluation of a hyponatremic patient is to assess volume status and identify it as hypovolemic, euvolemic or hypervolemic. The patient with hypovolemic hyponatremia has both total body sodium and water deficits, with the sodium deficit exceeding the water deficit. This occurs with large gastrointestinal and renal losses of water and solute when accompanied by free water or hypotonic fluid intake. In patients with hypervolemic hyponatremia, total body sodium is increased but total body water is increased even more than sodium, causing hyponatremia. These syndromes include congestive heart failure, nephrotic syndrome, and cirrhosis. They are all associated with impaired water excretion. Euvolemic hyponatremia is the most common dysnatremia in hospitalized patients. In these patients, by definition, no physical signs of increased total body sodium are detected. They may have a slight excess of volume but no edema [12]. (*Modified from* Halterman and Berl [12]; with permission.)

DRUGS ASSOCIATED WITH HYPONATREMIA

Antidiuretic hormone analogues
  Deamino-D-arginine vasopressin (DDAVP)
  Oxytocin
Drugs that enhance release of antidiuretic hormone
  Chlorpropamide
  Clofibrate
  Carbamazepine-oxycarbazepine
  Vincristine
  Nicotine
  Narcotics
  Antipsychotics
  Antidepressants
  Ifosfamide
Drugs that potentiate renal action of antidiuretic hormone
  Chlorpropamide
  Cyclophosphamide
  Nonsteroidal anti-inflammatory drugs
  Acetaminophen
Drugs that cause hyponatremia by unknown mechanisms
  Haloperidol
  Fluphenazine
  Amitriptyline
  Thioradazine
  Fluoxetine

FIGURE 1-17

Drugs that cause hyponatremia. Drug-induced hyponatremia is mediated by antidiuretic hormone analogues like deamino-D-arginine-vasopressin (DDAVP), or antidiuretic hormone release, or by potentiating the action of antidiuretic hormone. Some drugs cause hyponatremia by unknown mechanisms [13]. (*From* Veis and Berl [13]; with permission.)

CAUSES OF THE SYNDROME OF INAPPROPRIATE DIURETIC HORMONE SECRETION

Carcinomas	Pulmonary Disorders	Central Nervous System Disorders
Bronchogenic	Viral pneumonia	Encephalitis (viral or bacterial)
Duodenal	Bacterial pneumonia	Meningitis (viral, bacterial, tuberculous, fungal)
Pancreatic	Pulmonary abscess	
Thymoma	Tuberculosis	Head trauma
Gastric	Aspergillosis	Brain abscess
Lymphoma	Positive-pressure breathing	Brain tumor
Ewing's sarcoma		Guillain-Barré syndrome
Bladder	Asthma	Acute intermittent porphyria
Carcinoma of the ureter	Pneumothorax	Subarachnoid hemorrhage or subdural hematoma
Prostatic	Mesothelioma	Cerebellar and cerebral atrophy
Oropharyngeal	Cystic fibrosis	Cavernous sinus thrombosis
		Neonatal hypoxia
		Hydrocephalus
		Shy-Drager syndrome
		Rocky Mountain spotted fever
		Delirium tremens
		Cerebrovascular accident (cerebral thrombosis or hemorrhage)
		Acute psychosis
		Multiple sclerosis

FIGURE 1-18

Causes of the syndrome of inappropriate antidiuretic hormone secretion (SIADH). Though SIADH is the commonest cause of hyponatremia in hospitalized patients, it is a diagnosis of exclusion. It is characterized by a defect in osmoregulation of ADH in which plasma ADH levels are not appropriately suppressed for the degree of hypotonicity, leading to urine concentration by a variety of mechanisms. Most of these fall into one of three categories (*ie*, malignancies, pulmonary diseases, central nervous system disorders) [14].

DIAGNOSTIC CRITERIA FOR THE SYNDROME OF INAPPROPRIATE ANTIDIURETIC HORMONE SECRETION

Essential
Decreased extracellular fluid effective osmolality (< 270 mOsm/kg H_2O)
Inappropriate urinary concentration (> 100 mOsm/kg H_2O)
Clinical euvolemia
Elevated urinary sodium concentration ($U_{[Na]}$), with normal salt and H_2O intake
Absence of adrenal, thyroid, pituitary, or renal insufficiency or diuretic use

Supplemental
Abnormal H_2O load test (inability to excrete at least 90% of a 20–mL/kg H_2O load in 4 hrs or failure to dilute urinary osmolality to < 100 mOsm/kg)
Plasma antidiuretic hormone level inappropriately elevated relative to plasma osmolality
No significant correction of plasma sodium with volume expansion, but improvement after fluid restriction

FIGURE 1-19

Diagnostic criteria for the syndrome of inappropriate antidiuretic hormone secretion (SIADH). Clinically, SIADH is characterized by a decrease in the effective extracellular fluid osmolality, with inappropriately concentrated urine. Patients with SIADH are clinically euvolemic and are consuming normal amounts of sodium and water (H_2O). They have elevated urinary sodium excretion. In the evaluation of these patients, it is important to exclude adrenal, thyroid, pituitary, and renal disease and diuretic use. Patients with clinically suspected SIADH can be tested with a water load. Upon administration of 20 mL/kg of H_2O, patients with SIADH are unable to excrete 90% of the H_2O load and are unable to dilute their urine to an osmolality less than 100 mOsm/kg [15]. (*Modified from* Verbalis [15]; with permission.)

SIGNS AND SYMPTOMS OF HYPONATREMIA

Central Nervous System
Mild
  Apathy
  Headache
  Lethargy
Moderate
  Agitation
  Ataxia
  Confusion
  Disorientation
  Psychosis
Severe
  Stupor
  Coma
  Pseudobulbar palsy
  Tentorial herniation
  Cheyne-Stokes respiration
  Death

Gastrointestinal System
Anorexia
Nausea
Vomiting

Musculoskeletal System
Cramps
Diminished deep tendon reflexes

FIGURE 1-20

Signs and symptoms of hyponatremia. In evaluating hyponatremic patients, it is important to assess whether or not the patient is symptomatic, because symptoms are a better determinant of therapy than the absolute value itself. Most patients with serum sodium values above 125 mEq/L are asymptomatic. The rapidity with which hyponatremia develops is critical in the initial evaluation of such patients. In the range of 125 to 130 mEq/L, the predominant symptoms are gastrointestinal ones, including nausea and vomiting. Neuropsychiatric symptoms dominate the picture once the serum sodium level drops below 125 mEq/L, mostly because of cerebral edema secondary to hypotonicity. These include headache, lethargy, reversible ataxia, psychosis, seizures, and coma. Severe manifestations of cerebral edema include increased intracerebral pressure, tentorial herniation, respiratory depression and death. Hyponatremia-induced cerebral edema occurs principally with rapid development of hyponatremia, typically in patients managed with hypotonic fluids in the postoperative setting or those receiving diuretics, as discussed previously. The mortality rate can be as great as 50%. Fortunately, this rarely occurs. Nevertheless, neurologic symptoms in a hyponatremic patient call for prompt and immediate attention and treatment [16,17].

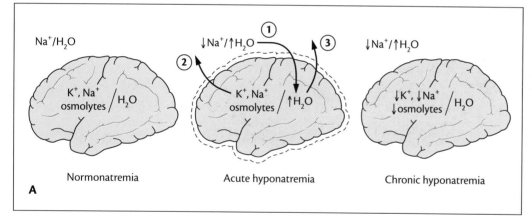

FIGURE 1-21

Cerebral adaptation to hyponatremia. **A,** Decreases in extracellular osmolality cause movement of water (H_2O) into the cells, increasing intracellular volume and thus causing tissue edema. This cellular edema within the fixed confines of the cranium causes increased intracranial pressure, leading to neurologic symptoms. To prevent this from happening, mechanisms geared toward volume regulation come into operation, to prevent cerebral edema from developing in the vast majority of patients with hyponatremia.

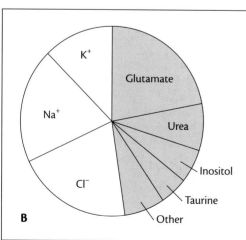

After induction of extracellular fluid hypo-osmolality, H_2O moves into the brain in response to osmotic gradients, producing cerebral edema (*middle panel, 1*). However, within 1 to 3 hours, a decrease in cerebral extracellular volume occurs by movement of fluid into the cerebrospinal fluid, which is then shunted back into the systemic circulation. This happens very promptly and is evident by the loss of extracellular and intracellular solutes (sodium and chloride ions) as early as 30 minutes after the onset of hyponatremia. As H_2O losses accompany the losses of brain solute (*middle panel, 2*), the expanded brain volume decreases back toward normal (*middle panel, 3*) [15]. **B,** Relative decreases in individual osmolytes during adaptation to chronic hyponatremia. Thereafter, if hyponatremia persists, other organic osmolytes such as phosphocreatine, myoinositol, and amino acids like glutamine, and taurine are lost. The loss of these solutes markedly decreases cerebral swelling. Patients who have had a slower onset of hyponatremia (over 72 to 96 hours or longer), the risk for osmotic demyelination rises if hyponatremia is corrected too rapidly [18,19]. Na+—sodium; K+—potassium; Cl-—chloride.

HYPONATREMIC PATIENTS AT RISK FOR NEUROLOGIC COMPLICATIONS

Complication	Persons at Risk
Acute cerebral edema	Postoperative menstruant females
	Elderly women taking thiazides
	Children
	Psychiatric polydipsic patients
	Hypoxemic patients
Osmotic demyelination syndrome	Alcoholics
	Malnourished patients
	Hypokalemic patients
	Burn victims
	Elderly women taking thiazide diuretics

FIGURE 1-22

Hyponatremic patients at risk for neurologic complications. Those at risk for cerebral edema include postoperative menstruant women, elderly women taking thiazide diuretics, children, psychiatric patients with polydipsia, and hypoxic patients. In women, and, in particular, menstruant ones, the risk for developing neurologic complications is 25 times greater than that for nonmenstruant women or men. The increased risk was independent of the rate of development, or the magnitude of the hyponatremia [21]. The osmotic demyelination syndrome or central pontine myelinolysis seems to occur when there is rapid correction of low osmolality (hyponatremia) in a brain already chronically adapted (more than 72 to 96 hours). It is rarely seen in patients with a serum sodium value greater than 120 mEq/L or in those who have hyponatremia of less than 48 hours' duration [20,21]. (*Adapted from* Lauriat and Berl [21]; with permission.)

SYMPTOMS OF CENTRAL PONTINE MYELINOLYSIS

Initial symptoms
Mutism
Dysarthria
Lethargy and affective changes

Classic symptoms
Spastic quadriparesis
Pseudobulbar palsy

Lesions in the midbrain, medulla oblongata, and pontine tegmentum
Pupillary and oculomotor abnormalities
  Altered sensorium
  Cranial neuropathies
Extrapontine myelinolysis
  Ataxia
  Behavioral abnormalities
  Parkinsonism
  Dystonia

FIGURE 1-23

Symptoms of central pontine myelinolysis. This condition has been described all over the world, in all age groups, and can follow correction of hyponatremia of any cause. The risk for development of central pontine myelinolysis is related to the severity and chronicity of the hyponatremia. Initial symptoms include mutism and dysarthria. More than 90% of patients exhibit the classic symptoms of myelinolysis (*ie*, spastic quadriparesis and pseudobulbar palsy), reflecting damage to the corticospinal and corticobulbar tracts in the basis pontis. Other symptoms occur on account of extension of the lesion to other parts of the midbrain. This syndrome follows a biphasic course. Initially, a generalized encephalopathy, associated with a rapid rise in serum sodium, occurs. This is followed by the classic symptoms 2 to 3 days after correction of hyponatremia, however, this pattern does not always occur [22]. (*Adapted from* Laureno and Karp [22]; with permission.)

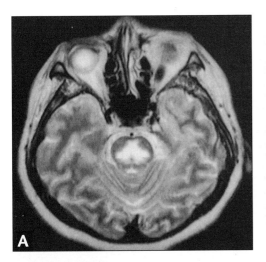
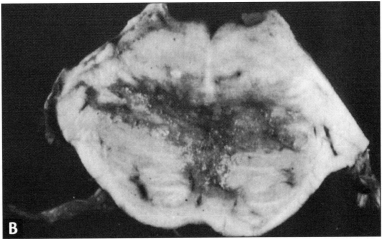

FIGURE 1-24

A, Imaging of central pontine myelinolysis. Brain imaging is the most useful diagnostic technique for central pontine myelinolysis. Magnetic resonance imaging (MRI) is more sensitive than computed tomography (CT). On CT, central pontine and extrapontine lesions appear as symmetric areas of hypodensity (not shown). On T2 images of MRI, the lesions appear as hyperintense and on T1 images, hypointense. These lesions do not enhance with gadolinium. They may not be apparent on imaging until 2 weeks into the illness. Other diagnostic tests are brainstem auditory evoked potentials, electroencephalography, and cerebrospinal fluid protein and myelin basic proteins [22]. B, Gross appearance of the pons in central pontine myelinolysis. (*From* Laureno and Karp [22]; with permission.)

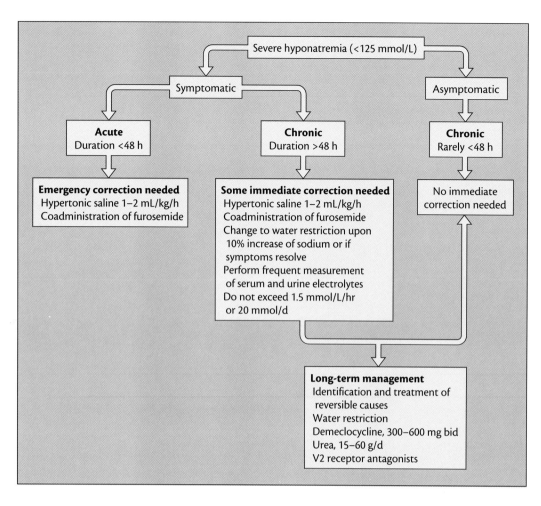

FIGURE 1-25

Treatment of severe euvolemic hyponatremia (<125 mmol/L). The evaluation of a hyponatremic patient involves an assessment of whether the patient is symptomatic, and if so, the duration of hyponatremia should be ascertained. The therapeutic approach to the hyponatremic patient is determined more by the presence or absence of symptoms than by the absolute level of serum sodium. Acutely hyponatremic patients are at great risk for permanent neurologic sequelae from cerebral edema if the hyponatremia is not promptly corrected. On the other hand, chronic hyponatremia carries the risk of osmotic demyelination syndrome if corrected too rapidly. The next step involves a determination of whether the patient has any risk factors for development of neurologic complications.

The commonest setting for acute, symptomatic hyponatremia is hospitalized, postoperative patients who are receiving hypotonic fluids. In these patients, the risk of cerebral edema outweighs the risk for osmotic demyelination. In the presence of seizures, obtundation, and coma, rapid infusion of 3% sodium chloride (4 to 6 mL/kg/h) or even 50 mL of 29.2% sodium chloride has been used safely. Ongoing careful neurologic monitoring is imperative [20].

A. GENERAL GUIDELINES FOR THE TREATMENT OF SYMPTOMATIC HYPONATREMIA*

Acute hyponatremia (duration < 48 hrs)

Increase serum sodium rapidly by approximately 2 mmol/L/h until symptoms resolve

Full correction probably safe but not necessary

Chronic hyponatremia (duration > 48 hrs)

Initial increase in serum sodium by 10% or 10 mmol/L

Perform frequent neurologic evaluations; correction rate may be reduced with improvement in symptoms

At no time should correction exceed rate of 1.5 mmol/L/h, or increments of 15 mmol/d

Measure serum and urine electrolytes every 1–2 h

*The sum of urinary cations ($U_{Na} + U_K$) should be less than the concentration of infused sodium, to ensure excretion of electrolyte-free water.

B. TREATMENT OF CHRONIC SYMPTOMATIC HYPONATREMIA

Calculate the net water loss needed to raise the serum sodium (S_{Na}) from 110 mEq/L to 120 mEq/L in a 50 kg person.

Example

Current S_{Na} × Total body water (TBW) = Desired S_{Na} × New TBW

Assume that TBW = 60% of body weight

Therefore TBW of patient = 50 × 0.6 = 30 L

New TBW = $\dfrac{110 \text{ mEq/L} \times 30 \text{ L}}{120 \text{ mEq/L}}$ = 27.5 L

Thus the electrolyte-free water loss needed to raise the S_{Na} to 120 mEq/L = Present TBW − New TBW = 2.5 L

Calculate the time course in which to achieve the desired correction (1 mEq/h)—in this case, 250 mL/h

Administer furosemide, monitor urine output, and replace sodium, potassium, and excess free water lost in the urine

Continue to monitor urine output and replace sodium, potassium, and excess free water lost in the urine

FIGURE 1-26

General guidelines for the treatment of symptomatic hyponatremia, **A.** Included herein are general guidelines for treatment of patients with acute and chronic symptomatic hyponatremia. In the treatment of chronic symptomatic hyponatremia, since cerebral water is increased by approximately 10%, a prompt increase in serum sodium by 10% or 10 mEq/L is permissible. Thereafter, the patient's fluids should be restricted. The total correction rate should not exceed 1.0 to 1.5 mEq/L/h, and the total increment in 24 hours should not exceed 15 mmol/d [12]. A specific example as to how to increase a patient's serum sodium is illustrated in **B.**

MANAGEMENT OPTIONS FOR CHRONIC ASYMPTOMATIC HYPONATREMIA

Treatment	Mechanism of Action	Dose	Advantages	Limitations
Fluid restriction	Decreases availability of free water	Variable	Effective and inexpensive	Noncompliance
Pharmacologic inhibition of antidiuretic hormone action				
Lithium	Inhibits the kidney's response to antidiuretic hormone	900–1200 mg/d	Unrestricted water intake	Polyuria, narrow therapeutic range, neurotoxicity
Demeclocycline	Inhibits the kidney's response to antidiurectic hormone	1200 mg/d initially; then, 300–900 mg/d	Effective; unrestricted water intake	Neurotoxicity, polyuria, photosensitivity, nephrotoxicity
V2-receptor antagonist	Antagonizes vasopressin action		Ongoing trials	
Increased solute intake				
Furosemide	Increases free water clearance	Titrate to optimal dose; coadminister 2–3 g sodium chloride	Effective	Ototoxicity, K+ and Mg2+ depletion
Urea	Osmotic diuresis	30–60 g/d	Effective; unrestricted water intake	Polyuria, unpalatable gastrointestinal symptoms

FIGURE 1-27

Management options for patients with chronic asymptomatic hyponatremia. If the patient has chronic hyponatremia and is asymptomatic, treatment need not be intensive or emergent. Careful scrutiny of likely causes should be followed by treatment. If the cause is determined to be the syndrome of inappropriate antidiuretic hormone (ADH) secretion, it must be treated as a chronic disorder. As summarized here, the treatment strategies involve fluid restriction, pharmacologic inhibition of ADH action, and increased solute intake. Fluid restriction is frequently successful in normalizing serum sodium and preventing symptoms [23].

MANAGEMENT OF NONEUVOLEMIC HYPONATREMIA

Hypovolemic hyponatremia
Volume restoration with isotonic saline
Identify and correct causes of water and sodium losses

Hypervolemic hyponatremia
Water restriction
Sodium restriction
Substitiute loop diuretics for thiazide diurectics
Treatment of timulus for sodium and water retention
V2-receptor antagonist

FIGURE 1-28

Management of noneuvolemic hyponatremia. Hypovolemic hyponatremia results from the loss of both water and solute, with relatively greater loss of solute. The nonosmotic release of antidiuretic hormone stimulated by decreased arterial circulating blood volume causes antidiuresis and perpetuates the hyponatremia. Most of these patients are asymptomatic. The keystone of therapy is isotonic saline administration, which corrects the hypovolemia and removes the stimulus of antidiuretic hormone to retain fluid. Hypervolemic hyponatremia occurs when both solute and water are increased, but water more than solute. This occurs with heart failure, cirrhosis and nephrotic syndrome. The cornerstones of treatment include fluid restriction, salt restriction, and loop diuretics [20]. (*Adapted from* Lauriat and Berl [20]; with permission.)

Approach to the Hypernatremic Patient

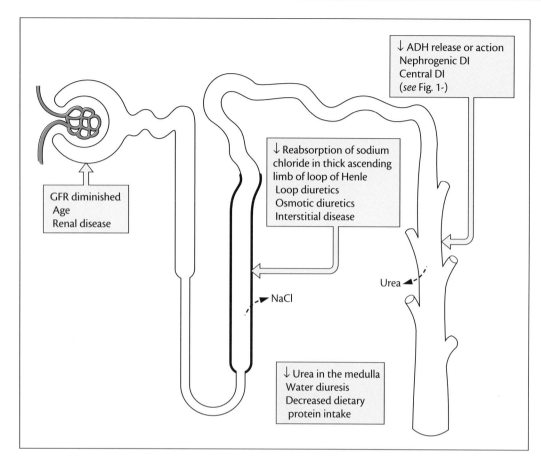

FIGURE 1-29

Pathogenesis of hypernatremia. The renal concentrating mechanism is the first line of defense against water depletion and hyperosmolality. When renal concentration is impaired, thirst becomes a very effective mechanism for preventing further increases in serum osmolality. The components of the normal urine concentrating mechanism are shown in Figure 1-2. Hypernatremia results from disturbances in the renal concentrating mechanism. This occurs in interstitial renal disease, with administration of loop and osmotic diuretics, and with protein malnutrition, in which less urea is available to generate the medullary interstitial tonicity.

Hypernatremia usually occurs only when hypotonic fluid losses occur in combination with a disturbance in water intake, typically in elders with altered consciousness, in infants with inadequate access to water, and, rarely, with primary disturbances of thirst [24]. GFR—glomerular filtration rate; ADH—antidiuretic hormone; DI—diabetes insipidus.

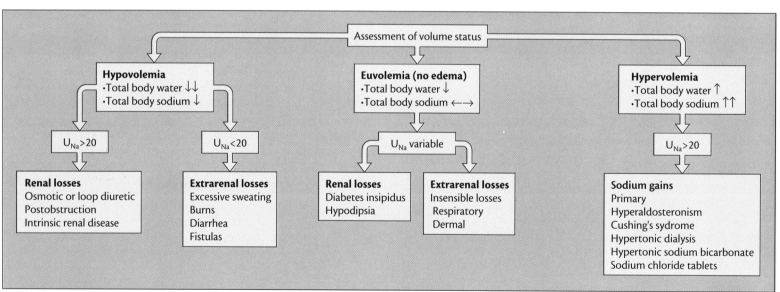

FIGURE 1-30

Diagnostic algorithm for hypernatremia. As for hyponatremia, the initial evaluation of the patient with hypernatremia involves assessment of volume status. Patients with hypovolemic hypernatremia lose both sodium and water, but relatively more water. On physical examination, they exhibit signs of hypovolemia. The causes listed reflect principally hypotonic water losses from the kidneys or the gastrointestinal tract.

Euvolemic hyponatremia reflects water losses accompanied by inadequate water intake. Since such hypodipsia is uncommon, hypernatremia usually supervenes in persons who have no access to water or who have a neurologic deficit that impairs thirst perception—the very young and the very old. Extrarenal water loss occurs from the skin

and respiratory tract, in febrile or other hypermetabolic states. Very high urine osmolality reflects an intact osmoreceptor–antidiuretic hormone–renal response. Thus, the defense against the development of hyperosmolality requires appropriate stimulation of thirst and the ability to respond by drinking water. The urine sodium (U_{Na}) value varies with the sodium intake. The renal water losses that lead to euvolemic hypernatremia are a consequence of either a defect in vasopressin production or release (central diabetes insipidus) or failure of the collecting duct to respond to the hormone (nephrogenic diabetes insipidus) [23]. (*Modified from* Halterman and Berl [12]; with permission.)

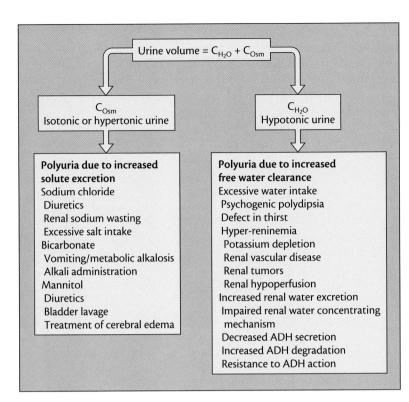

Urine volume = C_{H_2O} + C_{Osm}

C_{Osm}
Isotonic or hypertonic urine

C_{H_2O}
Hypotonic urine

Polyuria due to increased solute excretion
Sodium chloride
 Diuretics
 Renal sodium wasting
 Excessive salt intake
Bicarbonate
 Vomiting/metabolic alkalosis
 Alkali administration
Mannitol
 Diuretics
 Bladder lavage
 Treatment of cerebral edema

Polyuria due to increased free water clearance
Excessive water intake
 Psychogenic polydipsia
 Defect in thirst
Hyper-reninemia
 Potassium depletion
 Renal vascular disease
 Renal tumors
 Renal hypoperfusion
Increased renal water excretion
Impaired renal water concentrating
 mechanism
Decreased ADH secretion
Increased ADH degradation
Resistance to ADH action

FIGURE 1-31

Physiologic approach to polyuric disorders. Among euvolemic hypernatremic patients, those affected by polyuric disorders are an important subcategory. Polyuria is arbitrarily defined as urine output of more than 3 L/d. Urine volume can be conceived of as having two components: the volume needed to excrete solutes at the concentration of solutes in plasma (called the *osmolar clearance*) and the other being the *free water clearance*, which is the volume of solute-free water that has been added to (positive free water clearance [CH_2O]) or subtracted (negative CH_2O) from the isotonic portion of the urine osmolar clearance (Cosm) to create either a hypotonic or hypertonic urine.

Consumption of an average American diet requires the kidneys to excrete 600 to 800 mOsm of solute each day. The urine volume in which this solute is excreted is determined by fluid intake. If the urine is maximally diluted to 60 mOsm/kg of water, the 600 mOsm will need 10 L of urine for effective osmotic clearance. If the concentrating mechanism is maximally stimulated to 1200 mOsm/kg of water, osmotic clearance will occur in a minimum of 500 mL of urine. This flexibility is affected when drugs or diseases alter the renal concentrating mechanism.

Polyuric disorders can be secondary to an increase in solute clearance, free water clearance, or a combination of both. ADH—antidiuretic hormone.

WATER DEPRIVATION TEST

Diagnosis	Urine Osmolality with Water Deprivation (mOsm/kg H_2O)	Plasma Arginine Vasopressin (AVP) after Dehydration	Increase in Urine Osmolality with Exogenous AVP
Normal	> 800	> 2 pg/mL	Little or none
Complete central diabetes insipidus	< 300	Indetectable	Substantial
Partial central diabetes insipidus	300–800	< 1.5 pg/mL	> 10% of urine osmolality after water deprivation
Nephrogenic diabetes insipidus	< 300–500	> 5 pg/mL	Little or none
Primary polydipsia	> 500	< 5 pg/mL	Little or none

* Water intake is restricted until the patient loses 3%–5% of weight or until three consecutive hourly determinations of urinary osmolality are within 10% of each other. (Caution must be exercised to ensure that the patient does not become excessively dehydrated.) Aqueous AVP (5 U subcutaneous) is given, and urine osmolality is measured after 60 minutes. The expected responses are given above.

FIGURE 1-32

Water deprivation test. Along with nephrogenic diabetes insipidus and primary polydipsia, patients with central diabetes insipius present with polyuria and polydipsia. Differentiating between these entities can be accomplished by measuring vasopressin levels and determining the response to water deprivation followed by vasopressin administration [25]. (*From* Lanese and Teitelbaum [26]; with permission.)

CLINICAL FEATURES OF DIABETES INSIPIDUS

Abrupt onset
Equal frequency in both sexes
Rare in infancy, usual in second decade of life
Predilection for cold water
Polydipsia
Urine output of 3 to 15 L/d
Marked nocturia but no diurnal variation
Sleep deprivation leads to fatigue and irritability
Severe life-threatening hypernatremia can be associated with illness or water deprivation

FIGURE 1-33

Clinical features of diabetes insipidus. Other clinical features can distinguish compulsive water drinkers from patients with central diabetes insipidus. The latter usually has abrupt onset, whereas compulsive water drinkers may give a vague history of the onset. Unlike compulsive water drinkers, patients with central diabetes insipidus have a constant need for water. Compulsive water drinkers exhibit large variations in water intake and urine output. Nocturia is common with central diabetes insipidus and unusual in compulsive water drinkers. Finally, patients with central diabetes insipidus have a predilection for drinking cold water. Plasma osmolality above 295 mOsm/kg suggests central diabetes insipidus and below 270 mOsm/kg suggests compulsive water drinking [23].

CAUSES OF DIABETES INSIPIDUS

Central diabetes insipidus	Nephrogenic diabetes insipidus
Congenital	Congenital
Autosomal-dominant	X-linked
Autosomal-recessive	Autosomal-recessive
Acquired	Acquired
Post-traumatic	Renal diseases (medullary cystic disease, polycystic disease, analgesic nephropathy, sickle cell nephropathy, obstructive uro-pathy, chronic pyelonephritis, multiple myeloma, amyloidosis, sarcoidosis)
Iatrogenic	
Tumors (metastatic from breast, craniopharyngioma, pinealoma)	
Cysts	Hypercalcemia
Histiocytosis	Hypokalemia
Granuloma (tuberculosis, sarcoid)	Drugs (lithium compounds, demeclocycline, methoxyflurane, amphotericin, foscarnet)
Aneurysms	
Meningitis	
Encephalitis	
Guillain-Barré syndrome	
Idiopathic	

FIGURE 1-34

Causes of diabetes insipidus. The causes of diabetes insipidus can be divided into central and nephrogenic. Most (about 50%) of the central causes are idiopathic; the rest are caused by central nervous system involvement with infection, tumors, granuloma, or trauma. The nephrogenic causes can be congenital or acquired [23].

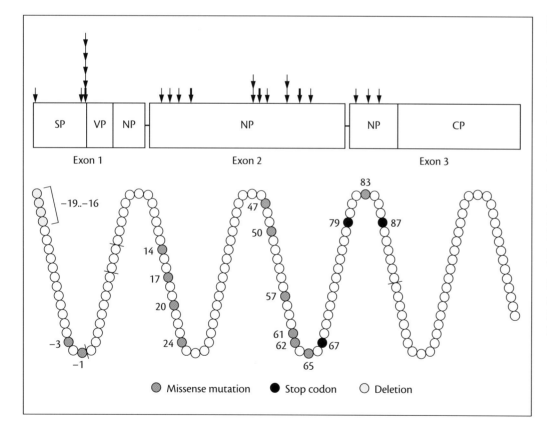

FIGURE 1-35

Congenital central diabetes insipidus (DI), autosomal-dominant form. This condition has been described in many families in Europe and North America. It is an autosomal dominant inherited disease associated with marked loss of cells in the supraoptic nuclei. Molecular biology techniques have revealed multiple point mutations in the vasopressin-neurophysin II gene. This condition usually presents early in life [25]. A rare autosomal-recessive form of central DI has been described that is characterized by DI, diabetes mellitus (DM), optic atrophy (OA), and deafness (DIDMOAD or Wolfram's syndrome). This has been linked to a defect in chromosome-4 and involves abnormalities in mitochondrial DNA [27]. SP—signal peptide; VP—vasopressin; NP—neurophysin; GP—glycoprotein.

Diseases of Water Metabolism

TREATMENT OF CENTRAL DIABETES INSIPIDUS

Condition	Drug	Dose
Complete central DI	dDAVP	10–20 (g intranasally q 12–24 h
Partial central DI	Vasopressin tannate	2–5 U IM q 24–48 h
	Aqueous vasopressin	5–10 U SC q 4–6 h
	Chlorpropamide	250–500 mg/d
	Clofibrate	500 mg tid–qid
	Carbamazepine	400–600 mg/d

FIGURE 1-36

Treatment of central diabetes insipidus (DI). Central DI may be treated with hormone replacement or drugs. In acute settings when renal water losses are extensive, aqueous vasopressin (pitressin) is useful. It has a short duration of action that allows for careful monitoring and avoiding complications like water intoxication. This drug should be used with caution in patients with underlying coronary artery disease and peripheral vascular disease, as it can cause vascular spasm and prolonged vasoconstriction. For the patient with established central DI, desmopressin acetate (dDAVP) is the agent of choice. It has a long half-life and does not have significant vasoconstrictive effects like those of aqueous vasopressin. It can be conveniently administered intranasally every 12 to 24 hours. It is usually tolerated well. It is safe to use in pregnancy and resists degradation by circulating vasopressinase. In patients with partial DI, agents that potentiate release of antidiuretic hormone can be used. These include chlorpropamide, clofibrate, and carbamazepine. They work effectively only if combined with hormone therapy, decreased solute intake, or diuretic administration [23].

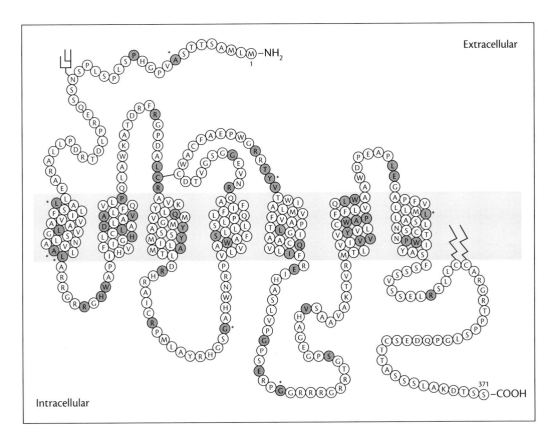

FIGURE 1-37

Congenital nephrogenic diabetes insipidus, X-linked–recessive form. This is a rare disease of male patients who do not concentrate their urine after administration of antidiuretic hormone. The pedigrees of affected families have been linked to a group of Ulster Scots who emigrated to Halifax, Nova Scotia in 1761 aboard the ship called "Hopewell." According to the Hopewell hypothesis, most North American patients with this disease are descendants of a common ancestor with a single gene defect. Recent studies, however, disproved this hypothesis [28]. The gene defect has now been traced to 87 different mutations in the gene for the vasopressin receptor (AVP-R2) in 106 presumably unrelated families [29]. (*From* Bichet, *et al.* [29]; with permission.)

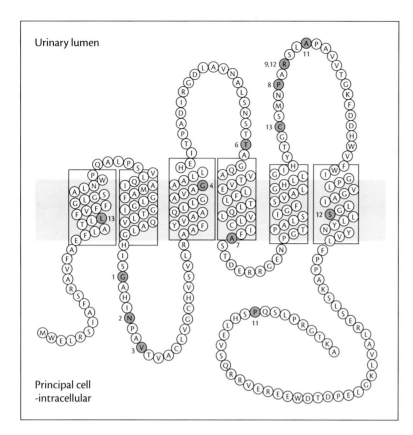

Urinary lumen

Principal cell
-intracellular

FIGURE 1-38

Congenital nephrogenic diabetes insipidus (NDI), autosomal-recessive form. In the autosomal recessive form of NDI, mutations have been found in the gene for the antiiuretic hormone (ADH)–sensitive water channel, AQP-2. This form of NDI is exceedingly rare as compared with the X-linked form of NDI [30]. Thus far, a total of 15 AQP-2 mutations have been described in total of 13 families [31]. The acquired form of NDI occurs in various kidney diseases and in association with various drugs, such as lithium and amphotericin B. (*From* Canfield *et al.* [31]; with permission.)

ACQUIRED NEPHROGENIC DIABETES INSIPIDUS: CAUSES AND MECHANISMS

Disease State	Defect in Generation of Medullary Interstitial Tonicity	Defect in cAMP Generation	Downregulation of AQP-2	Other
Chronic renal failure	✔	✔	✔	Downregulation of V_2 receptor message
Hypokalemia	✔	✔	✔	
Hypercalcemia	✔	✔		
Sickle cell disease	✔			
Protein malnutrition	✔		✔	
Demeclocycline		✔		
Lithium		✔	✔	
Pregnancy				Placental secretion of vasopressinase

FIGURE 1-39

Causes and mechanisms of acquired nephrogenic diabetes insidpidus. Acquired nephrogenic diabetes insipidus occurs in chronic renal failure, electrolyte imbalances, with certain drugs, in sickle cell disease and pregnancy. The exact mechanism involved has been the subject of extensive investigation over the past decade and has now been carefully elucidated for most of the etiologies.

PATIENT GROUPS AT INCREASED RISK FOR SEVERE HYPERNATREMIA

Elders and infants
Hospitalized patients receiving
  Hypertonic infusions
  Tube feedings
  Osmotic diuretics
  Lactulose
  Mechanical ventilation
Altered mental status
Uncontrolled diabetes mellitus
Underlying polyuria

FIGURE 1-40

Patient groups at increased risk for severe hypernatremia. Hypernatremia always reflects a hyperosmolar state. It usually occurs in a hospital setting (reported incidence 0.65% to 2.23% of all hospitalized patients) with very high morbidity and mortality (estimates of 42% to over 70%) [12].

SIGNS AND SYMPTOMS OF HYPERNATREMIA

Central Nervous System

Mild

Restlessness

Lethargy

Altered mental status

Irritability

Moderate

Disorientation

Confusion

Severe

Stupor

Coma

Seizures

Death

Respiratory System

Labored respiration

Gastrointestinal System

Intense thirst

Nausea

Vomiting

Musculoskeletal System

Muscle twitching

Spasticity

Hyperreflexia

FIGURE 1-41

Signs and symptoms of hypernatremia. Hypernatremia always reflects a hyperosmolar state; thus, central nervous system symptoms are prominent in affected patients [12].

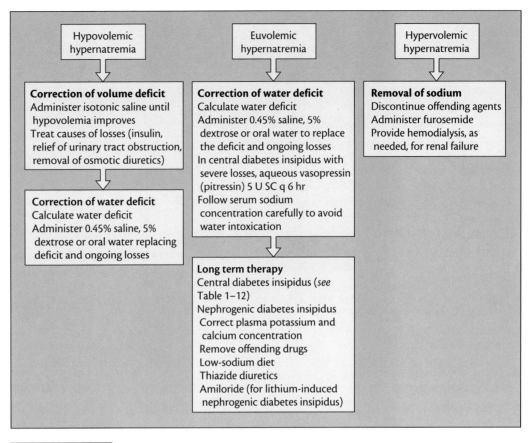

FIGURE 1-42

Management options for patients with hypernatremia. The primary goal in the treatment of hypernatremia is restoration of serum tonicity. Hypovolemic hypernatremia in the context of low total body sodium and orthostatic blood pressure changes should be managed with isotonic saline until blood pressure normalizes. Thereafter, fluid management generally involves administration of 0.45% sodium chloride or 5% dextrose solution. The goal of therapy for hypervolemic hypernatremias is to remove the excess sodium, which is achieved with diuretics plus 5% dextrose. Patients who have renal impairment may need dialysis. In euvolemic hypernatremic patients, water losses far exceed solute losses, and the mainstay of therapy is 5% dextrose. To correct the hypernatremia, the total body water deficit must be estimated. This is based on the serum sodium concentration and on the assumption that 60% of the body weight is water [24]. (*Modified from* Halterman and Berl [12]; with permission.)

GUIDELINES FOR THE TREATMENT OF SYMPTOMATIC HYPERNATREMIA*

Correct at a rate of 2 mmol/L/h

Replace half of the calculated water deficit over the first 12–24 hrs

Replace the remaining deficit over the next 24–36 hrs

Perform serial neurologic examinations (prescribed rate of correction can be decreased as symptoms improve)

Measure serum and urine electrolytes every 1–2 hrs

*If $U_{Na} + U_K$ is less than the concentration of P_{Na}, then water loss is ongoing and needs to be replaced.

FIGURE 1-43

Guidelines for the treatment of symptomatic hypernatremia. Patients with severe symptomatic hypernatremia are at high risk of dying and should be treated aggressively. An initial step is estimating the total body free water deficit, based on the weight (in kilograms) and the serum sodium. During correction of the water deficit, it is important to perform serial neurologic examinations.

References

1. Jacobson HR: Functional segmentation of the mammalian nephron. *Am J Physiol* 1981, 241:F203.

2. Goldberg M: Water control and the dysnatremias. In *The Sea Within Us*. Edited by Bricker NS. New York: Science and Medicine Publishing Co., 1975:20.

3. Kokko J, Rector F: Countercurrent multiplication system without active transport in inner medulla. *Kidney Int* 1972, 114.

4. Knepper MA, Roch-Ramel F: Pathways of urea transport in the mammalian kidney. *Kidney Int* 1987, 31:629.

5. Vander A: In *Renal Physiology*. New York: McGraw Hill, 1980:89.

6. Zimmerman E, Robertson AG: Hypothalamic neurons secreting vasopressin and neurophysin. *Kidney Int* 1976, 10(1):12.

7. Bichet DG: Nephrogenic and central diabetes insipidus. In *Diseases of the Kidney*, edn. 6. Edited by Schrier RW, Gottschalk CW. Boston: Little, Brown, and Co., 1997:2430

8. Bichet DG : Vasopressin receptors in health and disease. *Kidney Int* 1996, 49:1706.

9. Dunn FL, Brennan TJ, Nelson AE, Robertson GL: The role of blood osmolality and volume in regulating vasopressin secretion in the rat. *J Clin Invest* 1973, 52:3212.

10. Rose BD: Antidiuretic hormone and water balance. In *Clinical Physiology of Acid Base and Electrolyte Disorders*, edn. 4. New York: McGraw Hill, 1994.

11. Cogan MG: Normal water homeostasis. In *Fluid & Electrolytes, Physiology and Pathophysiology*. Edited by Cogan MG. Norwalk: Appleton & Lange, 1991:98.

12. Halterman R, Berl T: Therapy of dysnatremic disorders. In *Therapy in Nephrology and Hypertension*. Edited by Brady H, Wilcox C. Philadelphia: WB Saunders, 1998, in press.

13. Veis JH, Berl T, Hyponatremia: In *The Principles and Practice of Nephrology*, edn. 2. Edited by Jacobson HR, Striker GE, Klahr S. St.Louis: Mosby, 1995:890.

14. Berl T, Schrier RW: Disorders of water metabolism. In *Renal and Electrolyte Disorders*, edn 4. Philadelphia: Lippincott-Raven, 1997:52.

15. Verbalis JG: The syndrome of ianappropriate diuretic hormone secretion and other hypoosmolar disorders. In *Diseases of the Kidney*, edn. 6. Edited by Schrier RW, Gottschalk CW. Boston: Little, Brown, and Co., 1997:2393.

16. Berl T, Schrier RW: Disorders of water metabolism. In *Renal and Electrolyte Disorders*, edn. 4. Edited by Schrier RW. Philadelphia: Lippincott-Raven, 1997:54.

17. Berl T, Anderson RJ, McDonald KM, Schreir RW: Clinical Disorders of water metabolism. *Kidney Int* 1976, 10:117.

18. Gullans SR, Verbalis JG: Control of brain volume during hyperosmolar and hypoosmolar conditions. *Annu Rev Med* 1993, 44:289.

19. Zarinetchi F, Berl T: Evaluation and management of severe hyponatremia. *Adv Intern Med* 1996, 41:251.

20. Lauriat SM, Berl T: The Hyponatremic Patient: Practical focus on therapy. *J Am Soc Nephrol* 1997, 8(11):1599.

21. Ayus JC, Wheeler JM, Arieff AI: Postoperative hyponatremic encephalopathy in menstruant women. *Ann Intern Med* 1992,117:891.

22. Laureno R, Karp BI: Myelinolysis after correction of hyponatremia. *Ann Intern Med* 1997, 126:57.

23. Kumar S, Berl T: Disorders of serum sodium concentration. *Lancet* 1998. in press.

24. Cogan MG: Normal water homeostasis. In *Fluid & Electrolytes, Physiology and Pathophysiology*. Edited by Cogan MG. Norwalk: Appleton & Lange, 1991:94.

25. Rittig S, Robertson G, Siggaard C, *et al.*: Identification of 13 new mutations in the vasopressin-neurophysin II gene in 17 kindreds with familial autosomal dominant neurohypophyseal diabetes insipidus. *Am J Hum Genet* 1996, 58:107.

26. Lanese D, Teitelbaum I: Hypernatremia. In *The Principles and Practice of Nephrology*, edn. 2. Edited by Jacobson HR, Striker GE, Klahr S. St. Louis: Mosby, 1995:895.

27. Barrett T, Bundey S: Wolfram (DIDMOAD) syndrome. *J Med Genet* 1997, 29:1237.

28. Holtzman EJ, Ausiello DA: Nephrogenic Diabetes insipidus: Causes revealed. *Hosp Pract* 1994, Mar 15:89–104.

29. Bichet D, Oksche A, Rosenthal W: Congential Nephrogenic Diabetes Insipidus. *J Am Soc Nephrol* 1997, 8:1951.

30. Lieburg van, Verdjik M, Knoers N, *et al.*: Patients with autosomal nephrogenic diabetes insipidus homozygous for mutations in the aquaporin 2 water channel. *Am J Hum Genet* 1994, 55:648.

31. Canfield MC, Tamarappoo BK, Moses AM, *et al.*: Identification and characterization of aquaporin-2 water channel mutations causing nephrogenic diabetes insipidus with partial vasopressin response. *Hum Mol Genet* 1997, 6(11):1865.

Disorders of Sodium Balance

David H. Ellison

S odium is the predominant cation in extracellular fluid (ECF); the volume of ECF is directly proportional to the content of sodium in the body. Disorders of sodium balance, therefore, may be viewed as disorders of ECF volume. The body must maintain ECF volume within acceptable limits to maintain tissue perfusion because plasma volume is directly proportional to ECF volume. The plasma volume is a crucial component of the blood volume that determines rates of organ perfusion. Many authors suggest that ECF volume is maintained within narrow limits despite wide variations in dietary sodium intake. However, ECF volume may increase as much as 18% when dietary sodium intake is increased from very low to moderately high levels [1,2]. Such variation in ECF volume usually is well tolerated and leads to few short-term consequences. In contrast, the same change in dietary sodium intake causes only a 1% change in mean arterial pressure (MAP) in normal persons [3]. The body behaves as if the MAP, rather than the ECF volume, is tightly regulated. Under chronic conditions, the effect of MAP on urinary sodium excretion displays a remarkable gain; an increase in MAP of 1 mm Hg is associated with increases in daily sodium excretion of 200 mmol [4].

Guyton [4] demonstrated the importance of the kidney in control of arterial pressure. Endogenous regulators of vascular tone, hormonal vasoconstrictors, neural inputs, and other nonrenal mechanisms are important participants in short-term pressure homeostasis. Over the long term, blood pressure is controlled by renal volume excretion, which is adjusted to a set point. Increases in arterial pressure lead to natriuresis (called *pressure natriuresis*), which reduces blood volume. A decrease in blood volume reduces venous return to the heart and cardiac output. Urinary volume excretion exceeds dietary intake until the blood volume decreases sufficiently to return the blood pressure to the set point.

Disorders of sodium balance resulting from primary renal sodium retention lead only to modest volume expansion without edema because increases in MAP quickly return sodium excretion to baseline

CHAPTER

2

levels. Examples of these disorders include chronic renal failure and states of mineralocorticoid excess. In this case, the price of a return to sodium balance is hypertension. Disorders of sodium balance that result from secondary renal sodium retention, as in congestive heart failure, lead to more profound volume expansion owing to hypotension. In mild to moderates cases, volume expansion eventually returns the MAP to its set point; the price of sodium balance in this case is edema. In more severe cases, volume expansion never returns blood pressure to normal, and renal sodium retention is unremitting. In still other situations, such as nephrotic syndrome, volume expansion results from changes in both the renal set point and body volume distribution. In this case, the price of sodium balance may be both edema and hypertension. In each of these cases, renal sodium (and chloride) retention results from a discrepancy between the existing MAP and the renal set point.

The examples listed previously emphasize that disorders of sodium balance do not necessarily abrogate the ability to achieve sodium balance. When balance is defined as the equation of sodium intake and output, most patients with ECF expansion (and edema or hypertension) or ECF volume depletion achieve sodium balance. They do so, however, at the expense of expanded or contracted ECF volume. The *failure to achieve sodium balance at normal ECF volumes* characterizes these disorders.

Frequently, distinguishing disorders of sodium balance from disorders of water balance is useful. According to this scheme, disorders of water balance are disorders of body osmolality and usually are manifested by alterations in serum sodium concentration

(*see* Chapter 1). Disorders of sodium balance are disorders of ECF volume. This construct has a physiologic basis because water balance and sodium balance can be controlled separately and by distinct hormonal systems. It should be emphasized, however, that disorders of sodium balance frequently lead to or are associated with disorders of water balance. This is evident from Figure 2-24 in which hyponatremia is noted to be a sign of either ECF volume expansion or contraction. Thus, the distinction between disorders of sodium and water balance is useful in constructing differential diagnoses; however, the close interrelationships between factors that control sodium and water balance should be kept in mind.

The figures herein describe characteristics of sodium homeostasis in normal persons and also describe several of the regulatory systems that are important participants in controlling renal sodium excretion. Next, mechanisms of sodium transport along the nephron are presented, followed by examples of disorders of sodium balance that illuminate current understanding of their pathophysiology. Recently, rapid progress has been made in unraveling mechanisms of renal volume homeostasis. Most of the hormones that regulate sodium balance have been cloned and sequenced. Intracellular signaling mechanisms responsible for their effects have been characterized. The renal transport proteins that mediate sodium reabsorption also have been cloned and sequenced. The remaining challenges are to integrate this information into models that describe systemic volume homeostasis and to determine how alterations in one or more of the well-characterized systems lead to volume expansion or contraction.

Normal Extracellular Fluid Volume Homeostasis _____

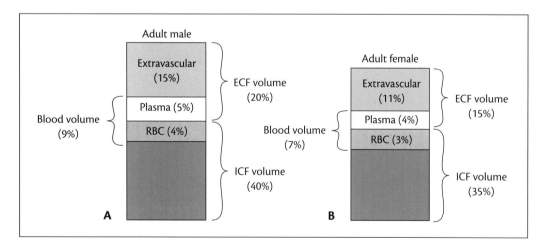

FIGURE 2-1

Fluid volumes in typical adult men and women, given as percentages of body weight. In men (**A**), total body water typically is 60% of body weight (Total body water = Extracellular fluid [ECF] volume + Intracellular fluid [ICF] volume). The ECF volume comprises the plasma volume and the extravascular volume. The ICF volume comprises the water inside erythrocytes (RBCs) and inside other cells. The blood volume comprises the plasma volume plus the RBC volume. Thus, the RBC volume is a unique component of ICF volume that contributes directly to cardiac output and blood pressure. Typically, water comprises a smaller percentage of the body weight in a woman (**B**) than in a man; thus, when expressed as a percentage of body weight, fluid volumes are smaller. Note, however, that the percentage of total body water that is intracellular is approximately 70% in both men and women [5].

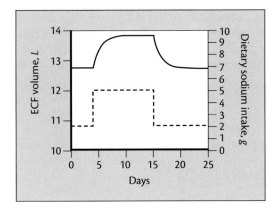

FIGURE 2-2

Effects of changes in dietary sodium (Na) intake on extracellular fluid (ECF) volume. The dietary intake of Na was increased from 2 to 5 g, and then returned to 2 g. The relationship between dietary Na intake (dashed line) and ECF volume (solid line) is derived from the model of Walser [1]. In this model the rate of Na excretion is assumed to be proportional to the content of Na in the body (A_t) above a zero point (A_0) at which Na excretion ceases. This relation can be expressed as $dA_t/dt = I - k(A_t - A_0)$, where I is the dietary Na intake and t is time. The ECF volume is approximated as the total body Na content divided by the plasma Na concentration. (This assumption is strictly incorrect because approximately 25% of Na is tightly bound in bone; however, this amount is nearly invariant and can be ignored in the current analysis.) According to this construct, when dietary Na intake changes from level 1 to level 2, the ECF volume approaches a new steady state exponentially with a time constant of k according to the following equation:

$$A_2 - A_1 = \frac{I_2}{k} + \frac{I_1 - I_2}{k} e^{-kt}$$

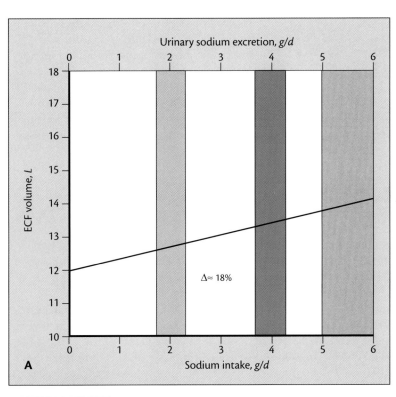

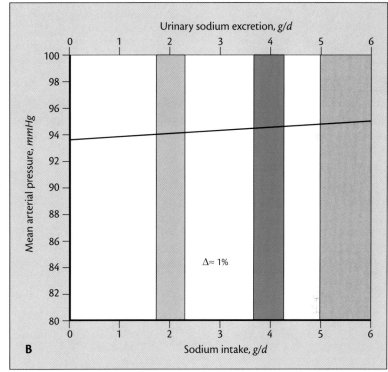

FIGURE 2-3

Relation between dietary sodium (Na), extracellular fluid (ECF) volume, and mean arterial pressure (MAP). A, Relation between the dietary intake of Na, ECF volume, and urinary Na excretion at steady state in a normal person. Note that 1 g of Na equals 43 mmol (43 mEq) of Na. At steady state, urinary Na excretion essentially is identical to the dietary intake of Na. As discussed in Figure 2-2, ECF volume increases linearly as the dietary intake of Na increases. At an ECF volume of under about 12 L, urinary Na excretion ceases. The gray bar indicates a normal dietary intake of Na when consuming a typical Western diet. The dark blue bar indicates the range of Na intake when consuming a "no added salt" diet. The light blue bar indicates that a "low-salt" diet generally contains about 2 g/d of Na. Note that increasing the dietary intake of Na from very low to normal levels leads to an 18% increase in ECF volume. B, Relation between the dietary intake of Na and MAP in normal persons. MAP is linearly dependent on Na intake; however, increasing dietary Na intake from very low to normal levels increases the MAP by only 1%. Thus, arterial pressure is regulated much more tightly than is ECF volume. (A, Data from Walser [1]; B, Data from Luft and coworkers [3].)

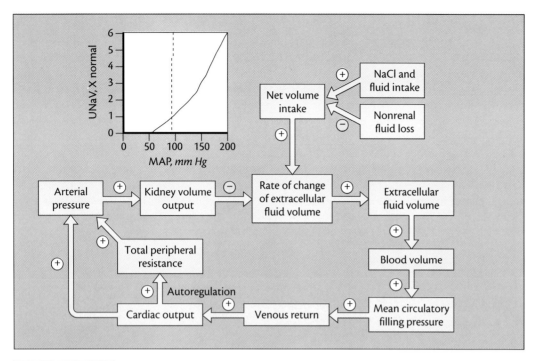

FIGURE 2-4

Schema for the kidney blood volume pressure feedback mechanism adapted from the work of Guyton and colleagues [6]. Positive relations are indicated by a plus sign; inverse relations are indicated by a minus sign. The block diagram shows that increases in extracellular fluid (ECF) volume result from increases in sodium chloride (NaCl) and fluid intake or decreases in kidney volume output. An increase in ECF volume increases the blood volume, thereby increasing the venous return to the heart and cardiac output. Increases in cardiac output increase arterial pressure both directly and by increasing peripheral vascular resistance (autoregulation). Increased arterial pressure is sensed by the kidney, leading to increased kidney volume output (pressure diuresis and pressure natriuresis), and thus returning the ECF volume to normal. The inset shows this relation between mean arterial pressure (MAP), renal volume, and sodium excretion [4]. The effects of acute increases in arterial pressure on urinary excretion are shown by the solid curve. The chronic effects are shown by the dotted curve; note that the dotted line is identical to the curve in Figure 2-3. Thus, when the MAP increases, urinary output increases, leading to decreased ECF volume and return to the original pressure set point. $U_{Na}V$—urinary sodium excretion volume.

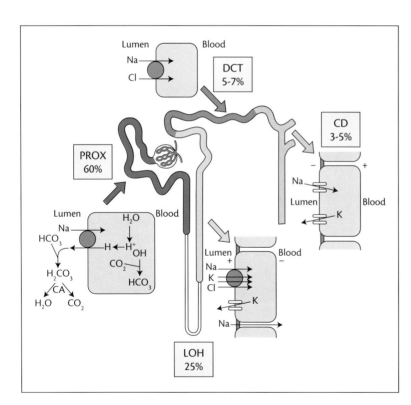

FIGURE 2-5

Sodium (Na) reabsorption along the mammalian nephron. About 25 moles of Na in 180 L of fluid daily is delivered into the glomerular filtrate of a normal person. About 60% of this load is reabsorbed along the proximal tubule (PROX), indicated in dark blue; about 25% along the loop of Henle (LOH), including the thick ascending limb indicated in light blue; about 5% to 7% along the distal convoluted tubule (DCT), indicated in dark gray; and 3% to 5% along the collecting duct (CD) system, indicated in light gray. All Na transporting cells along the nephron express the ouabain-inhibitable sodium-potassium adenosine triphosphatase (Na-K ATPase) pump at their basolateral (blood) cell surface. (The pump is not shown here for clarity.) Unique pathways are expressed at the luminal membrane that permit Na to enter cells. The most quantitatively important of these luminal Na entry pathways are shown here. These pathways are discussed in more detail in Figures 2-15 to 2-19. CA—carbonic anhydrase; Cl—chloride; CO_2—carbon dioxide; H—hydrogen; H_2CO_3—carbonic acid; HCO_3—bicarbonate; K—potassium; OH—hydroxyl ion.

Mechanisms of Extracellular Fluid Volume Control

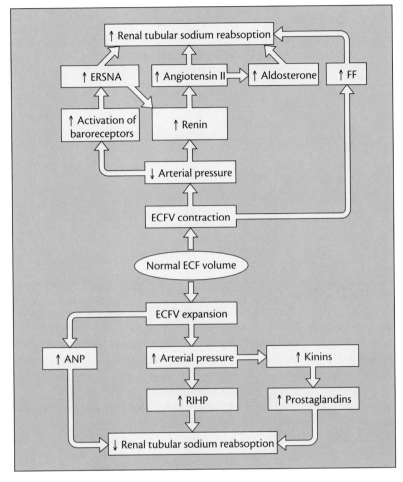

FIGURE 2-6

Integrated response of the kidneys to changes in extracellular fluid (ECF) volume. This composite figure illustrates natriuretic and antinatriuretic mechanisms. For simplicity, the systems are shown operating only in one direction and not all pathways are shown. The major antinatriuretic systems are the renin-angiotensin-aldosterone axis and increased efferent renal sympathetic nerve activity (ERSNA). The most important natriuretic mechanism is pressure natriuresis, because the level of renal perfusion pressure (RPP) determines the magnitude of the response to all other natriuretic systems. Renal interstitial hydrostatic pressure (RIHP) is a link between the circulation and renal tubular sodium reabsorption. Atrial natriuretic peptide (ANP) is the major systemic natriuretic hormone. Within the kidney, kinins and renomedullary prostaglandins are important modulators of the natriuretic response of the kidney. AVP—arginine vasopressin; FF—filtration fraction. (*Modified from* Gonzalez-Campoy and Knox [7].)

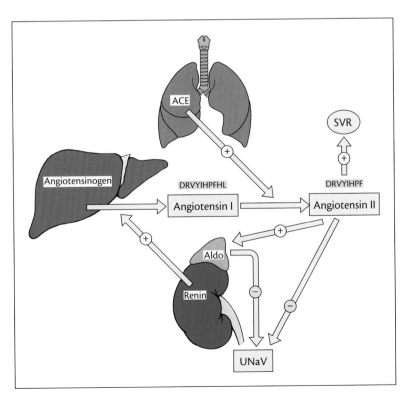

FIGURE 2-7

Overview of the renin-angiotensin-aldosterone system [8,9]. Angiotensinogen (or renin substrate) is a 56-kD glycoprotein produced and secreted by the liver. Renin is produced by the juxtaglomerular apparatus of the kidney, as shown in Figures 2-8 and 2-9. Renin cleaves the 10 N-terminal amino acids from angiotensinogen. This decapeptide (angiotensin I) is cleaved by angiotensin converting enzyme (ACE). The resulting angiotensin II comprises the 8 N-terminal amino acids of angiotensin I. The primary amino acid structures of angiotensins I and II are shown in single letter codes. Angiotensin II increases systemic vascular resistance (SVR), stimulates aldosterone secretion from the adrenal gland (indicated in gray), and increases sodium (Na) absorption by renal tubules, as shown in Figures 2-15 and 2-17. These effects decrease urinary Na (and chloride excretion; $U_{Na}V$).

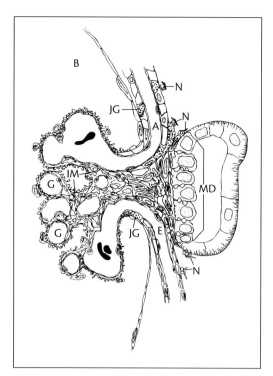

FIGURE 2-8

The juxtaglomerular (JG) apparatus. This apparatus brings into close apposition the afferent (A) and efferent (E) arterioles with the macula densa (MD), a specialized region of the thick ascending limb (TAL). The extraglomerular mesangium (EM), or lacis "Goormaghtigh apparatus (cells)," forms at the interface of these components. MD cells express the Na-K-2Cl (sodium-potassium-chloride) cotransporter (NKCC2) at the apical membrane [10,11]. By way of the action of this transporter, MD cells sense the sodium chloride concentration of luminal fluid. By way of mechanisms that are unclear, this message is communicated to JG cells located in and near the arterioles (especially the afferent arteriole). These JG cells increase renin secretion when the NaCl concentration in the lumen is low [12]. Cells in the afferent arteriole also sense vascular pressure directly, by way of the mechanisms discussed in Figure 2-9. Both the vascular and tubular components are innervated by sympathetic nerves (N). B—Bowman's space, G—glomerular capillary; IM—intraglomerular mesangium. (*From* Barajas [13]; with permission.)

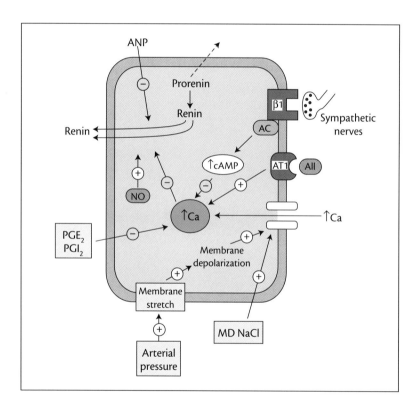

FIGURE 2-9

Schematic view of a (granular) juxtaglomerular cell showing secretion mechanisms of renin [8]. Renin is generated from prorenin. Renin secretion is inhibited by increases in and stimulated by decreases in intracellular calcium (Ca) concentrations. Voltage-sensitive Ca channels in the plasma membrane are activated by membrane stretch, which correlates with arterial pressure and is assumed to mediate baroreceptor-sensitive renin secretion. Renin secretion is also stimulated when the concentration of sodium (Na) and chloride (Cl) at the macula densa (MD) decreases [12,14]. The mediators of this effect are less well characterized; however, some studies suggest that the effect of Na and Cl in the lumen is more potent than is the baroreceptor mechanism [15]. Many other factors affect rates of renin release and contribute to the physiologic regulation of renin. Renal nerves, by way of β receptors coupled to adenylyl cyclase (AC), stimulate renin release by increasing the production of cyclic adenosine monophosphate (cAMP), which reduces Ca release. Angiotensin II (AII) receptors (AT1 receptors) inhibit renin release, as least in vitro. Prostaglandins E_2 and I_2 (PGE_2 and PGI_2, respectively) strongly stimulate renin release through mechanisms that remain unclear. Atrial natriuretic peptide (ANP) strongly inhibits renin secretion. Constitutive nitric oxide (NO) synthase is expressed by macula densa (MD) cells [16]. NO appears to stimulate renin secretion, an effect that may counteract inhibition of the renin gene by AII [17,18].

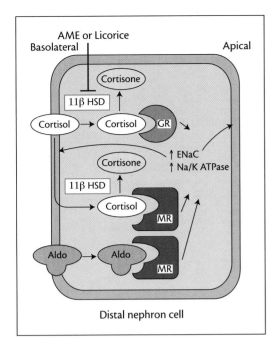

FIGURE 2-10

Mechanism of aldosterone action in the distal nephron [19]. Aldosterone, the predominant human mineralocorticoid hormone, enters distal nephron cells through the plasma membrane and interacts with its receptor (the mineralocorticoid receptor [MR], or Type I receptor). Interaction between aldosterone and this receptor initiates induction of new proteins that, by way of mechanisms that remain unclear, increase the number of sodium channels (ENaC) and sodium-potassium adenosine triphosphatase (Na-K ATPase) pumps at the cell surface. This increases transepithelial Na (and potassium) transport. Cortisol, the predominant human glucocorticoid hormone, also enters cells through the plasma membrane and interacts with its receptor (the glucocorticoid receptor [GR]). Cortisol, however, also interacts with mineralocorticoid receptors; the affinity of cortisol and aldosterone for mineralocorticoid receptors is approximately equal. In distal nephron cells, this interaction also stimulates electrogenic Na transport [20]. Cortisol normally circulates at concentrations 100 to 1000 times higher than the circulating concentration of aldosterone. In aldosterone-responsive tissues, such as the distal nephron, expression of the enzyme 11β-hydroxysteroid dehydrogenase (11β-HSD) permits rapid metabolism of cortisol so that only aldosterone can stimulate Na transport in these cells. An inherited deficiency of the enzyme 11β-HSD (the syndrome of apparent mineralocorticoid excess, AME), or inhibition of the enzyme by ingestion of licorice, leads to hypertension owing to chronic stimulation of distal Na transport by endogenous glucocorticoids [21].

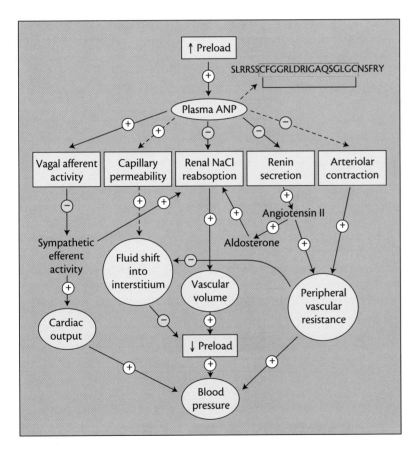

FIGURE 2-11

Control of systemic hemodynamics by the atrial natriuretic peptide (ANP) system. Increases in atrial stretch (PRELOAD) increase ANP secretion by cardiac atria. The primary amino acid sequence of ANP is shown in single letter code with its disulfide bond indicated by the lines. The amino acids highlighted in blue are conserved between ANP, brain natriuretic peptide, and C-type natriuretic peptide. ANP has diverse functions that include but are not limited to the following: stimulating vagal afferent activity, increasing capillary permeability, inhibiting renal sodium (Na) and water reabsorption, inhibiting renin release, and inhibiting arteriolar contraction. These effects reduce sympathetic nervous activity, reduce angiotensin II generation, reduce aldosterone secretion, reduce total peripheral resistance, and shift fluid out of the vasculature into the interstitium. The net effect of these actions is to decrease cardiac output, vascular volume, and peripheral resistance, thereby returning preload toward baseline. Many effects of ANP (indicated by solid arrows) are diminished in patients with edematous disorders (there is an apparent resistance to ANP). Effects indicated by dashed arrows may not be diminished in edematous disorders; these effects contribute to shifting fluid from vascular to extravascular tissue, leading to edema. This observation may help explain the association between elevated right-sided filling pressures and the tendency for Na retention [22]. (*Modified from* Brenner and coworkers [23].)

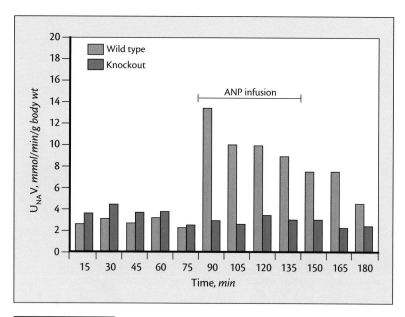

FIGURE 2-12

Mechanism of atrial natriuretic peptide (ANP) action on the kidney. Animals with disruption of the particulate form of guanylyl cyclase (GC) manifest increased mean arterial pressure that is independent of dietary intake of sodium chloride. To test whether ANP mediates its renal effects by way of the action of GC, ANP was infused into wild-type and GC-A–deficient mice. In wild-type animals, ANP led to prompt natriuresis. In GC-A–deficient mice, no effect was observed. $U_{Na}V$—urinary sodium excretion volume. (*Modified from* Kishimoto [24].)

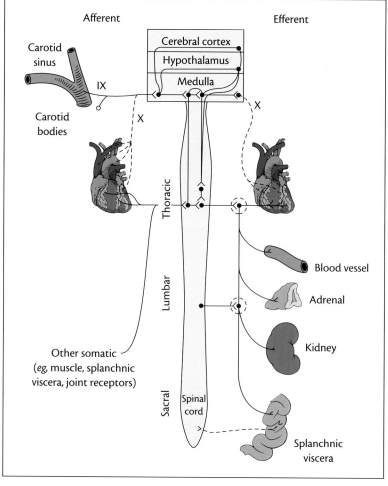

FIGURE 2-13

Schematic diagram of neural connections important in circulatory control. Although the system is bilaterally symmetric, afferent fibers are shown to the left and efferent fibers to the right. Sympathetic fibers are shown as solid lines and parasympathetic fibers as dashed lines. The heart receives both sympathetic and parasympathetic innervation. Sympathetic fibers lead to vasoconstriction and renal sodium chloride retention. X indicates the vagus nerve; IX indicates glossopharyngeal. (*From* Korner [25]; with permission.)

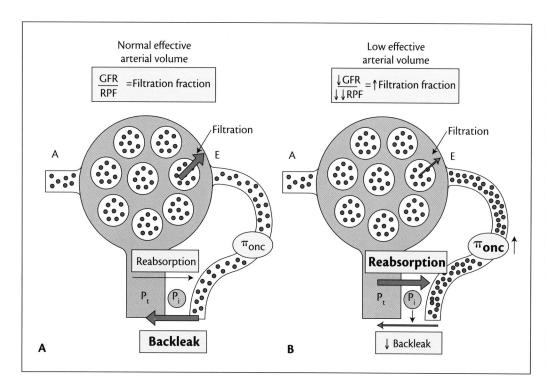

FIGURE 2-14

Cellular mechanisms of increased solute and water reabsorption by the proximal tubule in patients with "effective" arterial volume depletion. **A,** Normal effective arterial volume in normal persons. **B,** Low effective arterial volume in patients with both decreased glomerular filtration rates (GFR) and renal plasma flow (RPF). In contrast to normal persons, patients with low effective arterial volume have decreased GFR and RPF, yet the filtration fraction is increased because the RPF decreases more than does the GFR. The increased filtration fraction concentrates the plasma protein (indicated by the dots) in the peritubular capillaries leading to increased plasma oncotic pressure (π_{onc}). Increased plasma oncotic pressure reduces the amount of backleak from the peritubular capillaries. Simultaneously, the increase in filtration fraction reduces volume delivery to the

(*Legend continued on next page*)

FIGURE 2-14 *(continued)*

peritubular capillary, decreasing its hydrostatic pressure, and thereby reducing the renal interstitial hydrostatic pressure (P_i). Even though the proximal tubule hydrostatic pressure (P_t) may be reduced, owing to diminished GFR, the hydrostatic gradient from tubule to interstitium is increased, favoring increased volume reabsorption. A—afferent arteriole; E—efferent arteriole.

Mechanisms of Sodium and Chloride Transport along the Nephron

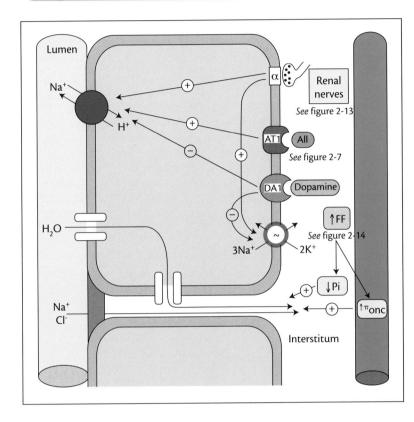

FIGURE 2-15

Cellular mechanisms and regulation of sodium chloride (NaCl) and volume reabsorption along the proximal tubule. The sodium-potassium adenosine triphosphate (Na-K ATPase) pump (shown as white circle with light blue outline) at the basolateral cell membrane keeps the intracellular Na concentration low; the K concentration high; and the cell membrane voltage oriented with the cell interior negative, relative to the exterior. Many pathways participate in Na entry across the luminal membrane. Only the sodium-hydrogen (Na-H) exchanger is shown because its regulation in states of volume excess and depletion has been characterized extensively. Activity of the Na-H exchanger is increased by stimulation of renal nerves, acting by way of α receptors and by increased levels of circulating angiotensin II (AII), as shown in Figures 2-7 and 2-13 [25–28]. Increased levels of dopamine (DA1) act to inhibit activity of the Na-H exchanger [29,30]. Dopamine also acts to inhibit activity of the Na-K ATPase pump at the basolateral cell membrane [30]. As described in Figure 2-14, increases in the filtration fraction (FF) lead to increases in oncotic pressure (π_{onc}) in peritubular capillaries and decreases in peritubular and interstitial hydrostatic pressure (P_i). These changes increase solute and volume absorption and decrease solute backflux. Water flows through water channels (Aquaporin-1) Na and Cl also traverse the paracellular pathway.

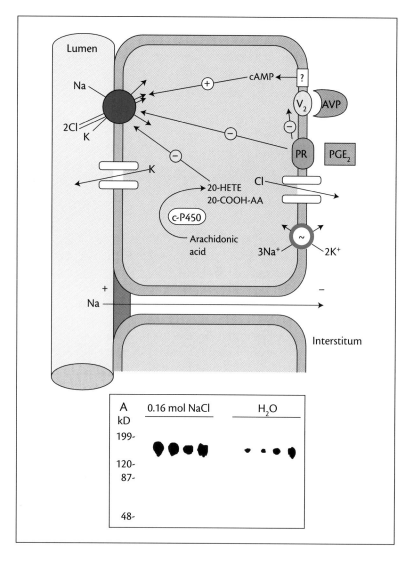

FIGURE 2-16

Cellular mechanisms and regulation of sodium (Na) and chloride (Cl) transport by thick ascending limb (TAL) cells. Na, Cl, and potassium (K) enter cells by way of the bumetanide-sensitive Na-K-2Cl cotransporter (NKCC2) at the apical membrane. K recycles back through apical membrane K channels (ROMK) to permit continued operation of the transporter. In this nephron segment, the asymmetric operations of the luminal K channel and the basolateral chloride channel generate a transepithelial voltage, oriented with the lumen positive. This voltage drives paracellular Na absorption. Although arginine vasopressin (AVP) is known to stimulate Na reabsorption by TAL cells in some species, data from studies in human subjects suggest AVP has minimal or no effect [31,32]. The effect of AVP is mediated by way of production of cyclic adenosine monophosphate (cAMP). Prostaglandin E_2 (PGE_2) and cytochrome P450 (c-P450) metabolites of arachidonic acid (20-HETE [hydroxy-eicosatetraenoic acid] and 20-COOH-AA) inhibit transepithelial NaCl transport, at least in part by inhibiting the Na-K-2Cl cotransporter [33–35]. PGE_2 also inhibits vasopressin-stimulated Na transport, in part by activating G_i and inhibiting adenylyl cyclase [36]. Increases in medullary NaCl concentration may activate transepithelial Na transport by increasing production of PGE_2. **Inset A,** Regulation of NKCC2 by chronic Na delivery. Animals were treated with 0.16 mol NaCl or water as drinking fluid for 2 weeks. The Western blot shows upregulation of NKCC2 in the group treated with saline [37]. G_i—inhibitory G protein; PR—prostaglandin receptor; V_2— AVP receptors. (*Modified from* Ecelbarger [37].)

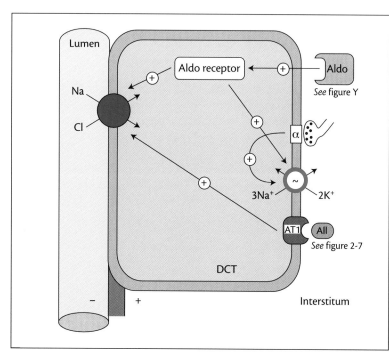

FIGURE 2-17

Mechanisms and regulation of sodium (Na) and chloride (Cl) transport by the distal nephron. As in other nephron segments, intracellular Na concentration is maintained low by the action of the Na-K ATPase (sodium-potassium adenosine triphosphatase) pump at the basolateral cell membrane. Na enters distal convoluted tubule (DCT) cells across the luminal membrane coupled directly to chloride by way of the thiazide-sensitive Na-Cl cotransporter. Activity of the Na-Cl cotransporter appears to be stimulated by both aldosterone and angiotensin II (AII) [38–40]. Transepithelial Na transport in this segment is also stimulated by sympathetic nerves acting by way of α receptors [41,42]. The DCT is impermeable to water.

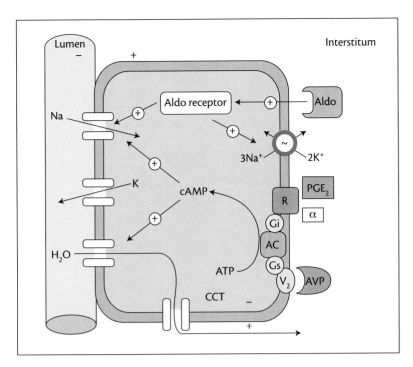

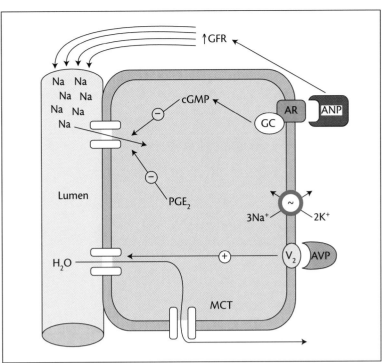

FIGURE 2-18

Principal cortical collecting tubule (CCT) cells. In these cells, sodium (Na) enters across the luminal membrane through Na channels (ENaC). The movement of cationic Na from lumen to cell depolarizes the luminal membrane, generating a transepithelial electrical gradient oriented with the lumen negative with respect to interstitium. This electrical gradient permits cationic potassium (K) to diffuse preferentially from cell to lumen through K channels (ROMK). Na transport is stimulated when aldosterone interacts with its intracellular receptor [43]. This effect involves both increases in the number of Na channels at the luminal membrane and increases in the number of Na-K ATPase (Sodium-potassium adenosine triphosphatase) pumps at the basolateral cell membrane. Arginine vasopressin (AVP) stimulates both Na absorption (by interacting with V_2 receptors and, perhaps, V_1 receptors) and water transport (by interacting with V_2 receptors) [44–46]. V_2 receptor stimulation leads to insertion of water channels (aquaporin 2) into the luminal membrane [47]. V_2 receptor stimulation is modified by PGE_2 and α_2 agonists that interact with a receptor that stimulates G_i [48]. AC—adenylyl cyclase; ATP—adenosine triphosphate; cAMP—cyclic adenosine monophosphate; CCT—cortical collecting tubule; G_i—inhibitory G protein; G_s—stimulatory G protein; R—Ri receptor.

FIGURE 2-19

Cellular mechanism of the medullary collecting tubule (MCT). Sodium (Na) and water are reabsorbed along the MCT. Atrial natriuretic peptide (ANP) is the best-characterized hormone that affects Na absorption along this segment [22]. Data on the effects of arginine vasopressin (AVP) and aldosterone are not as consistent [46,49]. Prostaglandin E_2 (PGE_2) inhibits Na transport by inner medullary collecting duct cells and may be an important intracellular mediator for the actions of endothelin and interleukin-1 [50,51]. ANP inhibits medullary Na transport by interacting with a G-protein–coupled receptor that generates cyclic guanosine monophosphate (cGMP). This second messenger inhibits a luminal Na channel that is distinct from the Na channel expressed by the principal cells of the cortical collecting tubule, as shown in Figure 2-18 [52,53]. Under normal circumstances, ANP also increases the glomerular filtration rate (GFR) and inhibits Na transport by way of the effects on the renin-angiotensin-aldosterone axis, as shown in Figures 2-7 to 2-10. These effects increase Na delivery to the MCT. The combination of increased distal Na delivery and inhibited distal reabsorption leads to natriuresis. In patients with congestive heart failure, distal Na delivery remains depressed despite high levels of circulating ANP. Thus, inhibition of apical Na entry does not lead to natriuresis, despite high levels of MCT cGMP. AR—ANP receptor; GC—guanylyl cyclase; K—potassium; V_2—receptors.

Causes, Signs, and Symptoms of Extracellular Fluid Volume Expansion and Contraction

CAUSES OF VOLUME EXPANSION

Primary renal sodium retention (with hypertension but without edema)
  Hyperaldosteronism (Conn's syndrome)
  Cushing's syndrome
  Inherited hypertension (Liddle's syndrome, glucocorticoid remediable hyperaldo-
    steronism, pseudohypoaldosteronism Type II, others)
  Renal failure
  Nephrotic syndrome (mixed disorder)

Secondary renal sodium retention
  Hypoproteinemia
    Nephrotic syndrome
    Protein-losing enteropathy
    Cirrhosis with ascites
  Low cardiac output
    Hemodynamically significant pericardial effusion
    Constrictive pericarditis
    Valvular heart disease with congestive heart failure
    Severe pulmonary disease
    Cardiomyopathies
  Peripheral vasodilation
    Pregnancy
    Gram-negative sepsis
    Anaphylaxis
    Arteriovenous fistula
    Trauma
    Cirrhosis
    Idiopathic edema (?)
    Drugs: minoxidil, diazoxide, calcium channel blockers (?)
  Increased capillary permeability
    Idiopathic edema (?)
    Burns
    Allergic reactions, including certain forms of angioedema
    Adult respiratory distress syndrome
    Interleukin-2 therapy
    Malignant ascites
  Sequestration of fluid ("3rd spacing," urine sodium concentration low)
    Peritonitis
    Pancreatitis
    Small bowel obstruction
    Rhabdomyolysis, crush injury
    Bleeding into tissues
    Venous occlusion

CAUSES OF VOLUME DEPLETION

Extrarenal losses (urine sodium concentration low)
  Gastrointestinal salt losses
    Vomiting
    Diarrhea
    Nasogastric or small bowel aspiration
    Intestinal fistulae or ostomies
    Gastrointestinal bleeding
  Skin and respiratory tract losses
    Burns
    Heat exposure
    Adrenal insufficiency
    Extensive dermatologic lesions
    Cystic fibrosis
    Pulmonary bronchorrhea
    Drainage of large pleural effusion

Renal losses (urine sodium concentration normal or elevated)
  Extrinsic
    Solute diuresis (glucose, bicarbonate, urea, mannitol, dextran, contrast dye)
    Diuretic agents
    Adrenal insufficiency
    Selective aldosterone deficiency
  Intrinsic
    Diuretic phase of oliguric acute renal failure
    Postobstructive diuresis
    Nonoliguric acute renal failure
    Salt-wasting nephropathy
      Medullary cystic disease
      Tubulointerstitial disease
      Nephrocalcinosis

FIGURE 2-21

In volume depletion, total body sodium is decreased.

FIGURE 2-20

In volume expansion, total body sodium (Na) content is increased. In primary renal Na retention, volume expansion is modest and edema does not develop because blood pressure increases until Na excretion matches intake. In secondary Na retention, blood pressure may not increase sufficiently to increase urinary Na excretion until edema develops.

CLINICAL SIGNS OF VOLUME EXPANSION

Edema
Pulmonary crackles
Ascites
Jugular venous distention
Hepatojugular reflux
Hypertension

FIGURE 2-22

Clinical signs of volume expansion.

CLINICAL SIGNS OF VOLUME DEPLETION

Orthostatic decrease in blood pressure and increase in pulse rate
Decreased pulse volume
Decreased venous pressure
Loss of axillary sweating
Decreased skin turgor
Dry mucous membranes

FIGURE 2-23

Clinical signs of volume depletion.

LABORATORY SIGNS OF VOLUME DEPLETION OR EXPANSION

Hypernatremia
Hyponatremia
Acid-base disturbances
Abnormal plasma potassium
Decrease in glomerular filtration rate
Elevated blood urea nitrogen–creatinine ratio
Low functional excretion of sodium (FE_{Na})

FIGURE 2-24

Note that laboratory test results for volume expansion and contraction are similar. Serum sodium (Na) concentration may be increased or decreased in either volume expansion or contraction, depending on the cause and intake of free water (*see* Chapter 1). Acid-base disturbances, such as metabolic alkalosis, and hypokalemia are common in both conditions. The similarity of the laboratory test results of volume depletion and expansion results from the fact that the "effective" arterial volume is depleted in both states despite dramatic expansion of the extracellular fluid volume in one.

Unifying Hypothesis of Renal Sodium Excretion

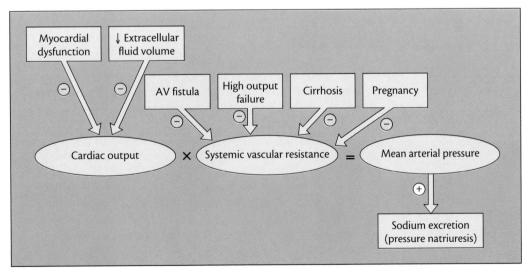

FIGURE 2-25

Summary of mechanisms of sodium (Na) retention in volume contraction and in depletion of the "effective" arterial volume. In secondary Na retention, Na retention results primarily from a reduction in mean arterial pressure (MAP). Some disorders decrease cardiac output, such as congestive heart failure owing to myocardial dysfunction; others decrease systemic vascular resistance, such as high-output cardiac failure, atriovenous fistulas, and cirrhosis. Because MAP is the product of systemic vascular resistance and cardiac output, all causes lead to the same result. As shown in Figures 2-3 and 2-4, small changes in MAP lead to large changes in urinary Na excretion. Although edematous disorders usually are characterized as resulting from contraction of the effective arterial volume, the MAP, as a determinant of renal perfusion pressure, may be the crucial variable (Figs. 2-26 and 2-28 provide supportive data). The mechanisms of edema in nephrotic syndrome are more complex and are discussed in Figures 2-36 to 2-39.

Mechanisms of Extracellular Fluid Volume Expansion in Congestive Heart Failure

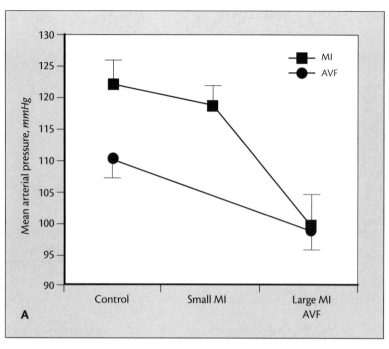

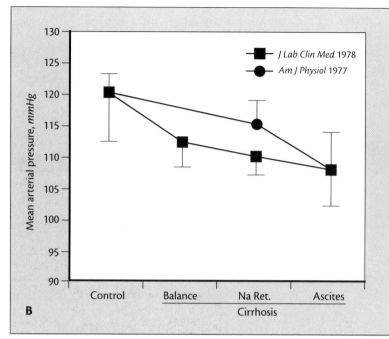

FIGURE 2-26

Role of renal perfusion pressure in sodium (Na) retention. **A,** Results from studies in rats that had undergone myocardial infarction (MI) or placement of an arteriovenous fistula (AVF) [54]. Rats with small and large MIs were identified. Both small and large MIs induced significant Na retention when challenged with Na loads. Renal Na retention occurred in the setting of mild hypotension. AVF also induced significant Na retention, which was associated with a decrease in mean arterial pressure (MAP) [55,56]. Figure 2-3 has shown that Na excretion decreases greatly for each mm Hg decrease in MAP. **B,** Results of two groups of experiments performed by Levy and Allotey [57,58] in

which experimental cirrhosis was induced in dogs by sporadic feeding with dimethylnitrosamine. Three cirrhotic stages were identified based on the pattern of Na retention. In the first, dietary Na intake was balanced by Na excretion. In the second, renal Na retention began, but still without evidence of ascites or edema. In the last, ascites were detected. Because Na was retained before the appearance of ascites, "primary" renal Na retention was inferred. An alternative interpretation of these data suggests that the modest decrease in MAP is responsible for Na retention in this model. Note that in both heart failure and cirrhosis, Na retention correlates with a decline in MAP.

FIGURE 2-27

Mechanism of sodium (Na) retention in high-output cardiac failure. Effects of high-output heart failure induced in dogs by arteriovenous (AV) fistula [59]. After induction of an AV fistula (day 0), plasma renin activity (PRA; thick solid line) increased greatly, correlating temporally with a reduction in urinary Na excretion ($U_{Na}V$; thin solid line). During this period, mean arterial pressure (MAP; dotted line) declined modestly. After day 5, the plasma atrial natriuretic peptide concentration (ANP; dashed line) increased because of volume expansion, returning urinary Na excretion to baseline levels. Thus, Na retention, mediated in part by the renin-angiotensin-aldosterone system, led to volume expansion. The volume expansion suppressed the renin-angiotensin-aldosterone system and stimulated ANP secretion, thereby returning Na excretion to normal. These experiments suggest that ANP secretion plays an important role in maintaining Na excretion in compensated congestive heart failure. This effect of ANP has been confirmed directly in experiments using anti-ANP antibodies [60]. AI—angiotensin I.

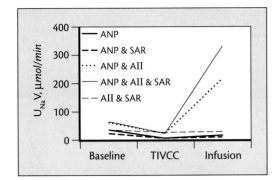

FIGURE 2-28

Mechanism of renal resistance to atrial natriuretic peptide (ANP) in experimental low-output heart failure. Low-output heart failure was induced in dogs by thoracic inferior vena caval constriction (TIVCC), which also led to a significant decrease in renal perfusion pressure (RPP) (from 127 to 120 mm Hg). ANP infusion into dogs with TIVCC did not increase urinary sodium (Na) excretion ($U_{Na}V$, ANP group). In contrast, when the RPP was returned to baseline by infusing angiotensin II (AII), urinary Na excretion increased greatly (ANP + AII). To exclude a direct effect of AII on urinary Na excretion, intrarenal saralasin (SAR) was infused to block renal AII receptors. SAR did not significantly affect the natriuresis induced by ANP plus AII. An independent effect of SAR on urinary Na excretion was excluded by infusing ANP plus SAR and AII plus SAR. These treatments were without effect. These results were interpreted as indicating that the *predominant* cause of resistance to ANP in dogs with low-output congestive heart failure is a reduction in RPP. (*Data from* Redfield and coworkers [61].)

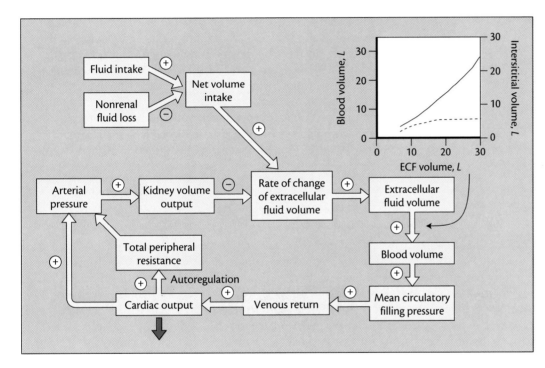

FIGURE 2-29

Mechanism of extracellular fluid (ECF) volume expansion in congestive heart failure. A primary decrease in cardiac output (indicated by dark blue arrow) leads to a decrease in arterial pressure, which decreases pressure natriuresis and volume excretion. These decreases expand the ECF volume. The inset graph shows that the ratio of interstitial volume (solid line) to plasma volume (dotted line) increases as the ECF volume expands because the interstitial compliance increases [62]. Thus, although expansion of the ECF volume increases blood volume and venous return, thereby restoring cardiac output toward normal, this occurs at the expense of a *disproportionate* expansion of interstitial volume, often manifested as edema.

Mechanisms of Extracellular Fluid Volume Expansion in Cirrhosis

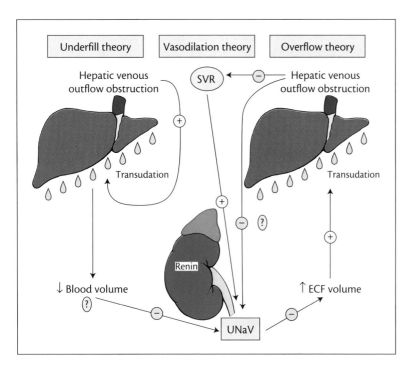

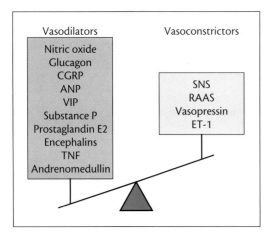

FIGURE 2-30

Three theories of ascites formation in hepatic cirrhosis. Hepatic venous outflow obstruction leads to portal hypertension. According to the *underfill theory*, transudation from the liver leads to reduction of the blood volume, thereby stimulating sodium (Na) retention by the kidney. As indicated by the question mark near the term *blood volume*, a low blood volume is rarely detected in clinical or experimental cirrhosis. Furthermore, this theory predicts that ascites would develop before renal Na retention, when the reverse generally occurs. According to the *overflow theory*, increased portal pressure stimulates renal Na retention through incompletely defined mechanisms. As indicated by the question mark near the arrow from hepatic venous outflow obstruction to $U_{Na}V$, the nature of the portal hypertension–induced signals for renal Na retention remains unclear. The *vasodilation theory* suggests that portal hypertension leads to vasodilation and relative arterial hypotension. Evidence for vasodilation in cirrhosis that precedes renal Na retention is now convincing, as shown in Figures 2-31 and 2-33 [63].

FIGURE 2-31

Alterations in cardiovascular hemodynamics in hepatic cirrhosis. Hepatic dysfunction and portal hypertension increase the production and impair the metabolism of several vasoactive substances. The overall balance of vasoconstriction and vasodilation shifts in favor of dilation. Vasodilation may also shift blood away from the central circulation toward the periphery and away from the kidneys. Some of the vasoactive substances postulated to participate in the hemodynamic disturbances of cirrhosis include those shown here. ANP—atrial natrivretic peptide; ET-1—endothelin-1; CGRP—calcitonin gene related peptide; RAAS—renin/angiotensin/aldosterone system; TNF—tumor necrosis factor; VIP— vasoactive intestinal peptide. (*Data from* Møller and Henriksen [64].)

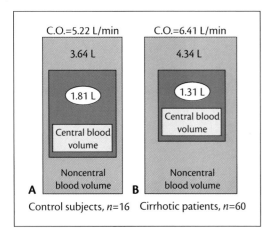

FIGURE 2-32

Effects of cirrhosis on central and noncentral blood volumes. The central blood volume is defined as the blood volume in the heart, lungs, and central arterial tree. Compared with control subjects (**A**), patients with cirrhosis (**B**) have decreased central and increased noncentral blood volumes. The higher cardiac output (CO) results from peripheral vasodilation. Perfusion of the kidney is reduced significantly in patients with cirrhosis. (*Data from* Hillarp and coworkers [65].)

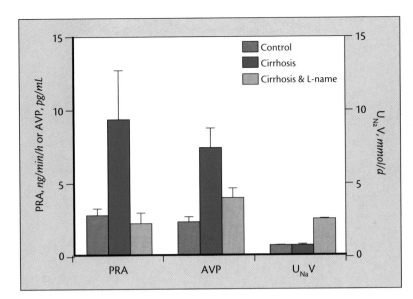

FIGURE 2-33

Contribution of nitric oxide to vasodilation and sodium (Na) retention in cirrhosis. Compared with control rats, rats having cirrhosis induced by carbon tetrachloride and phenobarbital exhibited increased plasma renin activity (PRA) and plasma arginine vasopressin (AVP) concentrations. At steady state, the urinary Na excretion ($U_{Na}V$) was similar in both groups. After treatment with L-NAME for 7 days, plasma renin activity decreased to normal levels, AVP concentrations decreased toward normal levels, and urinary Na excretion increased by threefold. These changes were associated with a normalization of mean arterial pressure and cardiac output. (Data compiled from Niederberger and coworkers [66,67] and Martin and Schrier [68].)

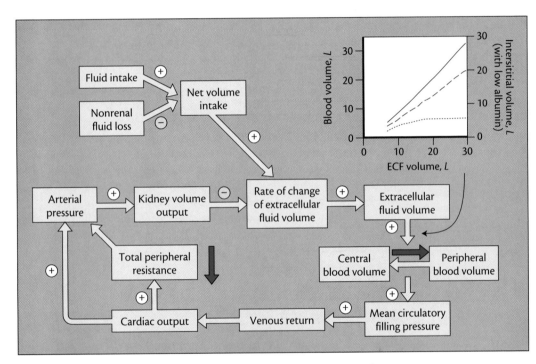

FIGURE 2-34

Mechanisms of sodium (Na) retention in cirrhosis. A primary decrease in systemic vascular resistance (indicated by dark blue arrow), induced by mediators shown in Figure 2-31, leads to a decrease in arterial pressure. The reduction in systemic vascular resistance, however, is not uniform and favors movement of blood from the central ("effective") circulation into the peripheral circulation, as shown in Figure 2-32. Hypoalbuminemia shifts the interstitial to blood volume ratio upward (compare the interstitial volume with normal [*dashed line*], and low [*solid line*], protein levels in the inset graph). Because cardiac output increases and venous return must equal cardiac output, dramatic expansion of the extracellular fluid (ECF) volume occurs.

Mechanisms of Extracellular Fluid Volume Expansion in Nephrotic Syndrome

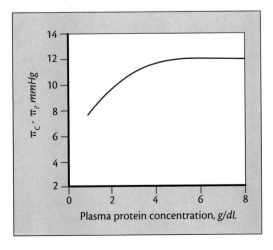

FIGURE 2-35

Changes in plasma protein concentration affect the net oncotic pressure difference across capillaries ($\pi_c - \pi_i$) in humans. Note that moderate reductions in plasma protein concentration have little effect on differences in transcapillary oncotic pressure. Only when plasma protein concentration decreases below 5 g/dL do changes become significant. (*Data from* Fadnes and coworkers [69].)

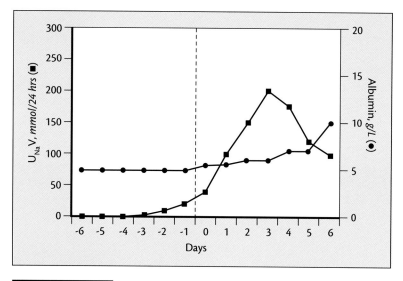

FIGURE 2-36

Time course of recovery from minimal change nephrotic syndrome in five children. Note that urinary Na excretion (squares) increases before serum albumin concentration increases. The data suggest that the natriuresis reflects a change in intrinsic renal Na retention. The data also emphasize that factors other than hypoalbuminemia must contribute to the Na retention that occurs in nephrosis. $U_{Na}V$—urinary Na excretion volume. (*Data from* Oliver and Owings [70].)

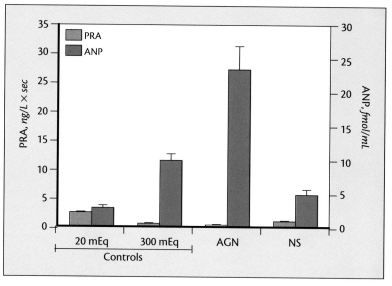

FIGURE 2-37

Plasma renin activity (PRA) and atrial natriuretic peptide (ANP) concentration in the nephrotic syndrome. Shown are PRA and ANP concentration (+standard error) in normal persons ingesting diets high (300 mEq/d) and low (20 mEq/d) in sodium (Na) and in patients with acute glomerulonephritis (AGN), predominantly post-streptococcal, or nephrotic syndrome (NS). Note that PRA is suppressed in patients with AGN to levels below those in normal persons on diets high in Na. PRA suppression suggests that primary renal NaCl retention plays an important role in the pathogenesis of volume expansion in AGN. Although plasma renin activity in patients with nephrotic syndrome is not suppressed to the same degree, the absence of PRA elevation in these patients suggests that primary renal Na retention plays a significant role in the pathogenesis of Na retention in NS as well. (*Data from* Rodrígeuez-Iturbe and coworkers [71].)

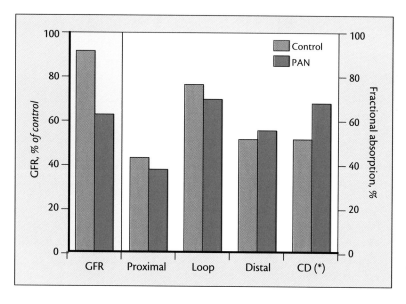

FIGURE 2-38

Sites of sodium (Na) reabsorption along the nephron in control and nephrotic rats (induced by puromycin aminonucleoside [PAN]). The glomerular filtration rates (GFR) in normal and nephrotic rats are shown by the hatched bars. Note the modest reduction in GFR in the nephrotic group, a finding that is common in human nephrosis. Fractional reabsorption rates along the proximal tubule, the loop of Henle, and the superficial distal tubule are indicated. The fractional reabsorption along the collecting duct (CD) is estimated from the difference between the end distal and urine deliveries. The data suggest that the predominant site of increased reabsorption is the collecting duct. Because superficial and deep nephrons may differ in reabsorptive rates, these data would also be consistent with enhanced reabsorption by deep nephrons. Asterisk—data inferred from the difference between distal and urine samples. (*Data from* Ichikawa and coworkers [72].)

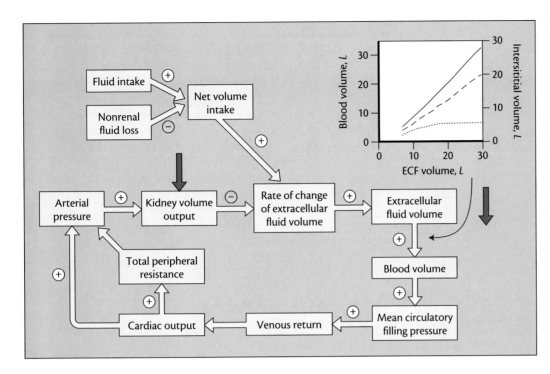

FIGURE 2-39

Mechanisms of extracellular fluid (ECF) volume expansion in nephrotic syndrome. Nephrotic syndrome is characterized by hypoalbuminemia, which shifts the relation between blood and interstitial volume upward (dashed to solid lines in inset). As discussed in Figure 2-35, these effects of hypoalbuminemia are evident when serum albumin concentrations decrease by more than half. In addition, however, hypoalbuminemia may induce vasodilation and arterial hypotension that lead to sodium (Na) retention, independent of transudation of fluid into the interstitium [73,74]. Unlike other states of hypoproteinemia and vasodilation, however, nephrotic syndrome usually is associated with normotension or hypertension. Coupled with the observation made in Figure 2-36 that natriuresis may take place before increases in serum albumin concentration in patients with nephrotic syndrome, these data implicate an important role for primary renal Na retention in this disorder (dark blue arrow). As suggested by Figure 2-37, the decrease in urinary Na excretion may play a larger role in patients with acute glomerulonephritis than in patients with minimal change nephropathy [71].

Extracellular Fluid Volume Homeostasis in Chronic Renal Failure

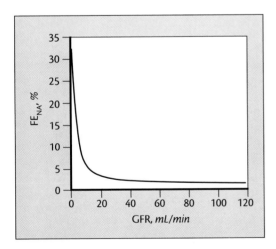

FIGURE 2-40

Relation between glomerular filtration rate (GFR) and fractional sodium (Na) excretion (FE_{Na}). The normal FE_{Na} is less than 1%. Adaptations in chronic renal failure maintain urinary Na excretion equal to dietary intake until end-stage renal disease is reached. To achieve this, the FE_{Na} must increase as the GFR decreases.

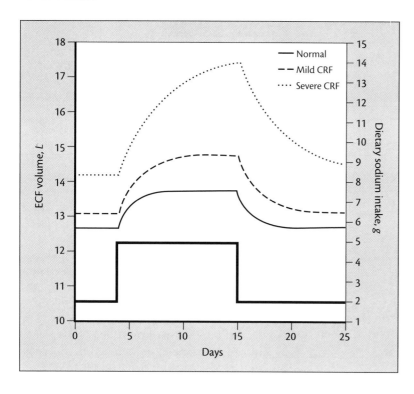

FIGURE 2-41

Effects of dietary sodium (Na) intake on extracellular fluid (ECF) volume in chronic renal failure (CRF) [75]. Compared with normal persons, patients with CRF have expanded ECF volume at normal Na intake. Furthermore, the time necessary to return to neutral balance on shifting from one to another level of Na intake is increased. Thus, whereas urinary Na excretion equals dietary intake of Na within 3 to 5 days in normal persons, this process may take up to 2 weeks in patients with CRF. This time delay means that not only are these patients susceptible to volume overload, but also to volume depletion. This phenomenon can be modeled simply by reducing the time constant (k) given in the equation in Figure 2-2, and leaving the set point (A_0) unchanged. The curves here represent time constants of 0.79 ± 0.05 day_{-1} (normal), 0.5 day_{-1} (mild CRF), and 0.25 day_{-1} (severe CRF).

References

1. Walser M: Phenomenological analysis of renal regulation of sodium and potassium balance. *Kidney Int* 1985, 27:837–841.

2. Simpson FO: Sodium intake, body sodium, and sodium excretion. *Lancet* 1990, 2:25–29.

3. Luft FC, Weinberger MH, Grim CE: Sodium sensitivity and resistance in normotensive humans. *Am J Med* 1982, 72:726–736.

4. Guyton AC: Blood pressure control: special role of the kidneys and body fluids. *Science* 1991, 252:1813–1816.

5. Lassiter WE: Regulation of sodium chloride distribution within the extracellular space. In *The Regulation of Sodium and Chloride Balance*. Edited by Seldin DW, Giebisch G. New York: Raven Press; 1990:23–58.

6. Hall JE, Jackson TE: The basic kidney-blood volume-pressure regulatory system: the pressure diuresis and natriuresis phenomena. In *Arterial Pressure and Hypertension*. Edited by Guyton AC. Philadelphia: WB Saunders Co, 1998:87–99.

7. Gonzalez-Campoy JM, Knox FG: Integrated responses of the kidney to alterations in extracellular fluid volume. In *The Kidney: Physiology and Pathophysiology*, edn 2. Edited by Seldin DW, Giebisch G. New York: Raven Press; 1992:2041–2097.

8. Hall JE, Brands MW: The renin-angiotensin-aldosterone systems. In *The Kidney: Physiology and Pathophysiology*, edn 2. Edited by Seldin DW, Giebisch G. New York: Raven Press; 1992:1455–1504.

9. Laragh JH, Sealey JE: The intergrated regulation of electrolyte balance and blood pressure by the renin system. In *The Regulation of Sodium and Chloride Balance*. Edited by Seldin DW, Giebisch G. New York: Raven Press, 1990:133–193.

10. Obermüller N, Kunchaparty S, Ellison DH, Bachmann S: Expression of the Na-K-2Cl cotransporter by macula densa and thick ascending limb cells of rat and rabbit nephron. *J Clin Invest* 1996, 98:635–640.

11. Lapointe J-Y, Bell PD, Cardinal J: Direct evidence for apical Na+:2Cl-:K+ cotransport in macula densa cells. *Am J Physiol* 1990, 258:F1466–F1469.

12. Briggs JP: Whys and the wherefores of juxtaglomerular apparatus functions. *Kidney Int* 1996, 49:1724–1726.

13. Barajas L: Architecture of the juxtaglomerular apparatus. In *Hypertension: Pathophysiology, Diagnosis and Treatment*. Edited by Laragh JH, Brenner BM. New York: Raven Press; 1990:XX–XX.

14. Skott O, Briggs JP: Direct demonstration of macula densa mediated renin secretion. *Science* 1987, 237:1618–1620.

15. Hall JE, Guyton AC: Changes in renal hemodynamics and renin release caused by increased plasma oncotic pressure. *Am J Physiol* 1976, 231:1550.

16. Bachmann S, Bosse HM, Mundel P: Topography of nitric oxide synthesis by localizing constitutive NO synthetases in mammalian kidney. *Am J Physiol* 1995, 268:F885–F898.

17. Johnson RA, Freeman RH: Renin release in rats during blockade of nitric oxide synthesis. *Am J Physiol* 1994, 266:R1723–R1729.

18. Schricker K, Hegyi I, Hamann M, *et al.*: Tonic stimulation of renin gene expression by nitric oxide is counteracted by tonic inhibition through angiotensin II. *Proc Natl Acad Sci USA* 1995, 92:8006–8010.

19. Funder JW: Mineralocorticoids, glucocorticoids, receptors and response elements. *Science* 1993, 259:1132–1133.

20. Náray-Fejes-Tóth A, Fejes-Tóth G: Glucocorticoid receptors mediate mineralocorticoid-like effects in cultured collecting duct cells. *Am J Physiol Renal Fluid Electrolyte Physiol* 1990, 259:F672–F678.

21. Mune T, Rogerson FM, Nikkila H, *et al.*: Human hypertension caused by mutations in the kidney isozyme of 11*beta*-hydroxysteroid dehydrogenase. *Nature Genet* 1995, 10:394–399.

22. Hollander W, Judson WE: The relationship of cardiovascular and renal hemodynamic function to sodium excretion in patients with severe heart disease but without edema. *J Clin Invest* 1956, 35:970–979.

23. Brenner BM, Ballermann BJ, Gunning ME, Zeidel ML: Diverse biological actions of atrial natriuretic peptide. *Physiol Rev* 1990, 70:665–700.

24. Kishimoto I, Dubois SK, Garbers DL: The heart communicates with the kidney exclusively through the guanylyl cyclase-A receptor: Acute handling of sodium and water in response to volume expansion. *Proc Natl Acad Sci USA* 1996, 93:6215–6219.

25. Korner PI: Integrative neural cardiovascular control. *Physiol Rev* 1971, 51:312–367.

26. Cogan MG: Neurogenic regulation of proximal bicarbonate and chloride reabsorption. *Am J Physiol* 1986, 250:F22–F26.

27. Geibel J, Giebisch G, Boron WF: Angiotensin II stimulates both Na+-H+ exchange and Na+/HCO_3 cotransport in the rabbit proximal tubule. *Proc Natl Acad Sci USA* 1990, 87:7917–7920.

28. Block RD, Zikos D, Fisher KA, *et al.*: Peterson DR: Activation of proximal tubular Na+-H+ exchanger by angiotensin II. *Am J Physiol* 1992, 263:F135–F143.

29. Bertorello A, Aperia A: Regulation of Na+-K+-ATPase activity in kidney proximal tubules: involvement of GTP binding proteins. *Am J Physiol* 1989, 256:F57–F62.

30. Aperia AC: Regulation of sodium transport. *Curr Opinion Nephrol Hypertens* 1995, 4:416–420.

31. Bouby N, Bankir L, Trinh-Trang-Tan MM, *et al.*: Selective ADH-induced hypertrophy of the medullary thick ascending limb in Brattleboro rats. *Kidney Int* 1985, 28:456–466.

32. Chabardès D, Gagnan-Brunette M, Imbert-Tébol M: Adenylate cyclase responsiveness to hormones in various portions of the human nephron. *J Clin Invest* 1980, 65:439–448.

33. Stokes JB: Effects of prostaglandin E_2 on chloride transport across the rabbit thick ascending limb of Henle. *J Clin Invest* 1979, 64:495–502.

34. Escalante B, Erlij D, Falck JR, McGiff JC: Effect of cytochrome P450 arachidonate metabolites on ion transport in rabbit kidney loop of Henle. *Science* 1991, 251:799–802.

35. Amlal H, Legoff C, Vernimmen C, *et al.*: Na(+)-K+(NH4+)-2Cl- cotransport in medullary thick ascending limb: control by PKA, PKC, and 20-HETE. *Am J Physiol* 1996, 271:C455–C463.

36. Culpepper RM, Adreoli TE: Interactions among prostaglandin E_2, antidiuretic hormone and cyclic adenosine monophosphate in modulating Cl- absorption in single mouse medullary thick ascending limbs of Henle. *J Clin Invest* 1983, 71:1588–1601.

37. Ecelbarger CA, Terris J, Hoyer JR, *et al.*: Localization and regulation of the rat renal Na+-K+-2Cl-, cotransporter, BSC-1. *Am J Physiol Renal Fluid Electrolyte Physiol* 1996, 271:F619–F628.

38. Chen Z, Vaughn DA, Blakeley P, Fanestil DD: Adrenocortical steroids increase renal thiazide diuretic receptor density and response. *J Am Soc Nephrol* 1994, 5:1361–1368.

39. Velázquez H, Bartiss A, Bernstein PL, Ellison DH: Adrenal steroids stimulate thiazide-sensitive NaCl transport by the rat renal distal tubule. *Am J Physiol* 1996, 39:F211–F219.

40. Wang T, Giebisch G: Effects of angiotensin II on electrolyte transport in the early and late distal tubule in rat kidney. *Am J Physiol Renal Fluid Electrolyte Physiol* 1996, 271:F143–F149.

41. Wang T, Chan YL: Neural control of distal tubular bicarbonate and fluid transport. *Am J Physiol* 1989, 257:F72–F76.

42. Bencsáth P, Szénási G, Takács L: Water and electrolyte transport in Henle's loop and distal tubule after renal sympathectomy in the rat. *Am J Physiol* 1985, 249:F308–F314.

43. Rossier BC, Palmer LG: Mechanisms of aldosterone action on sodium and potassium transport. In *The Kidney: Physiology and Pathophysiology*, edn 2. Edited by Seldin DW, Giebisch G. New York: Raven Press, 1992:1373–1409.

44. Breyer MD, Ando Y: Hormonal signalling and regulation of salt and water transport in the collecting duct. *Ann Rev Physiol* 1994, 56:711–739.

45. Schafer JA, Hawk CT: Regulation of Na+ channels in the cortical collecting duct by AVP and mineralocorticoids. *Int Kidney* 1992, 41:255–268.

46. Kudo LH, Van Baak AA, Rocha AS: Effects of vasopressin on sodium transport across inner medullary collecting duct. *Am J Physiol* 1990, 258:F1438–F1447.

47. Nielsen S, Chou C-L, Marples D, *et al.*: Vasopressin increases water permeability of kidney collecting duct by inducing translocation of aquaporin: CD water channels to plasma membrane. *Proc Natl Acad Sci USA* 1995, 92:1013–1017.

48. Schafer JA: Salt and water homeostasis: Is it just a matter of good bookkeeping? *J Am Soc Nephrol* 1994, 4:1933–1950.

49. Husted RF, Laplace JR, Stokes JB: Enhancement of electrogenic Na+ transport across rat inner medullary collecting duct cells in culture. *J Clin Invest* 1990, 86:498–506.

50. Zeidel ML, Jabs K, Kikeri D, Silva P: Kinins inhibit conductive Na+ uptake by rabbit inner medullary collecting duct cells. *Am J Physiol Renal Fluid Electrolyte Physiol* 1990, 258:F1584–F1591.

51. Zeidel ML: Hormonal regulation of inner medullary collecting duct sodium transport. *Am J Physiol Renal Fluid Electrolyte Physiol* 1993, 265:F159–F173.

52. Light DB, Ausiello DA, Stanton BA: Guanine nucleotide-binding protein, α_{i-3}, directly activates a cation channel in rat renal inner medullary collecting duct cells. *J Clin Invest* 1989, 84:352–356.

53. Light DB, Schwiebert EM, Karlson KH, Stanton BA: Atrial natriuretic peptide inhibits a cation channel in renal inner medullary collecting duct cells. *Science* 1989, 243:383–385.

54. Hostetter TH, Pfeffer JM, Pfeffer MA, *et al.*: Cardiorenal hemodynamics and sodium excretion in rats with myocardial dysfunction. *Am J Physiol* 1983, 245:H98–H103.

55. Villarreal D, Freeman RH, Brands MW: DOCA administration and atrial natriuretic factor in dogs with chronic heart failure. *Am J Physiol* 1989, 257:H739–H745.

56. Villarreal D, Freeman RH, Davis JO, *et al.*: Atrial natriuretic factor secretion in dogs with experimental high-output heart failure. *Am J Physiol* 1987, 252:H692–H696.

57. Levy M, Allotey JBK: Temporal relationsips between urinary salt retention and altered systemic hemodynamics in dogs with experimental cirrhosis. *J Lab Clin Med* 1978, 92:560–569.

58. Levy M: Sodium retention and ascites formation in dogs with experimental portal cirrhosis. *Am J Physiol* 1977, 233:F572–F585.

59. Villarreal D, Freeman RH, Johnson RA: Neurohumoral modulators and sodium balance in experimental heart failure. *Am J Physiol Heart Circ Physiol* 1993, 264:H1187–H1193.

60. Awazu M, Ichikawa I: Alterations in renal function in experimental congestive heart failure. *Sem Nephrology* 1994, 14:401–411.

61. Redfield MM, Edwards BS, Heublein DM, Burnett JC Jr: Restoration of renal response to atrial natriuretic factor in experimental low-output heart failure. *Am J Physiol* 1989, 257:R917–R923.

62. Manning RD Jr, Coleman TG, Samar RE: Autoregulation, cardiac output, total peripheral resistance and the "quantitative cascade" of the kidney-blood volume system for pressure control. In *Arterial Pressure and Hypertension*. Edited by Guyton AC. Philadelphia: WB Saunders Co; 1980:139–155.

63. Albillos A, Colombato LA, Groszmann RJ: Vasodilation and sodium retention in prehepatic portal hypertension. *Gastroenterology* 1992, 102:931–935.

64. Møller S, Henriksen JH: Circulatory abnormalities in cirrhosis with focus on neurohumoral aspects. *Sem Nephrol* 1997, 17:505–519.

65. Hillarp A, Zöller B, Dahlbäck M: Activated protein C resistance as a basis for venous thrombosis. *Am J Med* 1996, 101:534–540.

66. Niederberger M, Martin P-Y, Ginès P, *et al.*: Normalization of nitric oxide production corrects arterial vasodilation and hyperdynamic circulation in cirrhotic rats. *Gastroenterology* 1995, 109:1624–1630.

67. Niederberger M, Ginès P, Tsai P, *et al.*: Increased aortic cyclic guanosine monophosphate concentration in experimental cirrhosis in rats: evidence for a role of nitric oxide in the pathogenesis of arterial vasodilation in cirrhosis. *Hepatology* 1995, 21:1625–1631.

68. Martin P-Y, Schrier RW: Pathogenesis of water and sodium retention in cirrhosis. *Kidney Int* 1997, 51(suppl 59):S-43–S-49.

69. Fadnes HO, Pape JF, Sundsfjord JA: A study on oedema mechanism in nephrotic syndrome. *Scand J Clin Lab Invest* 1986, 46:533–538.

70. Oliver WJ, Owings CL: Sodium excretion in the nephrotic syndrome: relation to serum albumin concentration, glomerular filtration rate, and aldosterone secretion rate. *Am J Dis Child* 1967, 113:352–362.

71. Rodrígeuez-Iturbe B, Colic D, Parra G, Gutkowska J: Atrial natriuretic factor in the acute nephritic and nephrotic syndromes. *Kidney Int* 1990, 38:512–517.

72. Ichikawa I, Rennke HG, Hoyer JR, *et al.*: Role for intrarenal mechanisms in the impaired salt excretion of experimental nephrotic syndrome. *J Clin Invest* 1983, 71:91–103.

73. Manning RD Jr: Effects of hypoproteinemia on renal hemodynamics, arterial pressure, and fluid volume. *Am J Physiol* 1997, 252:F91–F98.

74. Manning RD Jr, Guyton AC: Effects of hypoproteinemia on fluid volumes and arterial pressure. *Am J Physiol* 1983, 245:H284–H293.

75. Mitch WE, Wilcox CS: Disorders of body fluids, sodium and potassium in chronic renal failure. *Am J Med* 1982, 72:536–550.

Disorders of Potassium Metabolism

Fredrick V. Osorio
Stuart L. Linas

Potassium, the most abundant cation in the human body, regulates intracellular enzyme function and neuromuscular tissue excitability. Serum potassium is normally maintained within the narrow range of 3.5 to 5.5 mEq/L. The intracellular-extracellular potassium ratio (K_i/K_e) largely determines neuromuscular tissue excitability [1]. Because only a small portion of potassium is extracellular, neuromuscular tissue excitability is markedly affected by small changes in extracellular potassium. Thus, the body has developed elaborate regulatory mechanisms to maintain potassium homeostasis. Because dietary potassium intake is sporadic and it cannot be rapidly excreted renally, short-term potassium homeostasis occurs via transcellular potassium shifts [2]. Ultimately, long-term maintenance of potassium balance depends on renal excretion of ingested potassium. The illustrations in this chapter review normal transcellular potassium homeostasis as well as mechanisms of renal potassium excretion.

With an understanding of normal potassium balance, disorders of potassium metabolism can be grouped into those that are due to altered intake, altered excretion, and abnormal transcellular distribution. The diagnostic algorithms that follow allow the reader to limit the potential causes of hyperkalemia and hypokalemia and to reach a diagnosis as efficiently as possible. Finally, clinical manifestations of disorders of potassium metabolism are reviewed, and treatment algorithms for hypokalemia and hyperkalemia are offered.

Recently, the molecular defects responsible for a variety of diseases associated with disordered potassium metabolism have been discovered [3–8]. Hypokalemia and Liddle's syndrome [3] and hyperkalemia and pseudohypoaldosteronism type I [4] result from mutations at different sites on the epithelial sodium channel in the distal tubules. The hypokalemia of Bartter's syndrome can be accounted for by two separate ion transporter defects in the thick ascending limb of Henle's loop [5]. Gitelman's syndrome, a clinical variant of Bartter's

CHAPTER

3

syndrome, is caused by a mutation in an ion cotransporter in a completely different segment of the renal tubule [6]. The genetic mutations responsible for hypokalemia in the syndrome of apparent mineralocorticoid excess [7] and glucocorticoid-remediable aldosteronism [8] have recently been elucidated and are illustrated below.

Overview of Potassium Physiology

PHYSIOLOGY OF POTASSIUM BALANCE: DISTRIBUTION OF POTASSIUM

ECF 350 mEq (10%)	ICF 3150 mEq (90%)
Plasma 15 mEq (0.4%)	Muscle 2650 mEq (76%)
Interstitial fluid 35 mEq (1%)	Liver 250 mEq (7%)
Bone 300 mEq (8.6%)	Erythrocytes 250 mEq (7%)
[K+] = 3.5–5.0 mEq/L	[K+] = 140–150 mEq/L
Urine 90–95 mEq/d	Urine 90–95 mEq/d
Stool 5–10mEq/d	Stool 5–10mEq/d
Sweat < 5 mEq/d	Sweat < 5 mEq/d

FIGURE 3-1

External balance and distribution of potassium. The usual Western diet contains approximately 100 mEq of potassium per day. Under normal circumstances, renal excretion accounts for approximately 90% of daily potassium elimination, the remainder being excreted in stool and (a negligible amount) in sweat. About 90% of total body potassium is located in the intracellular fluid (ICF), the majority in muscle. Although the extracellular fluid (ECF) contains about 10% of total body potassium, less than 1% is located in the plasma [9]. Thus, disorders of potassium metabolism can be classified as those that are due 1) to altered intake, 2) to altered elimination, or 3) to deranged transcellular potassium shifts.

FACTORS CAUSING TRANSCELLULAR POTASSIUM SHIFTS

Factor	Δ Plasma K+
Acid-base status	
Metabolic acidosis	
Hyperchloremic acidosis	↑↑
Organic acidosis	↔
Respiratory acidosis	↑
Metabolic alkalosis	↓
Respiratory alkalosis	↓
Pancreatic hormones	
Insulin	↓↓
Glucagon	↑
Catecholamines	
β-Adrenergic	↓
α-Adrenergic	↑
Hyperosmolarity	↑
Aldosterone	↓, ↔
Exercise	↑

FIGURE 3-2

Factors that cause transcellular potassium shifts.

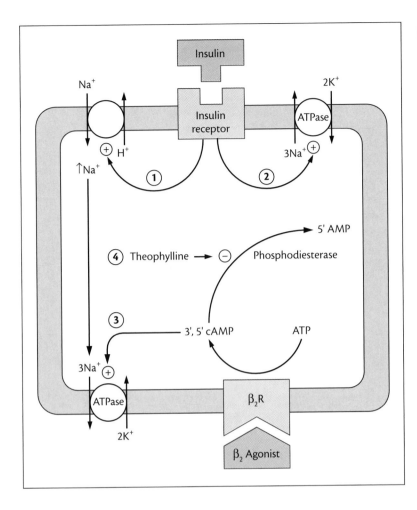

FIGURE 3-3

Extrarenal potassium homeostasis: insulin and catecholamines. Schematic representation of the cellular mechanisms by which insulin and β-adrenergic stimulation promote potassium uptake by extrarenal tissues. Insulin binding to its receptor results in hyperpolarization of cell membranes (1), which facilitates potassium uptake. After binding to its receptor, insulin also activates Na+-K+-ATPase pumps, resulting in cellular uptake of potassium (2). The second messenger that mediates this effect has not yet been identified. Catecholamines stimulate cellular potassium uptake via the β2 adrenergic receptor (β2R). The generation of cyclic adenosine monophosphate (3', 5' cAMP) activates Na+-K+-ATPase pumps (3), causing an influx of potassium in exchange for sodium [10]. By inhibiting the degradation of cyclic AMP, theophylline potentiates catecholamine-stimulated potassium uptake, resulting in hypokalemia (4).

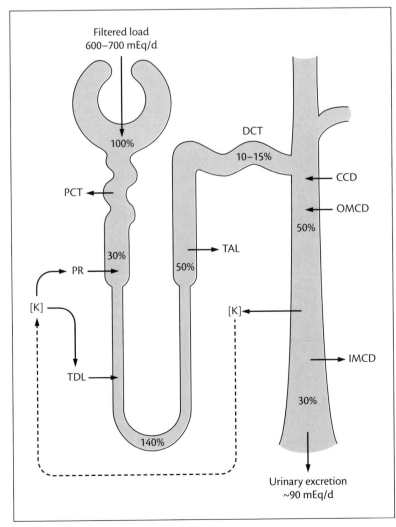

FIGURE 3-4

Renal potassium handling. More than half of filtered potassium is passively reabsorbed by the end of the proximal convoluted tubule (PCT). Potassium is then added to tubular fluid in the descending limb of Henle's loop (see below). The major site of active potassium reabsorption is the thick ascending limb of the loop of Henle (TAL), so that, by the end of the distal convoluted tubule (DCT), only 10% to 15% of filtered potassium remains in the tubule lumen. Potassium is secreted mainly by the principal cells of the cortical collecting duct (CCD) and outer medullary collecting duct (OMCD). Potassium reabsorption occurs via the intercalated cells of the medullary collecting duct (MCD). Urinary potassium represents the difference between potassium secreted and potassium reabsorbed [11]. During states of total body potassium depletion, potassium reabsorption is enhanced. Reabsorbed potassium initially enters the medullary interstitium, but then it is secreted into the pars recta (PR) and descending limb of the loop of Henle (TDL). The physiologic role of medullary potassium recycling may be to minimize potassium "backleak" out of the collecting tubule lumen or to enhance renal potassium secretion during states of excess total body potassium [12]. The percentage of filtered potassium remaining in the tubule lumen is indicated in the corresponding nephron segment.

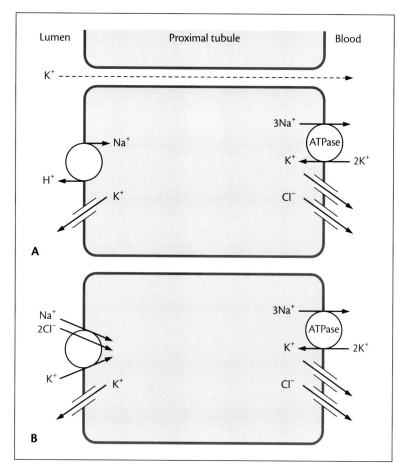

FIGURE 3-5

FIGURE 3-5

Cellular mechanisms of renal potassium transport: proximal tubule and thick ascending limb. **A,** Proximal tubule potassium reabsorption is closely coupled to proximal sodium and water transport. Potassium is reabsorbed through both paracellular and cellular pathways. Proximal apical potassium channels are normally almost completely closed. The lumen of the proximal tubule is negative in the early proximal tubule and positive in late proximal tubule segments. Potassium transport is not specifically regulated in this portion of the nephron, but net potassium reabsorption is closely coupled to sodium and water reabsorption. **B,** In the thick ascending limb of Henle's loop, potassium reabsorption proceeds by electroneutral Na^+-K^+-$2Cl^-$ cotransport in the thick ascending limb, the low intracellular sodium and chloride concentrations providing the driving force for transport. In addition, the positive lumen potential allows some portion of luminal potassium to be reabsorbed via paracellular pathways [11]. The apical potassium channel allows potassium recycling and provides substrate to the apical Na^+-K^+-$2Cl^-$ cotransporter [12]. Loop diuretics act by competing for the Cl^- site on this carrier.

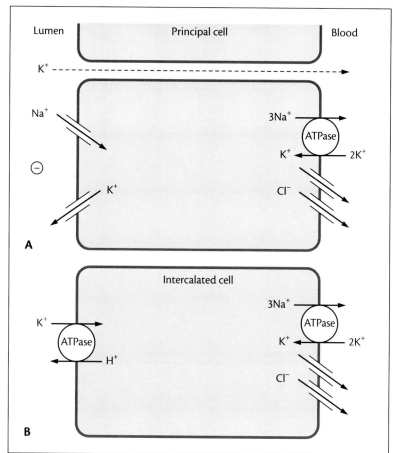

FIGURE 3-6

Cellular mechanisms of renal potassium transport: cortical collecting tubule. **A,** Principal cells of the cortical collecting duct: apical sodium channels play a key role in potassium secretion by increasing the intracellular sodium available to Na^+-K^+-ATPase pumps and by creating a favorable electrical potential for potassium secretion. Basolateral Na^+-K^+-ATPase creates a favorable concentration gradient for passive diffusion of potassium from cell to lumen through potassium-selective channels. **B,** Intercalated cells. Under conditions of potassium depletion, the cortical collecting duct becomes a site for net potassium reabsorption. The H^+-K^+-ATPase pump is regulated by potassium intake. Decreases in total body potassium increase pump activity, resulting in enhanced potassium reabsorption. This pump may be partly responsible for the maintenance of metabolic alkalosis in conditions of potassium depletion [11].

Hypokalemia: Diagnostic Approach

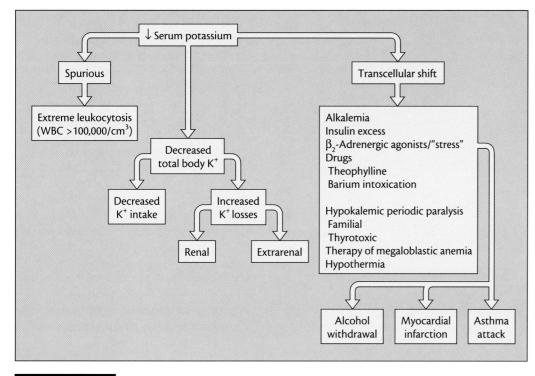

FIGURE 3-7

Overview of diagnostic approach to hypokalemia: hypokalemia without total body potassium depletion. Hypokalemia can result from transcellular shifts of potassium into cells without total body potassium depletion or from decreases in total body potassium. Perhaps the most dramatic examples occur in catecholamine excess states, as after administration of $\beta_2$adreneric receptor (β_2AR) agonists or during "stress." It is important to note

that, during some conditions (*eg*, ketoacidosis), transcellular shifts and potassium depletion exist simultaneously. Spurious hypokalemia results when blood specimens from leukemia patients are allowed to stand at room temperature; this results in leukocyte uptake of potassium from serum and artifactual hypokalemia. Patients with spurious hypokalemia do not have clinical manifestations of hypokalemia, as their in vivo serum potassium values are normal. Theophylline poisoning prevents cAMP breakdown (*see* Fig. 3-3). Barium poisoning from the ingestion of soluble barium salts results in severe hypokalemia by blocking channels for exit of potassium from cells. Episodes of hypokalemic periodic paralysis can be precipitated by rest after exercise, carbohydrate meal, stress, or administration of insulin. Hypokalemic periodic paralysis can be inherited as an autosomal-dominant disease or acquired by patients with thyrotoxicosis, especially Chinese males. Therapy of megaloblastic anemia is associated with potassium uptake by newly formed cells, which is occasionally of sufficient magnitude to cause hypokalemia [13].

```
                    Hypokalemia
                        │
                        ▼
            ┌─── Decreased total body K⁺ ───┐
            │                               │
            ▼                               ▼
   Extrarenal losses                  Renal losses
  (Urinary K⁺ <20mEq/L)            (Urinary K⁺ >20 mEq/L)
                                       (see Fig. 3–9)
   ┌────────┼────────┐
   ▼        ▼        ▼
Metabolic  Normal    Metabolic
acidosis   acid-base alkalosis
           status
   │        │        │
   ▼        ▼        ▼
```

Metabolic acidosis	Normal acid-base status	Metabolic alkalosis
Gastrointestinal losses	Decreased intake	Gastrointestinal losses
Diarrhea	Cutaneous losses	Laxative abuse
Laxative abuse	Gastrointestinal losses	Villous adenoma
Villous adenoma	Laxative abuse	Congenital chloride-losing diarrhea
Gastrointestinal fistulas	Villous adenoma	
	Geophagia	

FIGURE 3-8

Diagnostic approach to hypokalemia: hypokalemia with total body potassium depletion secondary to extrarenal losses. In the absence of redistribution, measurement of urinary potassium is helpful in determining whether hypokalemia is due to renal or to extrarenal potassium losses. The normal kidney responds to several (3 to 5) days of potassium depletion with appropriate renal potassium conservation. In the absence of severe polyuria, a "spot" urinary potassium

concentration of less than 20 mEq/L indicates renal potassium conservation. In certain circumstances (*eg*, diuretics abuse), renal potassium losses may not be evident once the stimulus for renal potassium wasting is removed. In this circumstance, urinary potassium concentrations may be deceptively low despite renal potassium losses. Hypokalemia due to colonic villous adenoma or laxative abuse may be associated with metabolic acidosis, alkalosis, or no acid-base disturbance. Stool has a relatively high potassium content, and fecal potassium losses could exceed 100 mEq per day with severe diarrhea. Habitual ingestion of clay (pica), encountered in some parts of the rural southeastern United States, can result in potassium depletion by binding potassium in the gut, much as a cation exchange resin does. Inadequate dietary intake of potassium, like that associated ith anorexia or a "tea and toast" diet, can lead to hypokalemia, owing to delayed renal conservation of potassium; however, progressive potassium depletion does not occur unless intake is well below 15 mEq of potassium per day.

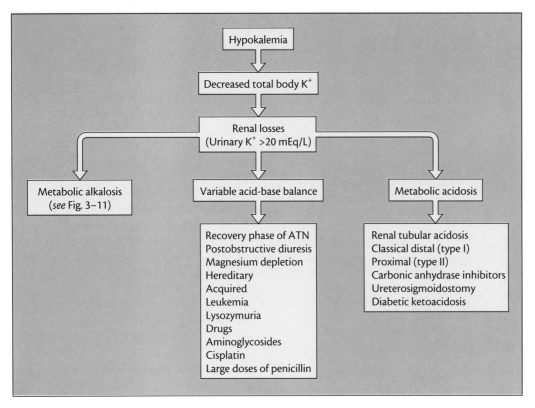

uropathy, presumably secondary to increased delivery of sodium and water to the distal nephrons. Patients with acute monocytic and myelomonocytic leukemias occasionally excrete large amounts of lysozyme in their urine. Lysozyme appears to have a direct kaliuretic effect on the kidneys (by an undefined mechanism). Penicillin in large doses acts as a poorly reabsorbable anion, resulting in obligate renal potassium wasting. Mechanisms for renal potassium wasting associated with aminoglycosides and cisplatin are ill-defined. Hypokalemia in type I renal tubular acidosis is due in part to secondary hyperaldosteronism, whereas type II renal tubular acidosis can result in a defect in potassium reabsorption in the proximal nephrons. Carbonic anhydrase inhibitors result in an acquired form of renal tubular acidosis. Ureterosigmoidostomy results in hypokalemia in 10% to 35% of patients, owing to the sigmoid colon's capacity for net potassium secretion. The osmotic diuresis associated with diabetic ketoacidosis results in potassium depletion, although patients may initially present with a normal serum potassium value, owing to altered transcellular potassium distribution.

FIGURE 3-9

Diagnostic approach to hypokalemia: hypokalemia due to renal losses with normal acid-base status or metabolic acidosis. Hypokalemia is occasionally observed during the diuretic recovery phase of acute tubular necrosis (ATN) or after relief of acute obstructive

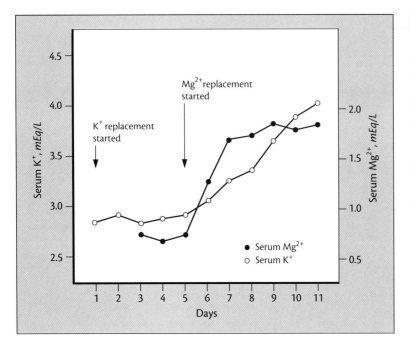

FIGURE 3-10

Hypokalemia and magnesium depletion. Hypokalemia and magnesium depletion can occur concurrently in a variety of clinical settings, including diuretic therapy, ketoacidosis, aminoglycoside therapy, and prolonged osmotic diuresis (as with poorly controlled diabetes mellitus). Hypokalemia is also a common finding in patients with congenital magnesium-losing kidney disease. The patient depicted was treated with cisplatin 2 months before presentation. Attempts at oral and intravenous potassium replacement of up to 80 mEq/day were unsuccessful in correcting the hypokalemia. Once serum magnesium was corrected, however, serum potassium quickly normalized [14].

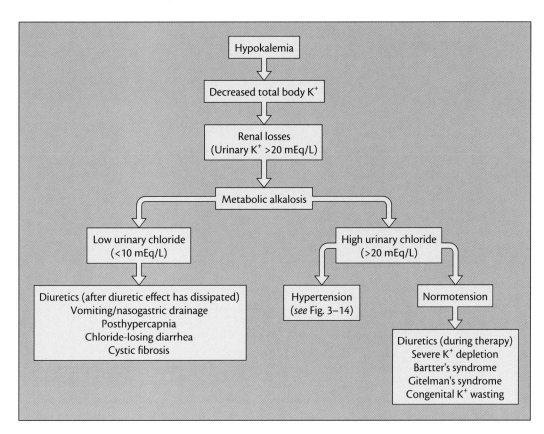

FIGURE 3-11

Diagnostic approach to hypokalemia: hypokalemia due to renal losses with metabolic alkalosis. The urine chloride value is helpful in distinguishing the causes of hypokalemia. Diuretics are a common cause of hypokalemia; however, after discontinuing diuretics, urinary potassium and chloride may be appropriately low. Urine diuretic screens are warranted for patients suspected of surreptious diuretic abuse. Vomiting results in chloride and sodium depletion, hyperaldosteronism, and renal potassium wasting. Posthypercapnic states are often associated with chloride depletion (from diuretics) and sodium avidity. If hypercapnia is corrected without replacing chloride, patients develop chloride-depletion alkalosis and hypokalemia.

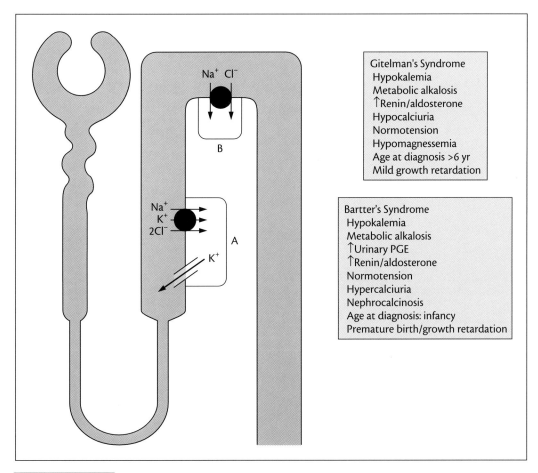

FIGURE 3-12

Mechanisms of hypokalemia in Bartter's syndrome and Gitelman's syndrome. **A**, A defective Na^+-K^+-$2Cl^-$ cotransporter in the thick ascending limb (TAL) of Henle's loop can account for virtually all features of Bartter's syndrome. Since approximately 30% of filtered sodium is reabsorbed by this segment of the nephron, defective sodium reabsorption

results in salt wasting and elevated renin and aldosterone levels. The hyperaldosteronism and increased distal sodium delivery account for the characteristic hypokalemic metabolic alkalosis. Moreover, impaired sodium reabsorption in the TAL results in the hypercalciuria seen in these patients, as approximately 25% of filtered calcium is reabsorbed in this segment in a process coupled to sodium reabsorption. Since potassium levels in the TAL are much lower than levels of sodium or chloride, luminal potassium concentrations are rate limiting for Na^+-K^+-$2Cl^-$ co-transporter activity. Defects in ATP-sensitive potassium channels would be predicted to alter potassium recycling and diminish Na^+-K^+-$2Cl^-$ cotransporter activity. Recently, mutations in the gene that encodes for the Na^+-K^+-$2Cl^-$ cotransporter and the ATP-sensitive potassium channel have been described in kindreds with Bartter's syndrome. Because loop diuretics interfere with the Na^+-K^+-$2Cl^-$ cotransporter, surreptitious diuretic abusers have a clinical presentation that is virtually indistinguishable from that of Bartter's syndrome. **B**, Gitelman's syndrome, which typically presents later in life and is associated with hypomagnesemia and hypocalciuria, is due to a defect in the gene encoding for the thiazide-sensitive Na^+-Cl^- cotransporter. The mild volume depletion results in more avid sodium and calcium reabsorption by the proximal nephrons.

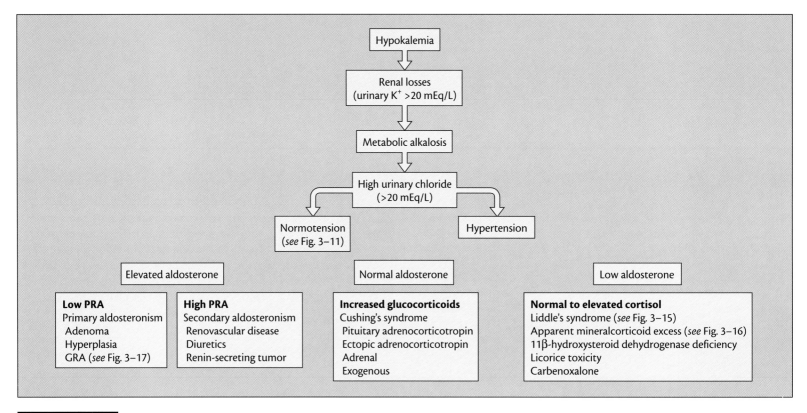

FIGURE 3-13

Diagnostic approach to hypokalemia: hypokalemia due to renal losses with hypertension and metabolic alkalosis.

FIGURE 3-14

Distinguishing characteristics of hypokalemia associated with hypertension and metabolic alkalosis.

CHARACTERISTICS OF HYPOKALEMIA WITH HYPERTENSION AND METABOLIC ALKALOSIS

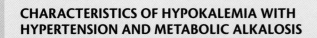

	Aldosterone	Renin	Response to Dexamethasone
Primary aldosteronism	↑	↓	—
11 β-hydroxysteroid dehydrogenase deficiency	↓	↓	+
Glucocorticoid remediable aldosteronism	↑	↓	+
Liddle's syndrome	↓→	↓	—

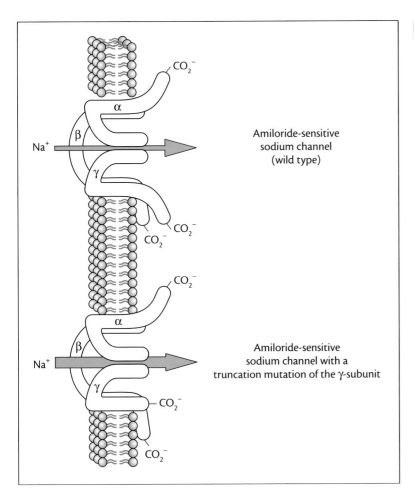

FIGURE 3-15

Mechanism of hypokalemia in Liddle's syndrome. The amiloride-sensitive sodium channel on the apical membrane of the distal tubule consists of homologous α, β, and γ subunits. Each subunit is composed of two transmembrane-spanning domains, an extracellular loop, and intracellular amino and carboxyl terminals. Truncation mutations of either the β or γ subunit carboxyl terminal result in greatly increased sodium conductance, which creates a favorable electrochemical gradient for potassium secretion. Although patients with Liddle's syndrome are not universally hypokalemic, they may exhibit severe potassium wasting with thiazide diuretics. The hypokalemia, hypertension, and metabolic alkalosis that typify Liddle's syndrome can be corrected with amiloride or triamterene or restriction of sodium.

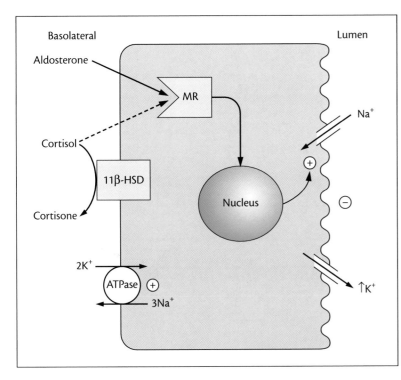

FIGURE 3-16

Mechanism of hypokalemia in the syndrome of apparent mineralo-corticoid excess (AME). Cortisol and aldosterone have equal affinity for the intracellular mineralocorticoid receptor (MR); however, in aldosterone-sensitive tissues such as the kidney, the enzyme 11 β-hydroxysteroid dehydrogenase (11 β-HSD) converts cortisol to cortisone. Since cortisone has a low affinity for the MR, the enzyme 11 β-HSD serves to protect the kidney from the effects of glucocorticoids. In hereditary or acquired AME, 11 β-HSD is defective or is inactiveted (by licorice or carbenoxalone). Cortisol, which is present at concentrations approximately 1000-fold that of aldosterone, becomes a mineralocorticoid. The hypermineralo-corticoid state results in increased transcription of subunits of the sodium channel and the $Na^+-K^+-ATPase$ pump. The favorable electrochemical gradient then favors potassium secretion [7,15].

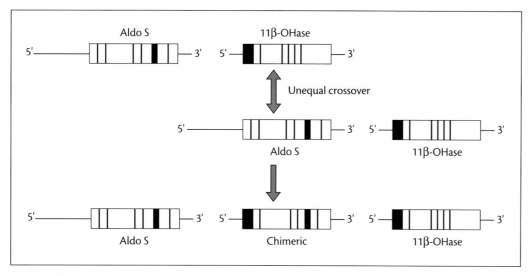

FIGURE 3-17

Genetics of glucocorticoid-remediable aldosteronism (GRA): schematic representation of unequal crossover in GRA. The genes for aldosterone synthase (Aldo S) and 11 β-hydroxylase (11 β-OHase) are normally expressed in separate zones of the adrenal cortex. Aldosterone is produced in the zona glomerulosa and cortisol, in the zona fasciculata. These enzymes have identical intron-extron structures and are closely linked on chromosome 8. If unequal crossover occurs, a new hybrid gene is produced that includes the 5' segment of the 11 β-OHase gene (ACTH-response element and the 11 β-OHase segment) plus the 3' segment of the Aldo S gene (aldosterone synthase segment). The chimeric gene is now under the contol of ACTH, and aldosterone secretion is enhanced, thus causing hypokalemia and hypertension. By inhibiting pituitary release of ACTH, glucocorticoid administration leads to a fall in aldosterone levels and correction of the clinical and biochemical abnormalities of GRA. The presence of Aldo S activity in the zona fasciculata gives rise to characteristic elevations in 18-oxidation products of cortisol (18-hydroxycortisol and 18-oxocortisol), which are diagnostic for GRA [8].

Hypokalemia: Clinical Manifestations

CLINICAL MANIFESTATIONS OF HYPOKALEMIA

Cardiovascular
  Abnormal electrocardiogram
  Predisposition for digitalis toxicity
  Atrial ventricular arrhythmias
  Hypertension
Neuromuscular
  Smooth muscle
    Constipation/ileus
    Bladder dysfunction
  Skeletal muscle
    Weakness/cramps
    Tetany
    Paralysis
    Myalgias/rhabdomyolysis

Renal/electrolyte
  Functional alterations
    Decreased glomerular filtration rate
    Decreased renal blood flow
    Renal concentrating defect
    Increased renal ammonia production
    Chloride wasting
    Metabolic alkalosis
    Hypercalciuria
    Phosphaturia
  Structural alterations
    Dilation and vacuolization of
      proximal tubules
    Medullary cyst formation
    Interstitial nephritis
Endocrine/metabolic
    Decreased insulin secretion
    Carbohydrate intolerance
    Increased renin
    Decreased aldosterone
    Altered prostaglandin synthesis
    Growth retardation

FIGURE 3-18

Clinical manifestations of hypokalemia.

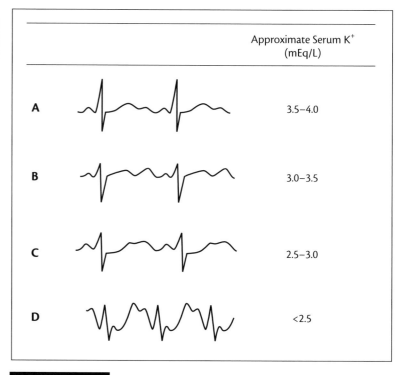

	Approximate Serum K+ (mEq/L)
A	3.5–4.0
B	3.0–3.5
C	2.5–3.0
D	<2.5

FIGURE 3-19

Electrocardiographic changes associated with hypokalemia. **A,** The U wave may be a normal finding and is not specific for hypokalemia. **B,** When the amplitude of the U wave exceeds that of the T wave, hypokalemia may be present. The QT interval may appear to be prolonged; however, this is often due to mistaking the QU interval for the QT interval, as the latter does not change in duration with hypokalemia. **C,** Sagging of the ST segment, flattening of the T wave, and a prominent U wave are seen with progressive hypokalemia. **D,** The QRS complex may widen slightly, and the PR interval is often prolonged with severe hypokalemia. Hypokalemia promotes the appearance of supraventricular and ventricular ectopic rhythms, especially in patients taking digitalis [16].

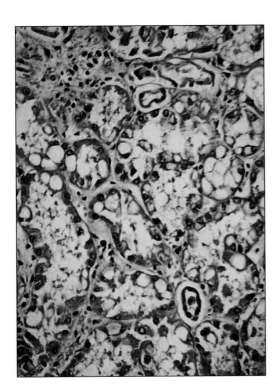

FIGURE 3-20

Renal lesions associated with hypokalemia. The predominant pathologic finding accompanying potassium depletion in humans is vacuolization of the epithelium of the proximal convoluted tubules. The vacoules are large and coarse, and staining for lipids is usually negative. The tubular vacuolation is reversible with sustained correction of the hypokalemia; however, in patients with long-standing hypokalemia, lymphocytic infiltration, interstitial scarring, and tubule atrophy have been described. Increased renal ammonia production may promote complement activation via the alternate pathway and can contribute to the interstitial nephritis [17,18].

Hypokalemia: Treatment

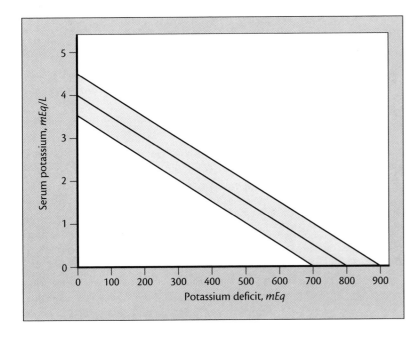

FIGURE 3-21

Treatment of hypokalemia: estimation of potassium deficit. In the absence of stimuli that alter intracellular-extracellular potassium distribution, a decrease in the serum potassium concentration from 3.5 to 3.0 mEq/L corresponds to a 5% reduction (~175 mEq) in total body potassium stores. A decline from 3.0 to 2.0 mEq/L signifies an additional 200 to 400-mEq deficit. Factors such as the rapidity of the fall in serum potassium and the presence or absence of symptoms dictate the aggressiveness of replacement therapy. In general, hypokalemia due to intracellular shifts can be managed by treating the underlying condition (hyperinsulinemia, theophylline intoxication). Hypokalemic periodic paralysis and hypokalemia associated with myocardial infarction (secondary to endogenous β-adrenergic agonist release) are best managed by potassium supplementation [19].

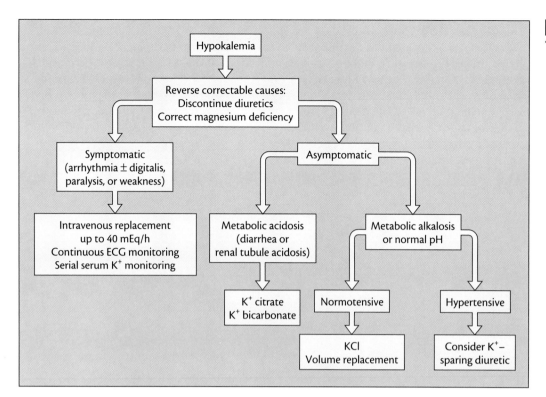

FIGURE 3-22

Treatment of hypokalemia.

Hyperkalemia: Diagnostic Approach

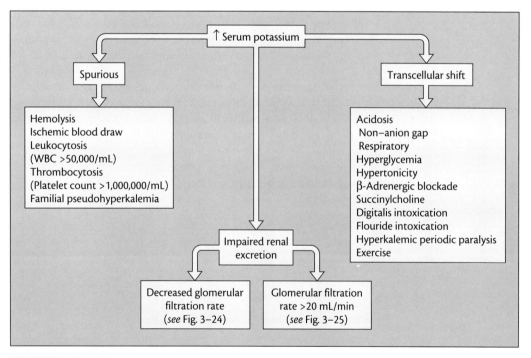

either leukocytes or platelets results in leakage of potassium from these cells. Familial pseudohyperkalemia is a rare condition of increased potassium efflux from red blood cells in vitro. Ischemia due to tight or prolonged tourniquet application or fist clenching increases serum potassium concentrations by as much as 1.0 to 1.6 mEq/L. Hyperkalemia can also result from decreases in K movement into cells or increases in potassium movement from cells. Hyperchloremic metabolic acidosis (in contrast to organic acid, anion-gap metabolic acidosis) causes potassium ions to flow out of cells. Hypertonic states induced by mannitol, hypertonic saline, or poor blood sugar control promote movement of water and potassium out of cells. Depolarizing muscle relaxants such as succinylcholine increase permeability of muscle cells and should be avoided by hyperkalemic patients. The mechanism of hyperkalemia with β-adrenergic blockade is illustrated in Figure 3-3. Digitalis impairs function of the Na^+-K^+-ATPase pumps and blocks entry of potassium into cells. Acute fluoride intoxication can be treated with cation-exchange resins or dialysis, as attempts at shifting potassium back into cells may not be successful.

FIGURE 3-23

Approach to hyperkalemia: hyperkalemia without total body potassium excess. Spurious hyperkalemia is suggested by the absence of electrocardiographic (ECG) findings in patients with elevated serum potassium. The most common cause of spurious hyperkalemia is hemolysis, which may be apparent on visual inspection of serum. For patients with extreme leukocytosis or thrombocytosis, potassium levels should be measured in plasma samples that have been promptly separated from the cellular components since extreme elevations in

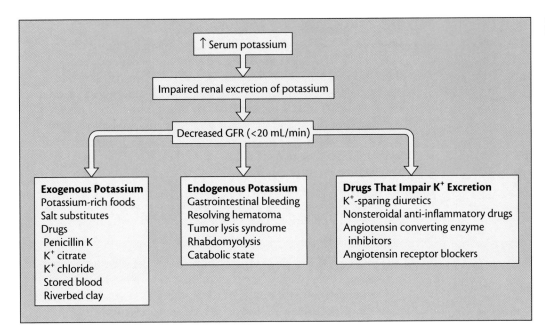

FIGURE 3-24

Approach to hyperkalemia: hyperkalemia with reduced glomerular filtration rate (GFR). Normokalemia can be maintained in patients who consume normal quantities of potassium until GFR decreases to less than 10 mL/min; however, diminished GFR predisposes patients to hyperkalemia from excessive exogenous or endogenous potassium loads. Hidden sources of endogenous and exogenous potassium—and drugs that predispose to hyperkalemia—are listed.

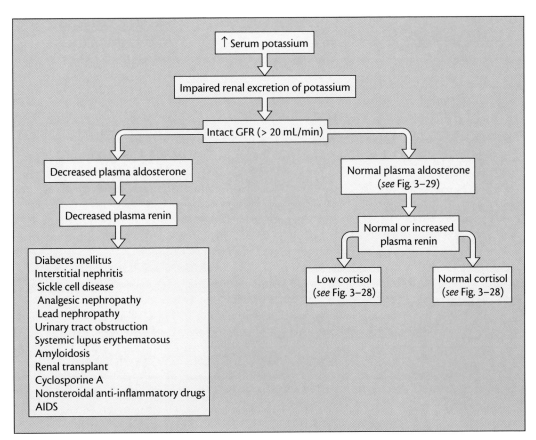

FIGURE 3-25

Approach to hyperkalemia: hyporeninemic hypoaldosteronism. Hyporeninemic hypoaldosteronism accounts for the majority of cases of unexplained hyperkalemia in patients with reduced glomerular filtration rate (GFR) whose level of renal insufficiency is not what would be expected to cause hyperkalemia. Interstitial renal disease is a feature of most of the diseases listed. The transtubular potassium gradient (*see* Fig. 3-26) can be used to distinguish between primary tubule defects and hyporeninemic hypoaldosteronism. Although the transtubular potassium gradient should be low in both disorders, exogenous mineralocorticoid would normalize transtubular potassium gradient in hyporeninemic hypoaldosteronism.

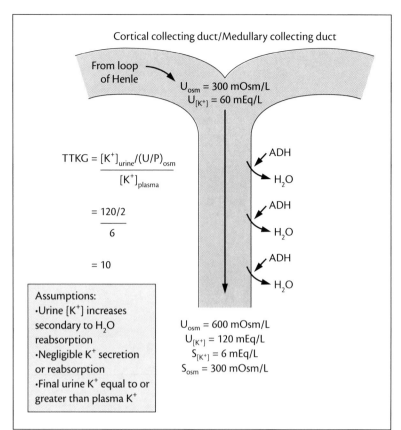

Cortical collecting duct/Medullary collecting duct

From loop of Henle

$U_{osm} = 300\ mOsm/L$
$U_{[K^+]} = 60\ mEq/L$

$$TTKG = \dfrac{[K^+]_{urine}/(U/P)_{osm}}{[K^+]_{plasma}}$$

$$= \dfrac{120/2}{6}$$

$$= 10$$

Assumptions:
- Urine $[K^+]$ increases secondary to H_2O reabsorption
- Negligible K^+ secretion or reabsorption
- Final urine K^+ equal to or greater than plasma K^+

ADH
H_2O
ADH
H_2O
ADH
H_2O

$U_{osm} = 600\ mOsm/L$
$U_{[K^+]} = 120\ mEq/L$
$S_{[K^+]} = 6\ mEq/L$
$S_{osm} = 300\ mOsm/L$

FIGURE 3-26

Physiologic basis of the transtubular potassium concentration gradient (TTKG). Secretion of potassium in the cortical collecting duct and outer medullary collecting duct accounts for the vast majority of potassium excreted in the urine. Potassium secretion in these segments is influenced mainly by aldosterone, plasma potassium concentrations, and the anion composition of the fluid in the lumen. Use of the TTKG assumes that negligible amounts of potassium are secreted or reabsorbed distal to these sites. The final urinary potassium concentration then depends on water reabsorption in the medullary collecting ducts, which results in a rise in the final urinary potassium concentration without addition of significant amounts of potassium to the urine. The TTKG is calculated as follows:

$$TTKG = ([K^+]urine/(U/P)osm)/[K^+]plasma$$

The ratio of $(U/P)_{osm}$ allows for "correction" of the final urinary potassium concentration for the amount of water reabsorbed in the medullary collecting duct. In effect, the TTKG is an index of the gradient of potassium achieved at potassium secretory sites, independent of urine flow rate. The urine must at least be iso-osmolal with respect to serum if the TTKG is to be meaningful [20].

CAUSES FOR HYPERKALEMIA WITH AN INAPPROPRIATELY LOW TTKG THAT IS UNRESPONSIVE TO MINERALOCORTICOID CHALLENGE

Potassium-sparing diuretics
  Amiloride
  Triamterene
  Spironolactone
Tubular resistance to aldosterone
  Interstitial nephritis
  Sickle cell disease
  Urinary tract obstruction
  Pseudohypoaldosteronism type I
Drugs
  Trimethoprim
  Pentamidine

Increased distal nephron potassium reabsorption
  Pseudohypoaldosteronism type II
  Urinary tract obstruction

FIGURE 3-27

Clinical application of the transtubular potassium gradient (TTKG). The TTKG in normal persons varies much but is genarally within the the range of 6 to 12. Hypokalemia from extrarenal causes results in renal potassium conservation and a TTKG less than 2. A higher value suggests renal potassium losses, as through hyperaldosteronism. The expected TTKG during hyperkalemia is greater than 10. An inappropriately low TTKG in a hyperkalemic patient suggests hypoaldosteronism or a renal tubule defect. Administration of the mineralocorticoid 9 α-fludrocortisone (0.05 mg) should cause TTKG to rise above 7 in cases of hypoaldosteronism. Circumstances are listed in which the TTKG would not increase after mineralocorticoid challenge, because of tubular resistance to aldosterone [21].

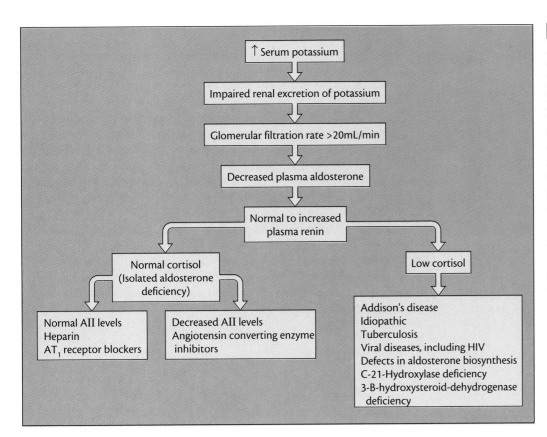

FIGURE 3-28

Approach to hyperkalemia: low aldosterone with normal to increased plasma renin. Heparin impairs aldosterone synthesis by inhibiting the enzyme 18-hydroxylase. Despite its frequent use, heparin is rarely associated with overt hyperkalemia; this suggests that other mechanisms (*eg*, reduced renal potassium secretion) must be present simultaneously for hyperkalemia to manifest itself. Both angiotensin-converting enzyme inhibitors and the angiotensin type 1 receptor blockers (AT$_1$) receptor blockers interfere with adrenal aldosterone synthesis. Generalized impairment of adrenal cortical function manifested by combined glucocorticoid and mineralocorticoid deficiencies are seen in Addison's disease and in defects of aldosterone biosynthesis.

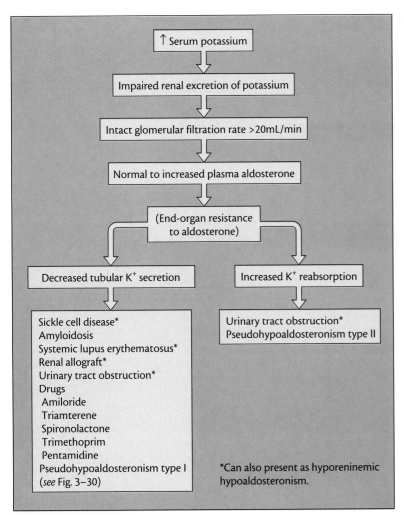

FIGURE 3-29

Approach to hyperkalemia: pseudohypoaldosteronism. The mechanism of decreased potassium excretion is caused either by failure to secrete potassium in the cortical collecting tubule or enhanced reabsorption of potassium in the medullary or papillary collecting tubules. Decreased secretion of potassium in the cortical and medullary collecting duct results from decreases in either apical sodium or potassium channel function or diminished basolateral Na$^+$-K$^+$-ATPase activity. Alternatively, potassium may be secreted normally but hyperkalemia can develop because potassium reabsorption is enhanced in the intercalated cells of the medullary collecting duct (*see* Fig. 3-4). The transtubule potassium gradient (TTKG) in both situations is inappropriately low and fails to normalize in response to mineralocorticoid replacement.

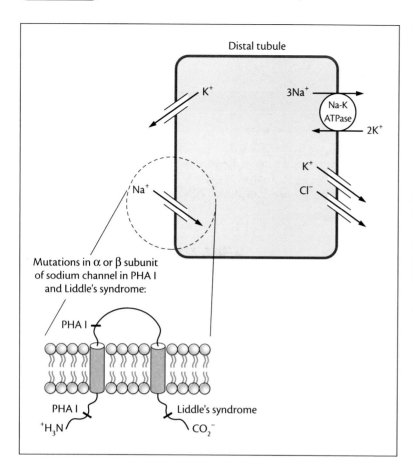

FIGURE 3-30

Mechanism of hyperkalemia in pseudohypoaldosteronism type I (PHA I). This rare autosomally transmitted disease is characterized by neonatal dehydration, failure to thrive, hyponatremia, hyperkalemia, and metabolic acidosis. Kidney and adrenal function are normal, and patients do not respond to exogenous mineralocorticoids. Genetic mutations responsible for PHA I occur in the α and β subunits of the amiloride-sensitive sodium channel of the collecting tubule. Frameshift or premature stop codon mutations in the cytoplasmic amino terminal or extracellular loop of either subunit disrupt the integrity of the sodium channel and result in loss of channel activity. Failure to reabsorb sodium results in volume depletion and activation of the renin-aldosterone axis. Furthermore, since sodium reabsorption is indirectly coupled to potassium and hydrogen ion secretion, hyperkalemia and metabolic acidosis ensue. Interestingly, when mutations are introduced into the cytoplasmic carboxyl terminal, sodium channel activity is increased and Liddle's syndrome is observed [4].

Hyperkalemia: Clinical Manifestations

CLINICAL MANIFESTATIONS OF HYPERKALEMIA

Cardiac	Renal electrolyte
Abnormal electrocardiogram	Decreased renal NH_4^+ production
Atrial/ventricular arrhythmias	Natriuresis
Pacemaker dysfunction	Endocrine
Neuromuscular	Increased aldosterone secretion
Paresthesias	Increased insulin secretion
Weakness	
Paralysis	

FIGURE 3-31

Clinical manifestations of hyperkalemia.

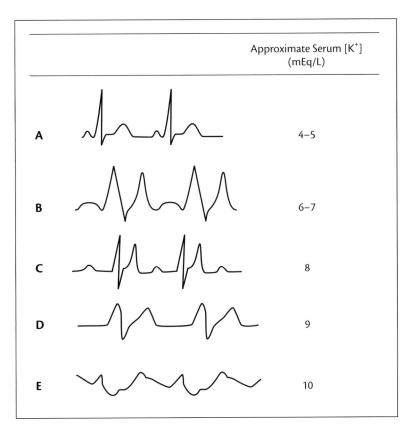

Approximate Serum [K$^+$]
(mEq/L)

A   4–5

B   6–7

C   8

D   9

E   10

FIGURE 3-32

Electrocardiographic (ECG) changes associated with hyperkalemia. **A,** Normal ECG pattern. **B,** Peaked, narrow-based T waves are the earliest sign of hyperkalemia. **C,** The P wave broadens and the QRS complex widens when the plamsa potassium level is above 7 mEq/L. **D,** With higher elevations in potassium, the P wave becomes difficult to identify. **E,** Eventually, an undulating sinusoidal pattern is evident. Although the ECG changes are depicted here as correlating to the severity of hyperkalemia, patients with even mild ECG changes may abruptly progress to terminal rhythm disturbances. Thus, hyperkalemia with any ECG changes should be treated as an emergency.

Hyperkalemia: Treatment

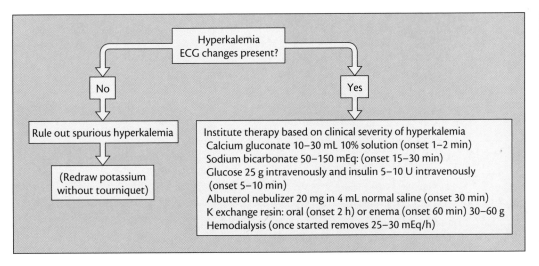

FIGURE 3-33

Treatment of hyperkalemia.

References

1. MacNight ADC: Epithelial transport of potassium. *Kidney Int* 1977, 11:391–397.

2. Bia MJ, DeFronzo RA: Extrarenal potassium homeostasis. *Am J Physiol* 1981, 240:F257–262.

3. Hansson JH, Nelson-Williams C, Suzuki H, *et al.*: Hypertension caused by a truncated epithelial sodium channel gamma subunit: Genetic heterogeneity of Liddle's syndrome. *Nature Genetics* 1995, 11:76–82.

4. Chang SS, Grunder S, Hanukoglu A, *et al.*: Mutations in subunits of the epithelial sodium channel cause salt wasting with hyperkalemic acidosis, pseudohypoaldosteronism type I. *Nature Genetics* 1996, 12:248–253.

5. Simon DB, Karet FE, Rodriguez-Soriano J, *et al.*: Genetic heterogeneity of Bartter's syndrome revealed by mutations in the K$^+$ channel, ROMK. *Nature Genetics* 1996, 14:152–156.

6. Pollack MR, Delaney VB, Graham RM, Hebert SC. Gitelman's syndrome (Bartter's variant) maps to the thiazide-sensitive co-transporter gene locus on chromosome 16q13 in a large kindred. *J Am Soc Nephrol* 1996, 7:2244–2248.

7. Sterwart PM, Krozowski ZS, Gupta A, *et al.*: Hypertension in the syndrome of apparent mineralocorticoid excess due to a mutation of the 11 (-hydroxysteroid dehydrogenase type 2 gene. *Lancet* 1996, 347:88–91.

8. Pascoe L, Curnow KM, Slutsker L, *et al.*: Glucocorticoid suppressable hyperaldosteronism results from hybrid genes created by unequal crossovers between CYP11B1 and CYP11B2. *Proc Natl Acad Sci USA* 1992, 89:8237–8331.

9. Welt LG, Blyth WB. Potassium in clinical medicine. In *A Primer on Potassium Metabolism.* Chicago: Searle & Co.; 1973.

10. DeFronzo RA: Regulation of extrarenal potassium homeostasis by insulin and catecholamines. In *Current Topics in Membranes and Transport*, vol. 28. Edited by Giebisch G. San Diego: Academic Press; 1987:299–329.

11. Giebisch G, Wang W: Potassium transport: from clearance to channels and pumps. *Kidney Int* 1996, 49:1642–1631.

12. Jamison RL: Potassium recycling. *Kidney Int* 1987, 31:695–703.

13. Nora NA, Berns AS: Hypokalemic, hypophosphatemic thyrotoxic periodic paralysis. *Am J Kidney Dis* 1989, 13:247–251.

14. Whang R, Flink EB, Dyckner T, *et al.*: Magnesium depletion as a cause of refractory potassium repletion. *Arch Int Med* 1985, 145:1686–1689.

15. Funder JW: Corticosteroid receptors and renal 11 β-hydroxysteroid dehydrogenase activity. *Semin Nephrol* 1990, 10:311–319.

16. Marriott HJL: Miscellaneous conditions: Hypokalemia. In *Practical Electrocardiography*, edn 8. Baltimore: Williams and Wilkins; 1988.

17. Riemanschneider TH, Bohle A: Morphologic aspects of low-potassium and low-sodium nephropathy. *Clin Nephrol* 1983, 19:271–279.

18. Tolins JP, Hostetter MK, Hostetter TH: Hypokalemic nephropathy in the rat: Role of ammonia in chronic tubular injury. *J Clin Invest* 1987, 79:1447–1458.

19. Sterns RH, Cox M, Fieg PU, *et al.*: Internal potassium balance and the control of the plasma potassium concentration. *Medicine* 1981, 60:339–344.

20. Kamel KS, Quaggin S, Scheich A, Halperin ML: Disorders of potassium homeostasis: an approach based on pathophysiology. *Am J Kidney Dis* 1994, 24:597–613.

21. Ethier JH, Kamel SK, Magner PO, *et al.*: The transtubular potassium concentration gradient in patients with hypokalemia and hyperkalemia. *Am J Kidney Dis* 1990, 15:309–315.

Divalent Cation Metabolism: Magnesium

James T. McCarthy

Rajiv Kumar

Magnesium is an essential intracellular cation. Nearly 99% of the total body magnesium is located in bone or the intracellular space. Magnesium is a critical cation and cofactor in numerous intracellular processes. It is a cofactor for adenosine triphosphate; an important membrane stabilizing agent; required for the structural integrity of numerous intracellular proteins and nucleic acids; a substrate or cofactor for important enzymes such as adenosine triphosphatase, guanosine triphosphatase, phospholipase C, adenylate cyclase, and guanylate cyclase; a required cofactor for the activity of over 300 other enzymes; a regulator of ion channels; an important intracellular signaling molecule; and a modulator of oxidative phosphorylation. Finally, magnesium is intimately involved in nerve conduction, muscle contraction, potassium transport, and calcium channels. Because turnover of magnesium in bone is so low, the short-term body requirements are met by a balance of gastrointestinal absorption and renal excretion. Therefore, the kidney occupies a central role in magnesium balance. Factors that modulate and affect renal magnesium excretion can have profound effects on magnesium balance. In turn, magnesium balance affects numerous intracellular and systemic processes [1–12].

In the presence of normal renal function, magnesium retention and hypermagnesemia are relatively uncommon. Hypermagnesemia inhibits magnesium reabsorption in both the proximal tubule and the loop of Henle. This inhibition of reabsorption leads to an increase in magnesium excretion and prevents the development of dangerous levels of serum magnesium, even in the presence of above-normal intake. However, in familial hypocalciuric hypercalcemia, there appears to be an abnormality of the thick ascending limb of the loop of Henle that prevents excretion of calcium. This abnormality may also extend to Mg. In familial hypocalciuric hypercalcemia, mild hypermagnesemia does not increase the renal excretion of magnesium. A similar abnormality may be caused by lithium [1,2,6,10]. The renal excretion of magnesium also is below normal in states of hypomagnesemia, decreased dietary magnesium, dehydration and volume depletion, hypocalcemia, hypothyroidism, and hyperparathyroidism [1,2,6,10].

CHAPTER

4

Magnesium Distribution

TOTAL BODY MAGNESIUM (MG) DISTRIBUTION

Location	Percent of Total	Mg Content, mmol*	Mg Content, mg*
Bone	53	530	12720
Muscle	27	270	6480
Soft tissue	19.2	192	4608
Erythrocyte	0.5	5	120
Serum	0.3	3	72
Total		1000	24000

*data typical for a 70 kg adult

FIGURE 4-1

Total distribution of magnesium (Mg) in the body. Mg (molecular weight, 24.305 D) is predominantly distributed in bone, muscle, and soft tissue. Total body Mg content is about 24 g (1 mol) per 70 kg. Mg in bone is adsorbed to the surface of hydroxyapatite crystals, and only about one third is readily available as an exchangeable pool. Only about 1% of the total body Mg is in the serum and interstitial fluid [1,2,8,9,11,12].

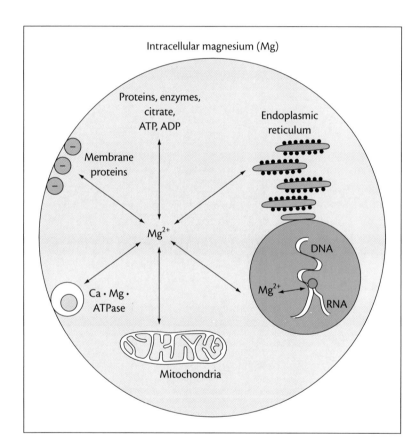

Intracellular magnesium (Mg)

FIGURE 4-2

Intracellular distribution of magnesium (Mg). Only 1% to 3% of the total intracellular Mg exists as the free ionized form of Mg, which has a closely regulated concentration of 0.5 to 1.0 mmol. Total cellular Mg concentration can vary from 5 to 20 mmol, depending on the type of tissue studied, with the highest Mg concentrations being found in skeletal and cardiac muscle cells. Our understanding of the concentration and distribution of intracellular Mg has been facilitated by the development of electron microprobe analysis techniques and fluorescent dyes using microfluorescence spectrometry. Intracellular Mg is predominantly complexed to organic molecules (*eg*, adenosine triphosphatase [ATPase], cell and nuclear membrane-associated proteins, DNA and RNA, enzymes, proteins, and citrates) or sequestered within subcellular organelles (mitochondria and endoplasmic reticulum). A heterogeneous distribution of Mg occurs within cells, with the highest concentrations being found in the perinuclear areas, which is the predominant site of endoplasmic reticulum. The concentration of intracellular free ionized Mg is tightly regulated by intracellular sequestration and complexation. Very little change occurs in the concentration of intracellular free Mg, even with large variations in the concentrations of total intracellular or extracellular Mg [1,3,11]. ADP—adenosine diphosphate; ATP—adenosine triphosphate; Ca^+—ionized calcium.

Intracellular Magnesium Metabolism

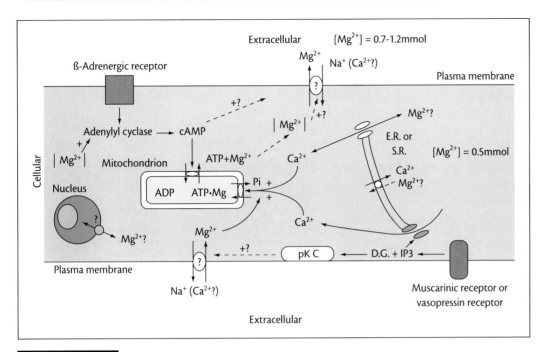

FIGURE 4-3

Regulation of intracellular magnesium (Mg²⁺) in the mammalian cell. Shown is an example of Mg²⁺ movement between intracellular and extracellular spaces and within intracellular compartments. The stimulation of adenylate cyclase activity (*eg*, through stimulation of β-adrenergic receptors) increases cyclic adenosine monophosphate (cAMP). The increase in cAMP induces extrusion of Mg from mitochondria by way of mitochondrial adenine nucleotide translocase, which exchanges 1 Mg²⁺-adenosine triphosphate (ATP) for adenosine diphosphate (ADP). This slight increase in cytosolic Mg²⁺ can then be extruded through the plasma membrane by way of a Mg-cation exchange mechanism, which may be activated by either cAMP or Mg. Activation of other cell receptors (*eg*, muscarinic receptor or vasopressin receptor) may alter cAMP levels or produce diacyl-

glycerol (DAG). DAG activates Mg influx by way of protein kinase C (pK C) activity. Mitochondria may accumulate Mg by the exchange of a cytosolic Mg²⁺-ATP for a mitochondrial matrix Pi molecule. This exchange mechanism is Ca²⁺-activated and bidirectional, depending on the concentrations of Mg²⁺-ATP and Pi in the cytosol and mitochondria. Inositol 1,4,5-trisphosphate (IP3) may also increase the release of Mg from endoplasmic reticulum or sarcoplasmic reticulum (ER or SR, respectively), which also has a positive effect on this Mg²⁺-ATP-Pi exchanger. Other potential mechanisms affecting cytosolic Mg include a hypothetical Ca²⁺-Mg²⁺ exchanger located in the ER and transport proteins that can allow the accumulation of Mg within the nucleus or ER. A balance must exist between passive entry of Mg into the cell and an active efflux mechanism because the concentration gradient favors the movement of extracellular Mg (0.7–1.2 mmol) into the cell (free Mg, 0.5 mmol). This Mg extrusion process may be energy-requiring or may be coupled to the movement of other cations. The cellular movement of Mg generally is not involved in the transepithelial transport of Mg, which is primarily passive and occurs between cells [1–3,7]. (*From* Romani and coworkers [3]; with permission.)

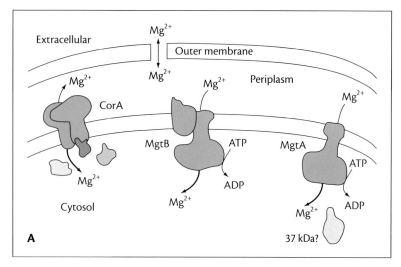

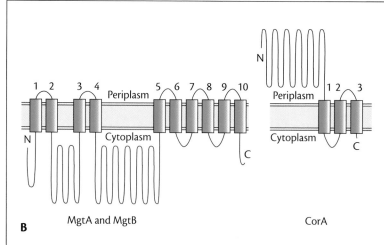

FIGURE 4-4

A, Transport systems of magnesium (Mg). Specific membrane-associated Mg transport proteins only have been described in bacteria such as *Salmonella*. Although similar transport proteins are believed to be present in mammalian cells based on nucleotide sequence analysis, they have not yet been demonstrated. Both MgtA and MgtB (molecular weight, 91 and 101 kDa, respectively) are members of the adenosine triphosphatase (ATPase) family of transport proteins. **B,** Both of these transport proteins have six C-terminal and four N-terminal membrane-spanning segments, with both the N- and C-terminals within the cytoplasm. Both proteins transport Mg with its electrochemical gradient, in contrast to other known ATPase proteins that usually transport ions against their chemical gradient. Low levels of extracellular Mg are capable of increasing transcription of these transport proteins, which increases transport of Mg into *Salmonella*. The CorA system has three membrane-spanning segments. This system mediates Mg influx; however, at extremely high extracellular Mg concentrations, this protein can also mediate Mg efflux. Another cell membrane Mg transport protein exists in erythrocytes (RBCs). This RBC Na^+-Mg^{2+} antiporter (not shown here) facilitates the outward movement of Mg from erythrocytes in the presence of extracellular Na^+ and intracellular adenosine triphosphate (ATP) [4,5]. ADP—adenosine diphosphate; C—carbon; N—nitrogen. (*From* Smith and Maguire [4]).

Gastrointestinal Absorption of Magnesium

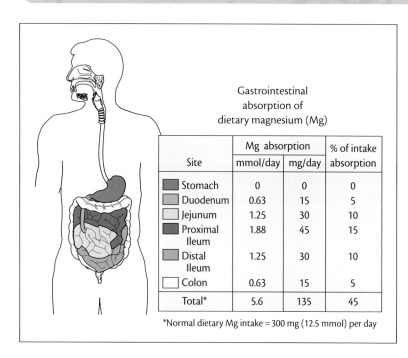

Gastrointestinal absorption of dietary magnesium (Mg)

Site	Mg absorption mmol/day	Mg absorption mg/day	% of intake absorption
Stomach	0	0	0
Duodenum	0.63	15	5
Jejunum	1.25	30	10
Proximal Ileum	1.88	45	15
Distal Ileum	1.25	30	10
Colon	0.63	15	5
Total*	5.6	135	45

*Normal dietary Mg intake = 300 mg (12.5 mmol) per day

FIGURE 4-5

Gastrointestinal absorption of dietary intake of magnesium (Mg). The normal adult dietary intake of Mg is 300 to 360 mg/d (12.5–15 mmol/d). A Mg intake of about 3.6 mg/kg/d is necessary to maintain Mg balance. Foods high in Mg content include green leafy vegetables (rich in Mg-containing chlorophyll), legumes, nuts, seafoods, and meats. Hard water contains about 30 mg/L of Mg. Dietary intake is the only source by which the body can replete Mg stores. Net intestinal Mg absorption is affected by the fractional Mg absorption within a specific segment of intestine, the length of that intestinal segment, and transit time of the food bolus. Approximately 40% to 50% of dietary Mg is absorbed. Both the duodenum and jejunum have a high fractional absorption of Mg. These segments of intestine are relatively short, however, and the transit time is rapid. Therefore, their relative contribution to total Mg absorption is less than that of the ileum. In the intact animal, most of the Mg absorption occurs in the ileum and colon. 1,25-dihydroxy-vitamin D_3 may mildly increase the intestinal absorption of Mg; however, this effect may be an indirect result of increased calcium absorption induced by the vitamin. Secretions of the upper intestinal tract contain approximately 1 mEq/L of Mg, whereas secretions from the lower intestinal tract contain 15 mEq/L of Mg. In states of nausea, vomiting, or nasogastric suction, mild to moderate losses of Mg occur. In diarrheal states, Mg depletion can occur rapidly owing to both high intestinal secretion and lack of Mg absorption [2,6,8–13].

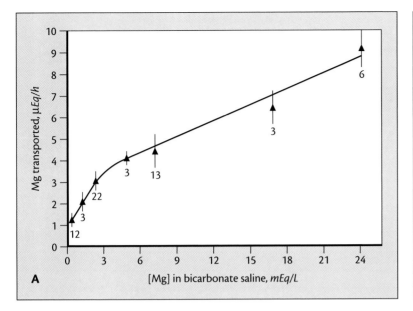

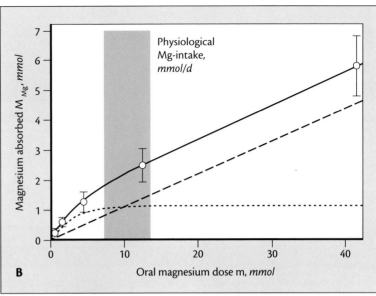

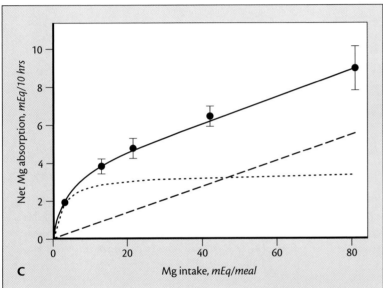

FIGURE 4-6

Intestinal magnesium (Mg) absorption. In rats, the intestinal Mg absorption is related to the luminal Mg concentration in a curvilinear fashion (**A**). This same phenomenon has been observed in humans (**B** and **C**). The hyperbolic curve (*dotted line* in **B** and **C**) seen at low doses and concentrations may reflect a saturable transcellular process; whereas the linear function (*dashed line* in **B** and **C**) at higher Mg intake may be a concentration-dependent passive intercellular Mg absorption. Alternatively, an intercellular process that can vary its permeability to Mg, depending on the luminal Mg concentration, could explain these findings (*see* Fig. 4-7) [13–15]. (**A**, *From* Kayne and Lee [13]; **B**, *from* Roth and Wermer [14]; **C**, *from* Fine and coworkers [15]; with permission.)

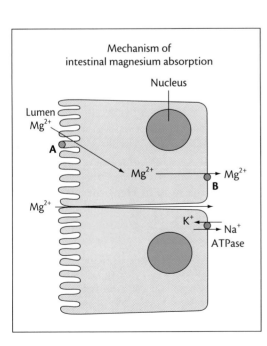

FIGURE 4-7

Proposed pathways for movement of magnesium (Mg) across the intestinal epithelium. Two possible routes exist for the absorption of Mg across intestinal epithelial cells: the transcellular route and the intercellular pathway. Although a transcellular route has not yet been demonstrated, its existence is inferred from several observations. No large chemical gradient exists for Mg movement across the cell membrane; however, a significant uphill electrical gradient exists for the exit of Mg from cells. This finding suggests the existence and participation of an energy-dependent mechanism for extrusion of Mg from intestinal cells. If such a system exists, it is believed it would consist of two stages. 1) Mg would enter the apical membrane of intestinal cells by way of a passive carrier or facilitated diffusion. 2) An active Mg pump in the basolateral section of the cell would extrude Mg. The intercellular movement of Mg has been demonstrated to occur by both gradient-driven and solvent-drag mechanisms. This intercellular path may be the only means by which Mg moves across the intestinal epithelium. The change in transport rates at low Mg concentrations would reflect changes in the "openness" of this pathway. High concentrations of luminal Mg (*eg*, after a meal) are capable of altering the morphology of the tight junction complex. High local Mg concentrations near the intercellular junction also can affect the activities of local membrane-associated proteins (*eg*, sodium-potassium adenosine triphosphate [Na-K ATPase]) near the tight junction and affect its permeability (*see* Fig. 4-6) [13–15].

Renal Handling of Magnesium

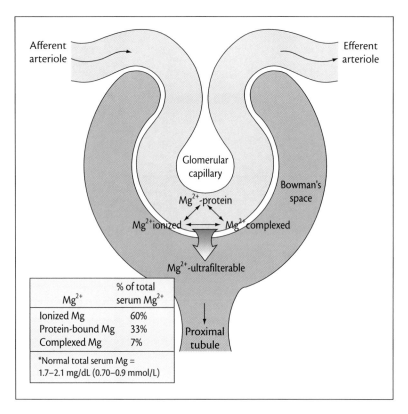

FIGURE 4-8

The glomerular filtration of magnesium (Mg). Total serum Mg consists of ionized, complexed, and protein bound fractions, 60%, 7%, and 33% of total, respectively. The complexed Mg is bound to molecules such as citrate, oxalate, and phosphate. The ultrafilterable Mg is the total of the ionized and complexed fractions. Normal total serum Mg is approximately 1.7 to 2.1 mg/dL (about 0.70–0.90 mmol/L) [1,2,7–9,11,12].

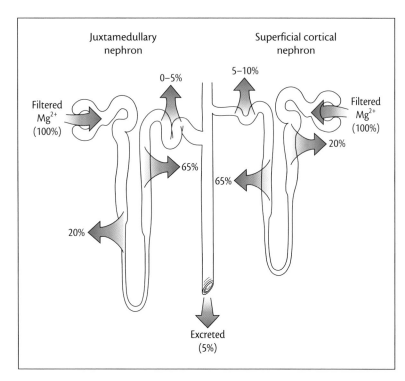

FIGURE 4-9

The renal handling of magnesium (Mg^{2+}). Mg is filtered at the glomerulus, with the ultrafilterable fraction of plasma Mg entering the proximal convoluted tubule (PCT). At the end of the PCT, the Mg concentration is approximately 1.7 times the initial concentra-

tion of Mg and about 20% of the filtered Mg has been reabsorbed. Mg reabsorption occurs passively through paracellular pathways. Hydrated Mg has a very large radius that decreases its intercellular permeability in the PCT when compared with sodium. The smaller hydrated radius of sodium is 50% to 60% reabsorbed in the PCT. No clear evidence exists of transcellular reabsorption or secretion of Mg within the mammalian PCT. In the pars recta of the proximal straight tubule (PST), Mg reabsorption can continue to occur by way of passive forces in the concentrating kidney. In states of normal hydration, however, very little Mg reabsorption occurs in the PST. Within the thin descending limb of the loop of Henle, juxtamedullary nephrons are capable of a small amount of Mg reabsorption in a state of antidiuresis or Mg depletion. This reabsorption does not occur in superficial cortical nephrons. No data exist regarding Mg reabsorption in the thin ascending limb of the loop of Henle. No Mg reabsorption occurs in the medullary portion of the thick ascending limb of the loop of Henle; whereas nearly 65% of the filtered load is absorbed in the cortical thick ascending limb of the loop of Henle in both juxtamedullary and superficial cortical nephrons. A small amount of Mg is absorbed in the distal convoluted tubule. Mg transport in the connecting tubule has not been well quantified. Little reabsorption occurs and no evidence exists of Mg secretion within the collecting duct. Normally, 95% of the filtered Mg is reabsorbed by the nephron. In states of Mg depletion the fractional excretion of Mg can decrease to less than 1%; whereas Mg excretion can increase in states of above-normal Mg intake, provided no evidence of renal failure exists [1,2,6–9,11,12].

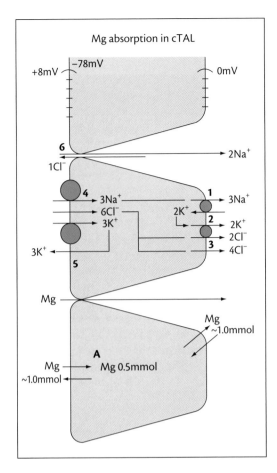

FIGURE 4-10

Magnesium (Mg) reabsorption in the cortical thick ascending limb (cTAL) of the loop of Henle. Most Mg reabsorption within the nephron occurs in the cTAL owing primarily to voltage-dependent Mg flux through the intercellular tight junction. Transcellular Mg movement occurs only in response to cellular metabolic needs. The sequence of events necessary to generate the lumen-positive electrochemical gradient that drives Mg reabsorption is as follows: 1) A basolateral sodium-potassium-adenosine triphosphatase (Na^+-K^+-ATPase) decreases intracellular sodium, generating an inside-negative electrical potential difference; 2) Intracellular K is extruded by an electroneutral K-Cl (chloride) cotransporter; 3) Cl is extruded by way of conductive pathways in the basolateral membrane; 4) The apical-luminal Na-2Cl-K (furosemide-sensitive) cotransport mechanism is driven by the inside-negative potential difference and decrease in intracellular Na; 5) Potassium is recycled back into the lumen by way of an apical K conductive channel; 6) Passage of approximately 2 Na molecules for every Cl molecule is allowed by the paracellular pathway (intercellular tight junction), which is cation permselective; 7) Mg reabsorption occurs passively, by way of intercellular channels, as it moves down its electrical gradient [1,2,6,7]. (*Adapted from* de Rouffignac and Quamme [1].)

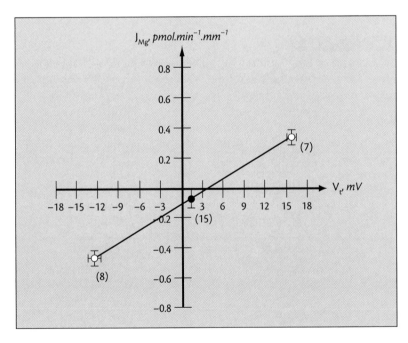

FIGURE 4-11

Voltage-dependent net magnesium (Mg) flux in the cortical thick ascending limb (cTAL). Within the isolated mouse cTAL, Mg flux (J_{Mg}) occurs in response to voltage-dependent mechanisms. With a relative lumen-positive transepithelial potential difference (V_t), Mg reabsorption increases (positive J_{Mg}). Mg reabsorption equals zero when no voltage-dependent difference exists, and Mg is capable of moving into the tubular lumen (negative J_{Mg}) when a lumen-negative voltage difference exists [1,16]. (*From* di Stefano and coworkers [16]).

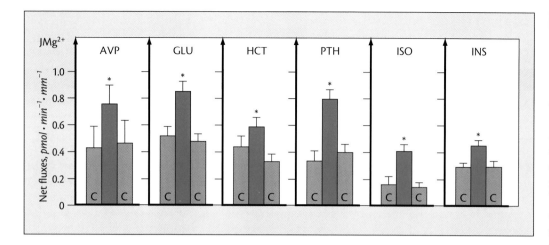

FIGURE 4-12

Effect of hormones on magnesium (Mg) transport in the cortical thick ascending limb (cTAL). In the presence of arginine vasopressin (AVP), glucagon (GLU), human calcitonin (HCT), parathyroid hormone (PTH), 1,4,5-isoproteronol (ISO), and insulin (INS), increases occur in Mg reabsorption from isolated segments of mouse cTALs. These hormones have no effect on medullary TAL segments. As already has been shown in Figure 4-3, these hormones affect intracellular "second messengers" and cellular Mg movement. These hormone-induced alterations can affect the paracellular permeability of the intercellular tight junction. These changes may also affect the transepithelial voltage across the cTAL. Both of these forces favor net Mg reabsorption in the cTAL [1,2,7,8]. Asterisk—significant change from preceding period; J_{Mg}—Mg flux; C—control, absence of hormone. (*Adapted from* de Rouffignac and Quamme [1].)

Magnesium Depletion

CAUSES OF MAGNESIUM (Mg) DEPLETION

Poor Mg intake	Other
Starvation	Lactation
Anorexia	Extensive burns
Protein calorie malnutrition	Exchange transfusions
No Mg in intravenous fluids	
Renal losses	
see Fig. 4-14	
Increased gastrointestinal Mg losses	
Nasogastric suction	
Vomiting	
Intestinal bypass for obesity	
Short-bowel syndrome	
Inflammatory bowel disease	
Pancreatitis	
Diarrhea	
Laxative abuse	
Villous adenoma	

FIGURE 4-13

The causes of magnesium (Mg) depletion. Depletion of Mg can develop as a result of low intake or increased losses by way of the gastrointestinal tract, the kidneys, or other routes [1,2,8–13].

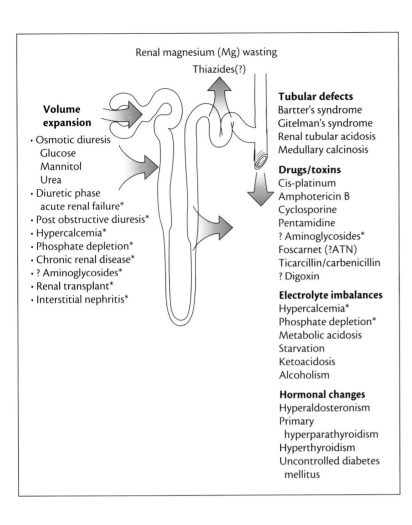

Renal magnesium (Mg) wasting

Thiazides(?)

Volume expansion
- Osmotic diuresis
  Glucose
  Mannitol
  Urea
- Diuretic phase
  acute renal failure*
- Post obstructive diuresis*
- Hypercalcemia*
- Phosphate depletion*
- Chronic renal disease*
- ? Aminoglycosides*
- Renal transplant*
- Interstitial nephritis*

Tubular defects
Bartter's syndrome
Gitelman's syndrome
Renal tubular acidosis
Medullary calcinosis

Drugs/toxins
Cis-platinum
Amphotericin B
Cyclosporine
Pentamidine
? Aminoglycosides*
Foscarnet (?ATN)
Ticarcillin/carbenicillin
? Digoxin

Electrolyte imbalances
Hypercalcemia*
Phosphate depletion*
Metabolic acidosis
Starvation
Ketoacidosis
Alcoholism

Hormonal changes
Hyperaldosteronism
Primary
  hyperparathyroidism
Hyperthyroidism
Uncontrolled diabetes
  mellitus

FIGURE 4-14

Renal magnesium (Mg) wasting. Mg is normally reabsorbed in the proximal tubule (PT), cortical thick ascending limb (cTAL), and distal convoluted tubule (DCT) (*see* Fig. 4-9). Volume expansion and osmotic diuretics inhibit PT reabsorption of Mg. Several renal diseases and electrolyte disturbances (asterisks) inhibit Mg reabsorption in both the PT and cTAL owing to damage to the epithelial cells and the intercellular tight junctions, plus disruption of the electrochemical forces that normally favor Mg reabsorption. Many drugs and toxins directly damage the cTAL. Thiazides have little direct effect on Mg reabsorption; however, the secondary hyperaldosteronism and hypercalcemia effect Mg reabsorption in CD and/or cTAL. Aminoglycosides accumulate in the PT, which affects sodium reabsorption, also leading to an increase in aldosterone. Aldosterone leads to volume expansion, decreasing Mg reabsorption. Parathyroid hormone has the direct effect of increasing Mg reabsorption in cTAL; however, hypercalcemia offsets this tendency. Thyroid hormone increases Mg loss. Diabetes mellitus increases Mg loss by way of both hyperglycemic osmotic diuresis and insulin abnormalities (deficiency and resistance), which decrease Mg reabsorption in the proximal convoluted tubule and cTAL, respectively. Cisplatin causes a Gitelman-like syndrome, which often can be permanent [1,2,8–12].

SIGNS AND SYMPTOMS OF HYPOMAGNESEMIA

Cardiovascular	Muscular
Electrocardiographic results	Cramps
Prolonged P-R and Q-T intervals,	Weakness
U waves	Carpopedal spasm
Angina pectoris	Chvostek's sign
?Congestive heart failure	Trousseau's sign
Atrial and ventricular arrhythmias	Fasciculations
?Hypertension	Tremulous
Digoxin toxicity	Hyperactive reflexes
Atherogenesis	Myoclonus
Neuromuscular	Dysphagia
Central nervous system	Skeletal
Seizures	Osteoporosis
Obtundation	Osteomalacia
Depression	
Psychosis	
Coma	
Ataxia	
Nystagmus	
Choreiform and athetoid movements	

FIGURE 4-15

Signs and symptoms of hypomagnesemia. Symptoms of hypomagnesemia can develop when the serum magnesium (Mg) level falls below 1.2 mg/dL. Mg is a critical cation in nerves and muscles and is intimately involved with potassium and calcium. Therefore, neuromuscular symptoms predominate and are similar to those seen in hypocalcemia and hypokalemia. Electrocardiographic changes of hypomagnesemia include an increased P-R interval, increased Q-T duration, and development of U waves. Mg deficiency increases the mortality of patients with acute myocardial infarction and congestive heart failure. Mg depletion hastens atherogenesis by increasing total cholesterol and triglyceride levels and by decreasing high-density lipoprotein cholesterol levels. Hypomagnesemia also increases hypertensive tendencies and impairs insulin release, which favor atherogenesis. Low levels of Mg impair parathyroid hormone (PTH) release, block PTH action on bone, and decrease the activity of renal 1-α-hydroxylase, which converts 25-hydroxy-vitamin D_3 into 1,25-dihydroxy-vitamin D_3, all of which contribute to hypocalcemia. Mg is an integral cofactor in cellular sodium-potassium-adenosine triphosphatase activity, and a deficiency of Mg impairs the intracellular transport of K and contributes to renal wasting of K, causing hypokalemia [6,8–12].

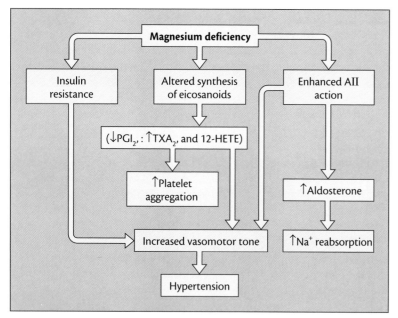

FIGURE 4-16

Mechanism whereby magnesium (Mg) deficiency could lead to hypertension. Mg deficiency does the following: increases angiotensin II (AII) action, decreases levels of vasodilatory prostaglandins (PGs), increases levels of vasoconstrictive PGs and growth factors, increases vascular smooth muscle cytosolic calcium, impairs insulin release, produces insulin resistance, and alters lipid profile. All of these results of Mg deficiency favor the development of hypertension and atherosclerosis [10,11]. Na+—ionized sodium; 12-HETE—hydroxy-eicosatetraenoic [acid]; TXA$_2$—thromboxane A2. (*From* Nadler and coworkers [17].)

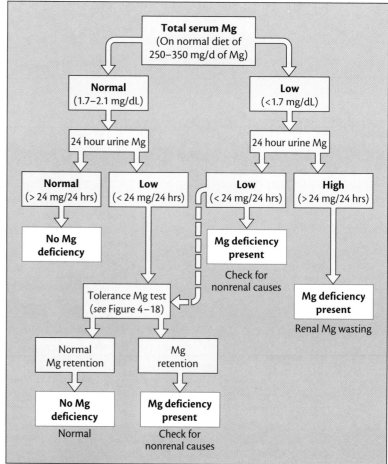

FIGURE 4-17

Evaluation in suspected magnesium (Mg) deficiency. Serum Mg levels may not always indicate total body stores. More refined tools used to assess the status of Mg in erythrocytes, muscle, lymphocytes, bone, isotope studies, and indicators of intracellular Mg, are not routinely available. Screening for Mg deficiency relies on the fact that urinary Mg decreases rapidly in the face of Mg depletion in the presence of normal renal function [2,6,8–15,18]. (*Adapted from* Al-Ghamdi and coworkers [11].)

FIGURE 4-18

The magnesium (Mg) tolerance test, in various forms [2,6,8–12,18], has been advocated to diagnose Mg depletion in patients with normal or near-normal serum Mg levels. All such tests are predicated on the fact that patients with normal Mg status rapidly excrete over 50% of an acute Mg load; whereas patients with depleted Mg retain Mg in an effort to replenish Mg stores. (*From* Ryzen and coworkers [18].)

MAGNESIUM (Mg) TOLERANCE TEST FOR PATIENTS WITH NORMAL SERUM MAGNESIUM

Time	Action
0 (baseline)	Urine (spot or timed) for molar Mg:Cr ratio
0–4 h	IV infusion of 2.4 mg (0.1 mmol) of Mg/kg lean body wt in 50 mL of 50% dextrose
0–24 h	Collect urine (staring with Mg infusion) for Mg and Cr
End	Calculate % Mg retained (%M)

$$\% \, M = 1 - \frac{(\text{24-h urine Mg}) - ([\text{Preinfusion urine Mg:Cr}] \times [\text{24-h urine Cr}])}{\text{Total Mg infused}} \times 100$$

Mg retained, %	Mg deficiency
>50	Definite
20–50	Probable
<20	None

Cr—creatinine; IV—intravenous; Mg—magnesium.

MAGNESIUM SALTS USED IN MAGNESIUM REPLACEMENT THERAPY

Magnesium salt	Chemical formula	Mg content, *mg/g*	Examples*	Mg content	Diarrhea
Gluconate	$Cl_2H_{22}MgO_{14}$	58	Magonate°	27-mg tablet 54 mg/5 mL	±
Chloride	$MgCl_2 . (H_2O)_6$	120	Mag-L-100	100-mg capsule	+
Lactate	$C_6H_{10}MgO_6$	120	MagTab SR*	84-mg caplet	+
Citrate	$C_{12}H_{10}Mg_3O_{14}$	53	Multiple	47–56 mg/5 mL	++
Hydroxide	$Mg(OH)_2$	410	Maalox°, Mylanta°, Gelusil° Riopan°	83 mg/ 5 mL and 63-mg tablet 96 mg/5 mL	++
Oxide	MgO	600	Mag-Ox 400° Uro-Mag° Beelith°	241-mg tablet 84.5-mg tablet 362-mg tablet	++
Sulfate	$MgSO_4 . (H_2O)_7$	100	IV IV Oral epsom salt	10%—9.9 mg/mL 50%—49.3 mg/mL 97 mg/g	++ ++
Milk of Magnesia			Phillips' Milk of Magnesia°	168 mg/ 5 mL	++

Data from McLean [9], Al-Ghamdi and coworkers [11], Oster and Epstein [19], and Physicians' Desk Reference [20].

*Magonate°, Fleming & Co, Fenton, MD; MagTab Sr°, Niche Pharmaceuticals, Roanoke, TX; Maalox°, Rhone-Poulenc Rorer Pharmaceutical, Collegeville, PA; Mylanta°, J & J-Merck Consumer Pharm, Ft Washinton, PA; Riopan°, Whitehall Robbins Laboratories, Madison, NJ; Mag-Ox 400° and Uro-Mag°, Blaine, Erlanger, KY; Beelith°, Beach Pharmaceuticals, Conestee, SC; Phillips' Milk of Magnesia, Bayer Corp, Parsippany, NJ.

FIGURE 4-19

Magnesium (Mg) salts that may be used in Mg replacement therapy.

GUIDELINES FOR MAGNESIUM (Mg) REPLACEMENT

Life-threatening event, *eg*, seizures and cardiac arrhythmia

I. 2–4 g MgSO₄ IV or IM stat
(2–4 vials [2 mL each] of 50% MgSO₄)
Provides 200–400 mg of Mg (8.3–16.7 mmol Mg)
Closely monitor:
  Deep tendon reflexes
  Heart rate
  Blood pressure
  Respiratory rate
  Serum Mg (<2.5 mmol/L [6.0 mg/dL])
  Serum K

II. IV drip over first 24 h to provide no more than 1200 mg (50 mmol) Mg/24 h

Subacute and chronic Mg replacement

I. 400–600 mg (16.7–25 mmol Mg daily for 2–5 d)
IV: continuous infusion
IM: painful
Oral: use divided doses to minimize diarrhea

FIGURE 4-20

Acute Mg replacement for life-threatening events such as seizures or potentially lethal cardiac arrhythmias has been described [8–12,19]. Acute increases in the level of serum Mg can cause nausea, vomiting, cutaneous flushing, muscular weakness, and hyporeflexia. As Mg levels increase above 6 mg/dL (2.5 mmol/L), electrocardiographic changes are followed, in sequence, by hyporeflexia, respiratory paralysis, and cardiac arrest. Mg should be administered with caution in patients with renal failure. In the event of an emergency the acute Mg load should be followed by an intravenous (IV) infusion, providing no more than 1200 mg (50 mmol) of Mg on the first day. This treatment can be followed by another 2 to 5 days of Mg repletion in the same dosage, which is used in less urgent situations. Continuous IV infusion of Mg is preferred to both intramuscular (which is painful) and oral (which causes diarrhea) administration. A continuous infusion avoids the higher urinary fractional excretion of Mg seen with intermittent administration of Mg. Patients with mild Mg deficiency may be treated with oral Mg salts rather than parenteral Mg and may be equally efficacious [8]. Administration of Mg sulfate may cause kaliuresis owing to excretion of the nonreabsorbable sulfate anion; Mg oxide administration has been reported to cause significant acidosis and hyperkalemia [19]. Parenteral Mg also is administered (often in a manner different from that shown here) to patients with preeclampsia, asthma, acute myocardial infarction, and congestive heart failure.

References

1. de Rouffignac C, Quamme G: Renal magnesium handling and its hormonal control. *Physiol Rev* 1994, 74:305–322.

2. Quamme GA: Magnesium homeostasis and renal magnesium handling. *Miner Electrolyte Metab* 1993, 19:218–225.

3. Romani A, Marfella C, Scarpa A: Cell magnesium transport and homeostasis: role of intracellular compartments. *Miner Electrolyte Metab* 1993, 19:282–289.

4. Smith DL, Maguire ME: Molecular aspects of Mg^{2+} transport systems. *Miner Electrolyte Metab* 1993, 19:266–276.

5. Roof SK, Maguire ME: Magnesium transport systems: genetics and protein structure (a review). *J Am Coll Nutr* 1994, 13:424–428.

6. Sutton RAL, Domrongkitchaiporn S: Abnormal renal magnesium handling. *Miner Electrolyte Metab* 1993, 19:232–240.

7. de Rouffignac C, Mandon B, Wittner M, di Stefano A: Hormonal control of magnesium handling. *Miner Electrolyte Metab* 1993, 19:226–231.

8. Whang R, Hampton EM, Whang DD: Magnesium homeostasis and clinical disorders of magnesium deficiency. *Ann Pharmacother* 1994, 28:220–226.

9. McLean RM: Magnesium and its therapeutic uses: a review. *Am J Med* 1994, 96:63–76.

10. Abbott LG, Rude RK: Clinical manifestations of magnesium deficiency. *Miner Electrolyte Metab* 1993, 19:314–322.

11. Al-Ghamdi SMG, Cameron EC, Sutton RAL: Magnesium deficiency: pathophysiologic and clinical overview. *Am J Kid Dis* 1994, 24:737–752.

12. Nadler JL, Rude RK: Disorders of magnesium metabolism. *Endocrinol Metab Clin North Am* 1995, 24:623–641.

13. Kayne LH, Lee DBN: Intestinal magnesium absorption. *Miner Electrolyte Metab* 1993, 19:210–217.

14. Roth P, Werner E: Intestinal absorption of magnesium in man. *Int J Appl Radiat Isotopes* 1979, 30:523–526.

15. Fine KD, Santa Ana CA, Porter JL, Fordtran JS: Intestinal absorption of magnesium from food and supplements. *J Clin Invest* 1991, 88:396–402.

16. di Stefano A, Roinel N, de Rouffignac C, Wittner M: Transepithelial Ca^+ and Mg^+ transport in the cortical thick ascending limb of Henle's loop of the mouse is a voltage-dependent process. *Renal Physiol Biochem* 1993, 16:157–166.

17. Nadler JL, Buchanan T, Natarajan R, *et al.*: Magnesium deficiency produces insulin resistance and increased thromboxane synthesis. *Hypertension* 1993, 21:1024–1029.

18. Ryzen E, Elbaum N, Singer FR, Rude RK: Parenteral magnesium tolerance testing in the evaluation of magnesium deficiency. *Magnesium* 1985, 4:137–147.

19. Oster JR, Epstein M: Management of magnesium depletion. *Am J Nephrol* 1988, 8:349–354.

20. *Physicians' Desk Reference* (PDR). Montvale, NJ: Medical Economics Company; 1996.

Vitamin D and Parathyroid Hormone Actions

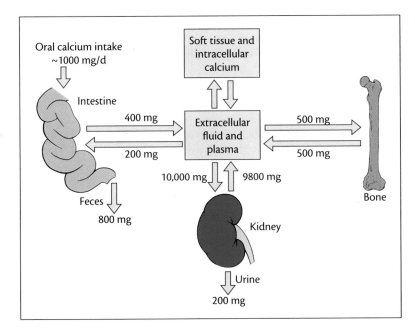

7-dehydrocholesterol

UV light   Skin

Vitamin D₃

Liver   25-hydroxylase

25-hydroxy-vitamin D₃

(+)	(−)	(+)
PTH	Hypercalcemia	1, 25(OH)₂D₃
PTHrP	Hyperphosphatemia	Hypercalcemia
Hypophosphatemia	1, 25(OH)₂D₃	Hyperphosphatemia
Hypocalcemia	Acidosis	
24R, 25(OH)₂D₃		
IGF-1		

Kidney   1-alpha-hydroxylase

24-hydroxylase   Kidney, intestine, other tissue

1, 25-hydroxy-vitamin D₃

24, 25-hydroxy-vitamin D₃

Various tissue enzymes

Hydroxylated and conjugated polar metabolites

FIGURE 5-3

Metabolism of vitamin D. The compound 7-dehydrocholesterol, through the effects of heat (37°C) and (UV) light (wavelength 280–305 nm), is converted into vitamin D₃ in the skin. Vitamin D₃ is then transported on vitamin D binding proteins (VDBP) to the liver. In the liver, vitamin D₃ is converted to 25-hydroxy-vitamin D₃ by the hepatic microsomal and mitochondrial cytochrome P450–containing vitamin D₃ 25-hydroxylase enzyme. The 25-hydroxy-vitamin D₃ is transported on VDBP to the proximal tubular cells of the kidney, where it is converted to 1,25-dihydroxy-vitamin D₃ by a 1-α-hydroxylase enzyme, which also is a cytochrome P450–containing enzyme. The genetic information for this enzyme is encoded on the 12q14 chromosome. Alternatively, 25-hydroxy-vitamin D₃ can be converted to 24R,25-dihydroxy-vitamin D₃, a relatively inactive vitamin D metabolite. 1,25-dihydroxy-vitamin D₃ can then be transported by VDBP to its most important target tissues in the distal tubular cells of the kidney, intestinal epithelial cells, parathyroid cells, and bone cells. VDBP is a 58 kD α-globulin that is a member of the albumin and α-fetoprotein gene family. The DNA sequence that encodes for this protein is on chromosome 4q11-13. 1,25-dihydroxy-vitamin D₃ is eventually metabolized to hydroxylated and conjugated polar metabolites in the enterohepatic circulation. Occasionally, 1,25-dihydroxy-vitamin D₃ also may be produced in extrarenal sites, such as monocyte-derived cells, and may have an antiproliferative effect in certain lymphocytes and keratinocytes [1,7–9]. (*Adapted from* Kumar [1].)

FIGURE 5-4

Calcium (Ca) flux between body compartments. Ca balance is a complex process involving bone, intestinal absorption of dietary Ca, and renal excretion of Ca. The parathyroid glands, by their production of parathyroid hormone, and the liver, through its participation in vitamin D metabolism, also are integral organs in the maintenance of Ca balance. (*From* Kumar [1]; with permission.)

Oral calcium intake ~1000 mg/d

Soft tissue and intracellular calcium

Intestine

400 mg → Extracellular fluid and plasma ← 500 mg (Bone)

200 mg ←   → 500 mg

Feces 800 mg

10,000 mg ↓ ↑ 9800 mg

Kidney

Bone

Urine 200 mg

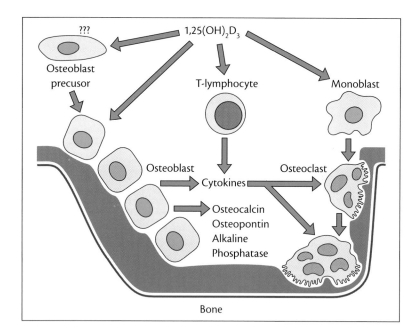

FIGURE 5-5

Effects of 1,25-dihydroxy-vitamin D_3 (calcitriol) on bone. In addition to the effects on parathyroid cells, the kidney, and intestinal epithelium, calcitriol has direct effects on bone metabolism. Calcitriol can promote osteoclast differentiation and activity from monocyte precursor cells. Calcitriol also promotes osteoblast differentiation into mature cells. (*From* Holick [8]; with permission.)

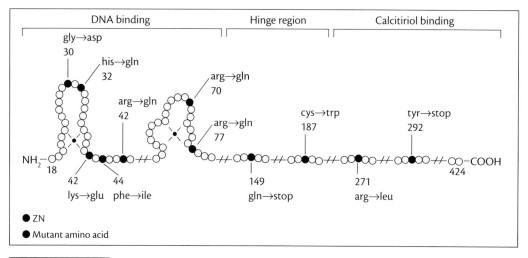

FIGURE 5-6

The vitamin D receptor (VDR). Within its target tissues, calcitriol binds to the VDR. The VDR is a 424 amino acid polypeptide. Its genomic information is encoded on the 12q12-14 chromosome, near the gene for the 1-α-hydroxylase enzyme. The VDR is found in the intestinal epithelium, parathyroid cells, kidney cells, osteoblasts, and thyroid cells. VDR also can be detected in keratinocytes, monocyte precursor cells, muscle cells, and numerous other tissues. The allele variations for the vitamin D receptor. Two allele variations exist for the vitamin D receptor (VDR): the b allele and the B allele. In general, normal persons with the b allele seem to have a higher bone mineral density [9]. Among patients on dialysis, those with the b allele may have higher levels of circulating parathyroid hormone (PTH) [7,9,10,11]. COOH—carboxy terminal; NH_2—amino terminal. (*From* Root [7]; with permission.)

FIGURE 5-7

Mechanism of action of 1-25-dihydroxy-vitamin D_3 ($1,25(OH)_2D_3$). $1,25(OH)_2D_3$ is transported to the target cell bound to the vitamin D–binding protein (VDBP). The free form of $1,25(OH)_2D_3$ enters the target cell and interacts with the vitamin D receptor (VDR) at the nucleus. This complex is phosphorylated and combined with the nuclear accessory factor (RAF). This forms a heterodimer, which then interacts with the vitamin D responsive element (VDRE). The VDRE then either promotes or inhibits the transcription of messenger RNA (mRNA) for proteins regulated by $1,25(OH)_2D_3$, such as Ca-binding proteins, the 25-hydroxy-vitamin D_3 24-hydroxylase enzyme, and parathyroid hormone. Pi—inorganic phosphate. (*Adapted from* Holick [8].)

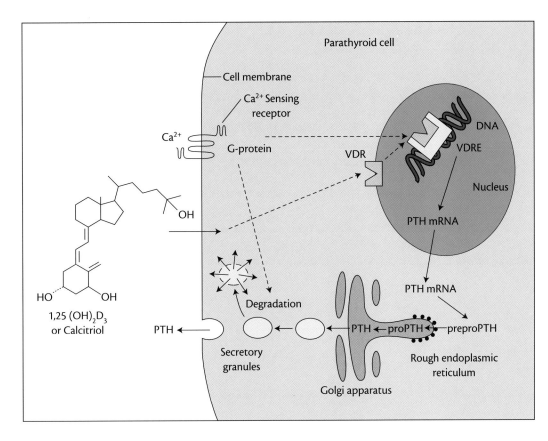

FIGURE 5-8

Metabolism of parathyroid hormone (PTH). The PTH gene is located on chromosome 11p15. PTH messenger RNA (mRNA) is transcribed from the DNA fragment and then translated into a 115 amino acid–containing molecule of prepro-PTH. In the rough endoplasmic reticulum, this undergoes hydrolysis to a 90 amino acid–containing molecule, pro-PTH, which undergoes further hydrolysis to the 84 amino acid–containing PTH molecule. PTH is then stored within secretory granules in the cytoplasm for release. PTH is metabolized by hepatic Kupffer cells and renal tubular cells. Transcription of the PTH gene is inhibited by 1,25-dihydroxy-vitamin D_3, calcitonin, and hypercalcemia. PTH gene transcription is increased by hypocalcemia, glucocorticoids, and estrogen. Hypercalcemia also can increase the intracellular degradation of PTH. PTH release is increased by hypocalcemia, β-adrenergic agonists, dopamine, and prostaglandin E_2. Hypomagnesemia blocks the secretion of PTH [7,12]. VDR—vitamin D receptor; VDRE—vitamin D responsive element. (*Adapted from* Tanaka and coworkers [12].)

	-2	-1	1	2	3	4	5	6	7	8	9	10	11	12	13

PTH (mw 9600) N— 1 — 34 — 84 —C

PTH-like peptide (mw 16,000) N— 1 — 141 —C

	-2	-1	1	2	3	4	5	6	7	8	9	10	11	12	13
PTH	LYS	ARG	SER	VAL	SER	GLU	ILE		GLN	LEU	MET	HIS	ASN	LEU	GLY	LYS
PTH-like peptide	LYS	ARG	ALA	VAL	SER	GLU	HIS		GLN	LEU	LEU	HIS	ASP	LYS	GLY	LYS

FIGURE 5-9

Parathyroid-hormone–related protein (PTHrP). PTHrP was initially described as the causative circulating factor in the humoral hypercalcemia of malignancy, particularly in breast cancer, squamous cell cancers of the lung, renal cell cancer, and other tumors. It is now clear that PTHrP can be expressed not only in cancer but also in many normal tissues. It may play an important role in the regulation of smooth muscle tone, transepithelial Ca transport (*eg*, in the mammary gland), and the differentiation of tissue and organ development [7,13]. Note the high degree of homology between PTHrP and PTH at the amino end of the polypeptides. MW—molecular weight; N—amino terminal; C—carboxy terminal. (*From* Root [7]; with permission.)

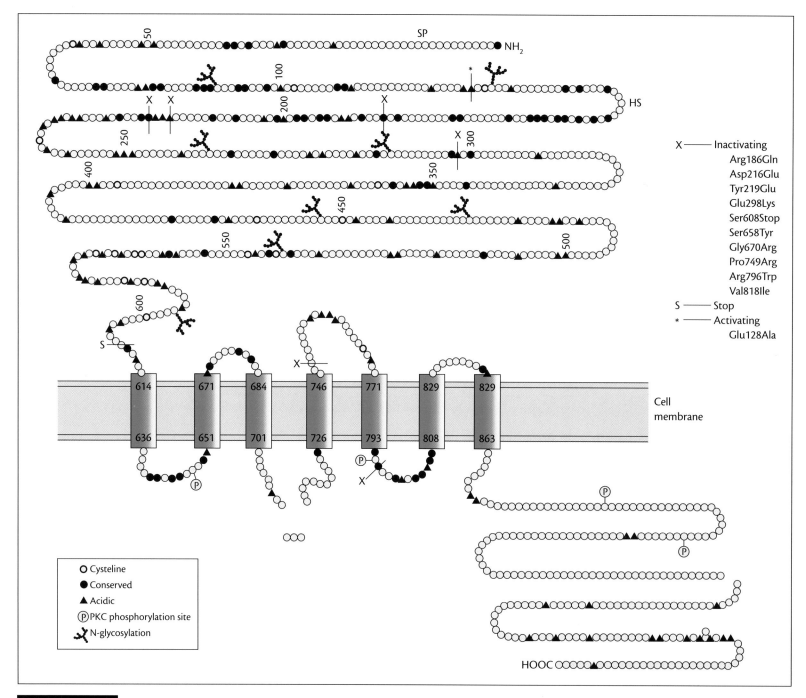

FIGURE 5-10

The calcium-ion sensing receptor (CaSR). The CaSR is a guanosine triphosphate (GTP) or G-protein–coupled polypeptide receptor. The human CaSR has approximately 1084 amino acid residues. The CaSR mediates the effects of Ca on parathyroid and renal tissues. CaSR also can be found in thyroidal C cells, brain cells, and in the gastrointestinal tract. The CaSR allows Ca to act as a first messenger on target tissues and then act by way of other second-messenger systems (*eg*, phospholipase enzymes and cyclic adenosine monophosphate). Within parathyroid cells, hypercalcemia increases CaSR-Ca binding, which activates the G-protein. The G-protein then activates the phospholipase C-β-1–phosphatidylinositol-4,5-biphosphate pathway to increase intracellular Ca, which then decreases translation of parathyroid hormone (PTH), decreases PTH secretion, and increases PTH degradation. The CaSR also is an integral part of Ca homeostasis within the kidney. The gene for CaSR is located on human chromosome 3q13 [3,4,7,14–16]. PKC—protein kinase C; HS—hydrophobic segment; NH₂—amino terminal. (*From* Hebert and Brown [4]; with permission.)

Gastrointestinal Absorption of Calcium

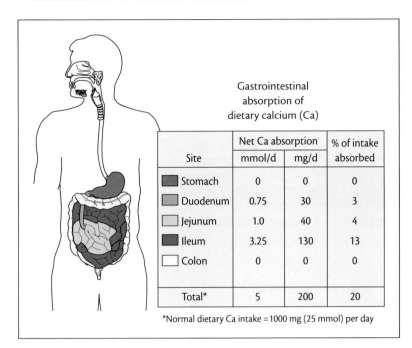

Gastrointestinal
absorption of
dietary calcium (Ca)

Site	Net Ca absorption		% of intake absorbed
	mmol/d	mg/d	
Stomach	0	0	0
Duodenum	0.75	30	3
Jejunum	1.0	40	4
Ileum	3.25	130	13
Colon	0	0	0
Total*	5	200	20

*Normal dietary Ca intake = 1000 mg (25 mmol) per day

FIGURE 5-11

Gastrointestinal absorption of dietary calcium (Ca). The normal recommended dietary intake of Ca for an adult is 800 to 1200 mg/d (20–30 mmol/d). Foods high in Ca content include milk, dairy products, meat, fish with bones, oysters, and many leafy green vegetables (*eg*, spinach and collard greens). Although serum Ca levels can be maintained in the normal range by bone resorption, dietary intake is the only source by which the body can replenish stores of Ca in bone. Ca is absorbed almost exclusively within the duodenum, jejunum, and ileum. Each of these intestinal segments has a high absorptive capacity for Ca, with their relative Ca absorption being dependent on the length of each respective intestinal segment and the transit time of the food bolus. Approximately 400 mg of the usual 1000 mg dietary Ca intake is absorbed by the intestine, and Ca loss by way of intestinal secretions is approximately 200 mg/d. Therefore, a net absorption of Ca is approximately 200 mg/d (20%). Biliary and pancreatic secretions are extremely rich in Ca. 1,25-dihydroxy-vitamin D_3 is an extremely important regulatory hormone for intestinal absorption of Ca [1,2,17,18].

FIGURE 5-12

Proposed pathways for calcium (Ca) absorption across the intestinal epithelium. Two routes exist for the absorption of Ca across the intestinal epithelium: the paracellular pathway and the transcellular route. The paracellular pathway is passive, and it is the predominant means of Ca absorption when the luminal concentration of Ca is high. This is a nonsaturable pathway and can account for one half to two thirds of total intestinal Ca absorption. The paracellular absorptive route may be indirectly influenced by 1,25-dihydroxy-vitamin D_3 $(1,25(OH)_2D_3)$ because it may be capable of altering the structure of intercellular tight junctions by way of activation of protein kinase C, making the tight junction more permeable to the movement of Ca. However, $1,25(OH)_2D_3$ primarily controls the active absorption of Ca. (1) Ca moves down its concentration gradient through a Ca channel or Ca transporter into the apical section of the microvillae. Because the intestinal concentration of Ca usually is 10^{-3} mol and the intracellular Ca concentration is 10^{-6} mol, a large concentration gradient favors the passive movement of Ca. Ca is rapidly and reversibly bound to the calmodulin-actin-myosin I complex. Ca may then move to the basolateral area of the cell by way of microvesicular transport, or ionized Ca may diffuse to this area of the cell. (2) As the calmodulin complex becomes saturated with Ca, the concentration gradient for the movement of Ca into the microvillae is not as favorable, which slows Ca absorption. (3) Under the influence of calcitriol, intestinal epithelial cells increase their synthesis of calbindin. (4) Ca binds to calbindin, thereby unloading the Ca-calmodulin complexes, which then remove Ca from the microvillae region. This decrease in Ca concentration again favors the movement of Ca into the microvillae. As the calbindin-Ca complex dissociates, the free intracellular Ca is actively extruded from the cell by either the Ca-adenosine triphosphatase (ATPase) or Na-Ca exchanger. Calcitriol may also increase the synthesis of the plasma membrane Ca-ATPase, thereby aiding in the active extrusion of Ca into the lamina propria [2,7,9,17,18].

Renal Handling of Calcium

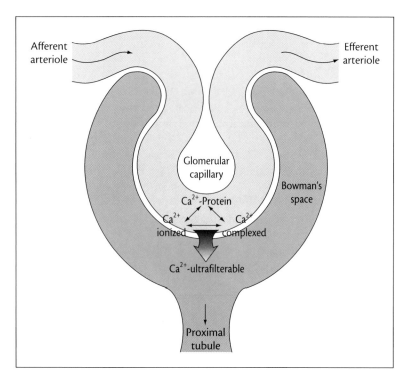

FIGURE 5-13

Glomerular filtration of calcium (Ca). Total serum Ca consists of ionized, protein bound, and complexed fractions (47.5%, 46.0%, and 6.5%, respectively). The complexed Ca is bound to molecules such as phosphate and citrate. The ultrafilterable Ca equals the total of the ionized and complexed fractions. Normal total serum Ca is approximately 8.9 to 10.1 mg/dL (about 2.2–2.5 mmol/L). Ca can be bound to albumin and globulins. For each 1.0 gm/dL decrease in serum albumin, total serum Ca decreases by 0.8 mg/dL; for each 1.0 gm/dL decrease in serum globulin fraction, total serum Ca decreases by 0.12 mg/dL. Ionized Ca is also affected by pH. For every 0.1 change in pH, ionized Ca changes by 0.12 mg/dL. Alkalosis decreases the ionized Ca [1,6,7].

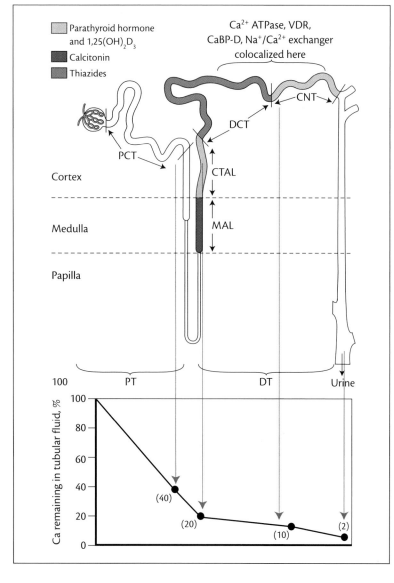

FIGURE 5-14

Renal handling of calcium (Ca). Ca is filtered at the glomerulus, with the ultrafilterable fraction (UF_{Ca}) of plasma Ca entering the proximal tubule (PT). Within the proximal convoluted tubule (PCT) and the proximal straight tubule (PST), isosmotic reabsorption of Ca occurs such that at the end of the PST the UF_{Ca} to TF_{Ca} ratio is about 1.1 and 60% to 70% of the filtered Ca has been reabsorbed. Passive paracellular pathways account for about 80% of Ca reabsorption in this segment of the nephron, with the remaining 20% dependent on active transcellular Ca movement. No reabsorption of Ca occurs within the thin segment of the loop of Henle. Ca is reabsorbed in small amounts within the medullary segment of the thick ascending limb (MAL) of the loop of Henle and calcitonin (CT) stimulates Ca reabsorption here. However, the cortical segments (cTAL) reabsorb about 20% of the initially filtered load of Ca. Under normal conditions, most of the Ca reabsorption in the cTAL is passive and paracellular, owing to the favorable electrochemical gradient. Active transcellular Ca transport can be stimulated by both parathyroid hormone (PTH) and 1,25-dihydroxy-vitamin D_3 ($1,25(OH)_2D_3$) in the cTAL. In the early distal convoluted tubule (DCT), thiazide-activated Ca transport occurs. The DCT is the primary site in the nephron at which Ca reabsorption is regulated by PTH and $1,25(OH)_2D_3$. Active transcellular Ca transport must account for Ca reabsorption in the DCT, because the transepithelial voltage becomes negative, which would not favor passive movement of Ca out of the tubular lumen. About 10% of the filtered Ca is reabsorbed in the DCT, with another 3% to 10% of filtered Ca reabsorbed in the connecting tubule (CNT) by way of mechanisms similar to those in the DCT [1,2,6, 7,18]. ATPase—adenosine triphosphatase; CaBP-D—Ca-binding protein D; DT—distal tubule; VDR—vitamin D receptor. (*Adapted from* Kumar [1].)

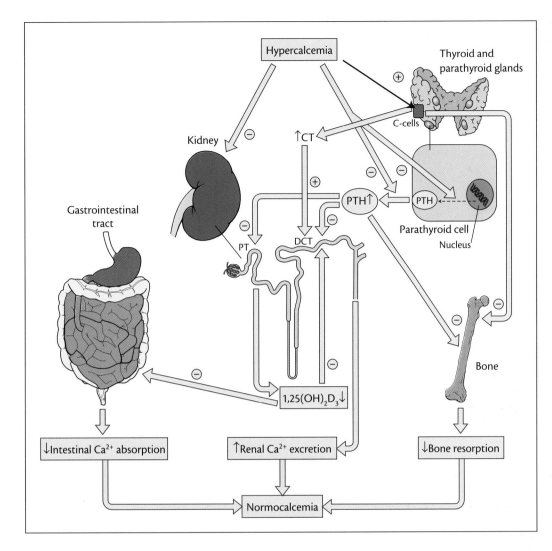

FIGURE 5-19

Physiologic response to hypercalcemia. Hypercalcemia directly inhibits both parathyroid hormone (PTH) release and synthesis. The decrease in PTH and hypercalcemia decrease the activity of the 1-α-hydroxylase enzyme located in the proximal tubular (PT) cells of the nephron, which in turn, decreases the synthesis of 1,25-dihydroxy-vitamin D_3 (1,25(OH)$_2$D$_3$). Hypercalcemia stimulates the C cells in the thyroid gland to increase synthesis of calcitonin (CT). Bone resorption by osteoclasts is blocked by the increased CT and decreased PTH. Decreased levels of PTH and 1,25(OH)$_2$D$_3$ inhibit Ca reabsorption in the distal convoluted tubules (DCT) of the nephrons and overwhelm the effects of CT, which augment Ca reabsorption in the medullary thick ascending limb leading to an increase in renal Ca excretion. The decrease in 1,25(OH)$_2$D$_3$ decreases gastrointestinal (GI) tract absorption of dietary Ca. All of these effects tend to return serum Ca to normal levels [1].

FIGURE 5-20

Causes of hypercalcemia (increase in ionized plasma calcium).

CAUSES OF HYPERCALCEMIA

Excess parathyroid hormone (PTH) production
Primary hyperparathyroidism
"Tertiary" hyperparathyroidism*

Excess 1,25-dihydroxy-vitamin D$_3$ (1,25(OH)$_2$D$_3$)
Vitamin D intoxication
Sarcoidosis and granulomatous diseases
Severe hypophosphatemia
Neoplastic production of 1,25(OH)$_2$D$_3$ (lymphoma)

Increased bone resorption
Metastatic (osteolytic) tumors (*eg*, breast, colon, prostate)
Humoral hypercalcemia
  PTH-related protein (*eg*, squamous cell lung, renal cell cancer)
  Osteoclastic activating factor (myeloma)
  1,25 (OH)$_2$D$_3$ (lymphoma)
  Prostaglandins
Hyperthyroidism
Immobilization
Paget disease
Vitamin A intoxication

Increased intestinal absorption of calcium
Vitamin D intoxication
Milk-alkali syndrome*

Decreased renal excretion of calcium
Familial hypocalciuric hypercalcemia
Thiazides

Impaired bone formation and incorporation of calcium
Aluminum intoxication*
Adynamic ("low-turnover") bone disease*
Corticosteroids

*Occurs in renal failure.

AVAILABLE THERAPY FOR HYPERCALCEMIA*

Agent	Mechanism of action
Saline and loop diuretics	Increase renal excretion of calcium
Corticosteroids	Block 1,25-dihydroxy-vitamin D_3 synthesis and bone resorption
Ketoconazole	Blocks P450 system, decreases 1, 25-dihydroxy-vitamin D_3
Oral or intravenous phosphate	Complexes calcium
Calcitonin	Inhibits bone resorption
Mithramycin	Inhibits bone resorption
Bisphosphonates	Inhibit bone resorption

*Always identify and treat the primary cause of hypercalcemia.

FIGURE 5-21

Therapy available for the treatment of hypercalcemia.

Secondary Hyperparathyroidism

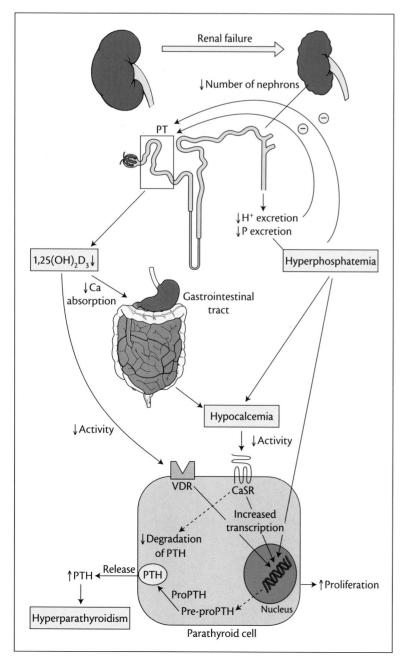

FIGURE 5-22

Pathogenesis of secondary hyperparathyroidism (HPT) in chronic renal failure (CRF). Decreased numbers of proximal tubular (PT) cells, owing to loss of renal mass, cause a quantitative decrease in synthesis of 1,25-dihydroxy-vitamin D_3 $(1,25(OH)_2D_3)$. Loss of renal mass also impairs renal phosphate (P) and acid (H^+) excretion. These impairments further decrease the activity of the 1-α-hydroxylase enzyme in the remaining PT cells, further contributing to the decrease in levels of $1,25(OH)_2D_3$. $1,25(OH)_2D_3$ deficiency decreases intestinal absorption of calcium (Ca), leading to hypocalcemia, which is augmented by the direct effect of hyperphosphatemia. Hypocalcemia and hyperphosphatemia stimulate PTH release and synthesis and can recruit inactive parathyroid cells into activity and PTH production. Hypocalcemia also may decrease intracellular degradation of PTH. The lack of $1,25(OH)_2D_3$, which would ordinarily feed back to inhibit the transcription of prepro-PTH and exert an antiproliferative effect on parathyroid cells, allows the increased PTH production to continue. In CRF there may be decreased expression of the Ca-sensing receptor (CaSR) in parathyroid cells, making them less sensitive to levels of plasma Ca. Patients with the b allele or the bb genotype vitamin D receptor (VDR) may be more susceptible to HPT, because the VDR-$1,25(OH)_2D_3$ complex is less effective at suppressing PTH production and cell proliferation. The deficiency of $1,25(OH)_2D_3$ may also decrease VDR synthesis, making parathyroid cells less sensitive to $1,25(OH)_2D_3$. Although the PTH receptor in bone cells is downregulated in CRF (*ie*, for any level of PTH, bone cell activity is lower in CRF patients than in normal persons), the increased plasma levels of PTH may have harmful effects on other systems (*eg*, cardiovascular system, nervous system, and integument) by way of alterations of intracellular Ca. Current therapeutic methods used to decrease PTH release in CRF include correction of hyperphosphatemia, maintenance of normal to high-normal levels of plasma Ca, administration of $1,25(OH)_2D_3$ orally or intravenously, and administration of a Ca-ion sensing receptor (CaSR) agonist [14–16,19–22].

Calcium and Vitamin D Preparations

CALCIUM CONTENT OF ORAL CALCIUM PREPARATIONS

Calcium (Ca) salt	Tablet size, *mg*	Elemental Ca, *mg, %*
Carbonate	1250	500 (40)
Acetate	667	169 (25)
Citrate	950	200 (21)
Lactate	325	42 (13)
Gluconate	500	4.5 (9)

Fractional intestinal absorption of Ca may differ between Ca salts.

Data from McCarthy and Kumar [19] and *Physicians' Desk Reference* [23].

FIGURE 5-23

Calcium (Ca) content of oral Ca preparations.

VITAMIN D PREPARATIONS AVAILABLE IN THE UNITED STATES

	Ergocalciferol (Vitamin D$_2$)	Calcifediol (25-hydroxy-vitamin D$_3$)	Dihydrotachysterol	Calcitriol (1,25-dihydroxy-vitamin D$_3$)
Commercial name	Calciferol	Calderol® (Organon, Inc, West Orange, NJ)	DHT Intensol® (Roxane Laboratories, Columbus, OH)	Rocaltrol® (Roche Laboratories, Nutley, NJ)
				Calcijex® (Abbott Laboratories, Abbott Park, NJ)
Oral preparations	50,000 IU tablets	20- and 50-µg capsules	0.125-, 0.2-, 0.4-mg tablets	0.25- and 0.50-µg capsules
Usual daily dose				
Hypoparathyroidism	50,000–500,000 IU	20–200 µg	0.2–1.0 mg	0.25–5.0 µg
Renal failure	Not used	20–40 µg*	0.2-0.4 mg*	0.25–0.50 µg
Time until increase in serum calcium†	4–8 wk	2–4 wk	1–2 wk	4–7 d
Time for reversal of toxic effects	17–60 d	7–30 d	3–14 d	2–10 d

*Not currently advised in patients with chronic renal failure.

†In patients with hypoparathyroidism who have normal renal function.

Data from McCarthy and Kumar [19] and *Physicians' Desk Reference* [23].

FIGURE 5-24

Vitamin D preparations.

References

1. Kumar R: Calcium metabolism. In *The Principles and Practice of Nephrology.* Edited by Jacobson HR, Striker GE, Klahr S. St. Louis: Mosby-Year Book; 1995, 964–971.

2. Johnson JA, Kumar R: Renal and intestinal calcium transport: roles of vitamin D and vitamin D-dependent calcium binding proteins. *Semin Nephrol* 1994, 14:119–128.

3. Hebert SC, Brown EM, Harris HW: Role of the Ca^{2+}-sensing receptor in divalent mineral ion homeostasis. *J Exp Biol* 1997, 200:295–302.

4. Hebert SC, Brown EM: The scent of an ion: calcium-sensing and its roles in health and disease. *Curr Opinion Nephrol Hypertens* 1996, 5:45–53.

5. Berridge MJ: Elementary and global aspects of calcium signalling. *J Exp Biol* 1997, 200:315–319.

6. Friedman PA, Gesek FA: Cellular calcium transport in renal epithelia: measurement, mechanisms, and regulation. *Physiol Rev* 1995, 75:429–471.

7. Root AW: Recent advances in the genetics of disorders of calcium homeostasis. *Adv Pediatr* 1996, 43:77–125.

8. Holick MF: Defects in the synthesis and metabolism of vitamin D. *Exp Clin Endocrinol* 1995, 103:219–227.

9. Kumar R: Calcium transport in epithelial cells of the intestine and kidney. *J Cell Biochem* 1995, 57:392–398.

10. White CP, Morrison NA, Gardiner EM, Eisman JA: Vitamin D receptor alleles and bone physiology. *J Cell Biochem* 1994, 56:307–314.

11. Fernandez E, Fibla J, Betriu A, *et al.*: Association between vitamin D receptor gene polymorphism and relative hypoparathyroidism in patients with chronic renal failure. *J Am Soc Nephrol* 1997, 8:1546–1552.

12. Tanaka Y, Funahashi J, Imai T, *et al.*: Parathyroid function and bone metabolic markers in primary and secondary hyperparathyroidism. *Sem Surg Oncol* 1997, 13:125–133.

13. Philbrick WM, Wysolmerski JJ, Galbraith S, *et al.*: Defining the roles of parathyroid hormone-related protein in normal physiology. *Physiol Rev* 1996, 76:127–173.

14. Goodman WG, Belin TR, Salusky IB: *In vivo>* assessments of calcium-regulated parathyroid hormone release in secondary hyperparathyroidism [editorial review]. *Kidney Int* 1996, 50:1834–1844.

15. Chattopadhyay N, Mithal A, Brown EM: The calcium-sensing receptor: a window into the physiology and pathophysiology of mineral ion metabolism. *Endocrine Rev* 1996, 17:289–307.

16. Nemeth EF, Steffey ME, Fox J: The parathyroid calcium receptor: a novel therapeutic target for treating hyperparathyroidism. *Pediatr Nephrol* 1996, 10:275–279.

17. Wasserman RH, Fullmer CS: Vitamin D and intestinal calcium transport: facts, speculations and hypotheses. *J Nutr* 1995, 125:1971S–1979S.

18. Johnson JA, Kumar R: Vitamin D and renal calcium transport. *Curr Opinion Nephrol Hypertens* 1994, 3:424–429.

19. McCarthy JT, Kumar R: Renal osteodystrophy. In *The Principles and Practice of Nephrology.* Edited by Jacobson HR, Striker GE, Klahr S. St. Louis: Mosby-Year Book; 1995, 1032–1045.

20. Felsenfeld AJ: Considerations for the treatment of secondary hyperparathyroidism in renal failure. *J Am Soc Nephrol* 1997, 8:993–1004.

21. Parfitt AM. The hyperparathyroidism of chronic renal failure: a disorder of growth. *Kidney Int* 1997, 52:3–9.

22. Salusky IB, Goodman WG: Parathyroid gland function in secondary hyperparathyroidism. *Pediatr Nephrol* 1996, 10:359–363.

23. *Physicians' Desk Reference* (PDR). Montvale NJ: Medical Economics Company; 1996.

Disorders of Acid-Base Balance

Horacio J. Adrogué
Nicolaos E. Madias

Maintenance of acid-base homeostasis is a vital function of the living organism. Deviations of systemic acidity in either direction can impose adverse consequences and when severe can threaten life itself. Acid-base disorders frequently are encountered in the outpatient and especially in the inpatient setting. Effective management of acid-base disturbances, commonly a challenging task, rests with accurate diagnosis, sound understanding of the underlying pathophysiology and impact on organ function, and familiarity with treatment and attendant complications [1].

Clinical acid-base disorders are conventionally defined from the vantage point of their impact on the carbonic acid-bicarbonate buffer system. This approach is justified by the abundance of this buffer pair in body fluids; its physiologic preeminence; and the validity of the isohydric principle in the living organism, which specifies that all the other buffer systems are in equilibrium with the carbonic acid-bicarbonate buffer pair. Thus, as indicated by the Henderson equation, $[H^+] = 24 \times PaCO_2/[HCO_3^-]$ (the equilibrium relationship of the carbonic acid-bicarbonate system), the hydrogen ion concentration of blood ($[H^+]$, expressed in nEq/L) at any moment is a function of the prevailing ratio of the arterial carbon dioxide tension ($PaCO_2$, expressed in mm Hg) and the plasma bicarbonate concentration ($[HCO_3^-]$, expressed in mEq/L). As a corollary, changes in systemic acidity can occur only through changes in the values of its two determinants, $PaCO_2$ and the plasma bicarbonate concentration. Those acid-base disorders initiated by a change in $PaCO_2$ are referred to as respiratory disorders; those initiated by a change in plasma bicarbonate concentration are known as metabolic disorders. There are four cardinal acid-base disturbances: respiratory acidosis, respiratory alkalosis, metabolic acidosis, and metabolic alkalosis. Each can be encountered alone, as a simple disorder, or can be a part of a mixed-disorder, defined as the simultaneous presence of two or more simple

CHAPTER

6

acid-base disturbances. Mixed acid-base disorders are frequently observed in hospitalized patients, especially in the critically ill.

The clinical aspects of the four cardinal acid-base disorders are depicted. For each disorder the following are

illustrated: the underlying pathophysiology, secondary adjustments in acid-base equilibrium in response to the initiating disturbance, clinical manifestations, causes, and therapeutic principles.

Respiratory Acidosis

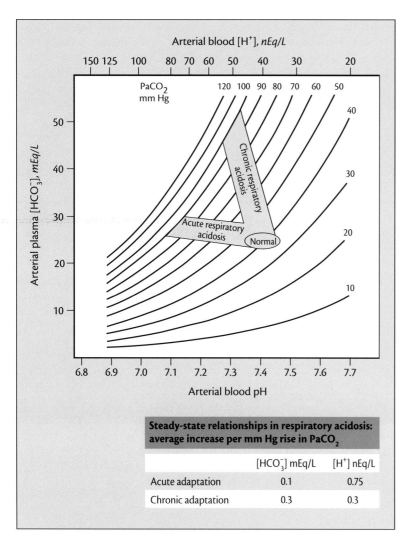

Arterial blood [H$^+$], *nEq/L*

Steady-state relationships in respiratory acidosis: average increase per mm Hg rise in PaCO$_2$

	[HCO$_3^-$] mEq/L	[H$^+$] nEq/L
Acute adaptation	0.1	0.75
Chronic adaptation	0.3	0.3

FIGURE 6-1

Quantitative aspects of adaptation to respiratory acidosis. Respiratory acidosis, or primary hypercapnia, is the acid-base disturbance initiated by an increase in arterial carbon dioxide tension (PaCO$_2$) and entails acidification of body fluids. Hypercapnia elicits adaptive increments in plasma bicarbonate concentration that should be viewed as an integral part of respiratory acidosis. An immediate increment in plasma bicarbonate occurs in response to hypercapnia. This acute adaptation is complete within 5 to 10 minutes from the onset of hypercapnia and originates exclusively from acidic titration of the nonbicarbonate buffers of the body (hemoglobin, intracellular proteins and phosphates, and to a lesser extent plasma proteins). When hypercapnia is sustained, renal adjustments markedly amplify the secondary increase in plasma bicarbonate, further ameliorating the resulting acidemia. This chronic adaptation requires 3 to 5 days for completion and reflects generation of new bicarbonate by the kidneys as a result of upregulation of renal acidification [2]. Average increases in plasma bicarbonate and hydrogen ion concentrations per mm Hg increase in PaCO$_2$ after completion of the acute or chronic adaptation to respiratory acidosis are shown. Empiric observations on these adaptations have been used for construction of 95% confidence intervals for graded degrees of acute or chronic respiratory acidosis represented by the areas in color in the acid-base template. The black ellipse near the center of the figure indicates the normal range for the acid-base parameters [3]. Note that for the same level of PaCO$_2$, the degree of acidemia is considerably lower in chronic respiratory acidosis than it is in acute respiratory acidosis. Assuming a steady state is present, values falling within the areas in color are consistent with but not diagnostic of the corresponding simple disorders. Acid-base values falling outside the areas in color denote the presence of a mixed acid-base disturbance [4].

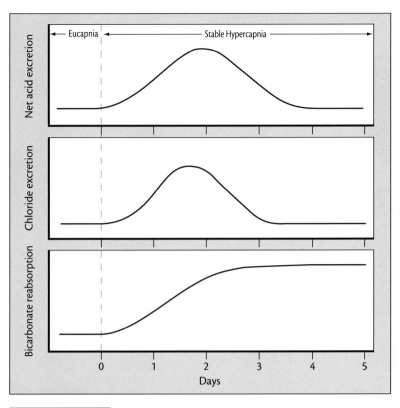

FIGURE 6-2

Renal acidification response to chronic hypercapnia. Sustained hypercapnia entails a persistent increase in the secretory rate of the renal tubule for hydrogen ions (H^+) and a persistent decrease in the reabsorption rate of chloride ions (Cl^-). Consequently, net acid excretion (largely in the form of ammonium) transiently exceeds endogenous

acid production, leading to generation of new bicarbonate ions (HCO_3^-) for the body fluids. Conservation of these new bicarbonate ions is ensured by the gradual augmentation in the rate of renal bicarbonate reabsorption, itself a reflection of the hypercapnia-induced increase in the hydrogen ion secretory rate. A new steady state emerges when two things occur: the augmented filtered load of bicarbonate is precisely balanced by the accelerated rate of bicarbonate reabsorption and net acid excretion returns to the level required to offset daily endogenous acid production. The transient increase in net acid excretion is accompanied by a transient increase in chloride excretion. Thus, the resultant ammonium chloride (NH_4Cl) loss generates the hypochloremic hyperbicarbonatemia characteristic of chronic respiratory acidosis. Hypochloremia is sustained by the persistently depressed chloride reabsorption rate. The specific cellular mechanisms mediating the renal acidification response to chronic hypercapnia are under active investigation. Available evidence supports a parallel increase in the rates of the luminal sodium ion–hydrogen ion (Na^+-H^+) exchanger and the basolateral Na^+-$3HCO_3^-$ cotransporter in the proximal tubule. However, the nature of these adaptations remains unknown [5]. The quantity of the H^+-adenosine triphosphatase (ATPase) pumps does not change in either cortex or medulla. However, hypercapnia induces exocytotic insertion of H^+-ATPase–containing subapical vesicles to the luminal membrane of proximal tubule cells as well as type A intercalated cells of the cortical and medullary collecting ducts. New H^+-ATPase pumps thereby are recruited to the luminal membrane for augmented acidification [6,7]. Furthermore, chronic hypercapnia increases the steady-state abundance of mRNA coding for the basolateral Cl^-—HCO_3^- exchanger (band 3 protein) of type A intercalated cells in rat renal cortex and medulla, likely indicating increased band 3 protein levels and therefore augmented basolateral anion exchanger activity [8].

SIGNS AND SYMPTOMS OF RESPIRATORY ACIDOSIS

Central Nervous System	Respiratory System	Cardiovascular System
Mild to moderate hypercapnia	Breathlessness	Mild to moderate hypercapnia
Cerebral vasodilation	Central and peripheral cyanosis	Warm and flushed skin
Increased intracranial pressure	(especially when breathing	Bounding pulse
Headache	room air)	Well maintained cardiac
Confusion	Pulmonary hypertension	output and blood pressure
Combativeness		Diaphoresis
Hallucinations		Severe hypercapnia
Transient psychosis		Cor pulmonale
Myoclonic jerks		Decreased cardiac output
Flapping tremor		Systemic hypotension
Severe hypercapnia		Cardiac arrhythmias
Manifestations of pseudotumor cerebri		Prerenal azotemia
Stupor		Peripheral edema
Coma		
Constricted pupils		
Depressed tendon reflexes		
Extensor plantar response		
Seizures		
Papilledema		

FIGURE 6-3

Signs and symptoms of respiratory acidosis. The effects of respiratory acidosis on the central nervous system are collectively known as hypercapnic encephalopathy. Factors responsible for its development include the magnitude and time course of the hypercapnia, severity of the acidemia, and degree of attendant hypoxemia. Progressive narcosis and coma may occur in patients receiving uncontrolled oxygen therapy in whom levels of arterial carbon dioxide tension ($PaCO_2$) may reach or exceed 100 mm Hg. The hemodynamic consequences of carbon dioxide retention reflect several mechanisms, including direct impairment of myocardial contractility, systemic vasodilation caused by direct relaxation of vascular smooth muscle, sympathetic stimulation, and acidosis-induced blunting of receptor responsiveness to catecholamines. The net effect is dilation of systemic vessels, including the cerebral circulation; whereas vasoconstriction might develop in the pulmonary and renal circulations. Salt and water retention commonly occur in chronic hypercapnia, especially in the presence of cor pulmonale. Mechanisms at play include hypercapnia-induced stimulation of the renin-angiotensin-aldosterone axis and the sympathetic nervous system, elevated levels of cortisol and antidiuretic hormone, and increased renal vascular resistance. Of course, coexisting heart failure amplifies most of these mechanisms [1,2].

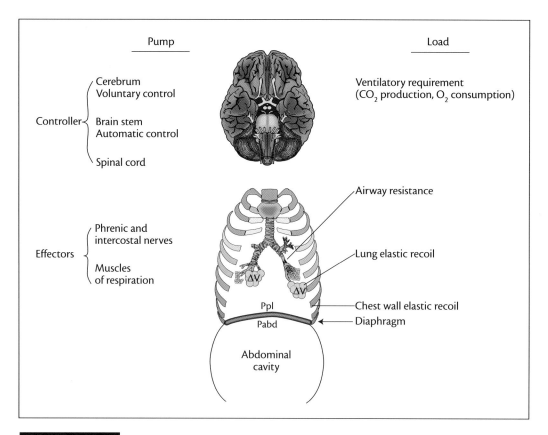

FIGURE 6-4

Main components of the ventilatory system. The ventilatory system is responsible for maintaining the arterial carbon dioxide tension ($PaCO_2$) within normal limits by adjusting minute ventilation ($\dot{v}$) to match the rate of carbon dioxide production. The main elements of ventilation are the respiratory pump, which generates a pressure gradient responsible for air flow, and the loads that oppose such action. The machinery of the respiratory pump includes the cerebrum, brain stem, spinal cord, phrenic and intercostal nerves, and the muscles of respiration. Inspiratory muscle contraction lowers pleural pressure (Ppl) thereby inflating the lungs (ΔV). The diaphragm, the most important inspiratory muscle, moves downward as a piston at the floor of the thorax, raising abdominal pressure (Pabd). The inspiratory decrease in Ppl by the respiratory pump must be sufficient to counterbalance the opposing effect of the combined loads, including the airway flow resistance, and the elastic recoil of the lungs and chest wall. The ventilatory requirement influences the load by altering the frequency and depth of the ventilatory cycle. The strength of the respiratory pump is evaluated by the pressure generated ($\Delta P = Ppl - Pabd$).

DETERMINANTS AND CAUSES OF CARBON DIOXIDE RETENTION

Respiratory Pump		Load	
Depressed Central Drive	**Abnormal Neuromuscular Transmission**	**Increased Ventilatory Demand**	**Lung Stiffness**
Acute	Acute	High carbohydrate diet	Acute
General anesthesia	High spinal cord injury	Sorbent-regenerative hemodialysis	Severe bilateral pneumonia
Sedative overdose	Guillain-Barré syndrome	Pulmonary thromboembolism	or bronchopneumonia
Head trauma	Status epilepticus	Fat, air pulmonary embolism	Acute respiratory
Cerebrovascular accident	Botulism	Sepsis	distress syndrome
Central sleep apnea	Tetanus	Hypovolemia	Severe pulmonary edema
Cerebral edema	Crisis in myasthenia gravis		Atelectasis
Brain tumor	Hypokalemic myopathy	**Augmented Airway Flow Resistance**	Chronic
Encephalitis	Familial periodic paralysis	Acute	Severe chronic pneumonitis
Brainstem lesion	Drugs or toxic agents *eg*, curare,	Upper airway obstruction	Diffuse infiltrative disease *eg*,
Chronic	succinylcholine, aminoglycosides,	Coma-induced hypopharyngeal obstruction	alveolar proteinosis
Sedative overdose	organophosphorus	Aspiration of foreign body or vomitus	Interstitial fibrosis
Methadone or heroin addiction	Chronic	Laryngospasm	
Sleep disordered breathing	Poliomyelitis	Angioedema	**Chest Wall Stiffness**
Brain tumor	Multiple sclerosis	Obstructive sleep apnea	Acute
Bulbar poliomyelitis	Muscular dystrophy	Inadequate laryngeal intubation	Rib fractures with flail chest
Hypothyroidism	Amyotrophic lateral sclerosis	Laryngeal obstruction after intubation	Pneumothorax
	Diaphragmatic paralysis	Lower airway obstruction	Hemothorax
	Myopathic disease *eg*, polymyositis	Generalized bronchospasm	Abdominal distention
		Airway edema and secretions	Ascites
	Muscle Dysfunction	Severe episode of spasmodic asthma	Peritoneal dialysis
	Acute	Bronchiolitis of infants and adults	Chronic
	Fatigue	Chronic	Kyphoscoliosis, spinal arthritis
	Hyperkalemia	Upper airway obstruction	Obesity
	Hypokalemia	Tonsillar and peritonsillar hypertrophy	Fibrothorax
	Hypoperfusion state	Paralysis of vocal cords	Hydrothorax
	Hypoxemia	Tumor of the cords or larynx	Chest wall tumor
	Malnutrition	Airway stenosis after prolonged intubation	
	Chronic	Thymoma, aortic aneurysm	
	Myopathic disease *eg*, polymyositis	Lower airway obstruction	
		Airway scarring	
		Chronic obstructive lung disease *eg*, bronchitis,	
		bronchiolitis, bronchiectasis, emphysema	

FIGURE 6-5

Determinants and causes of carbon dioxide retention. When the respiratory pump is unable to balance the opposing load, respiratory acidosis develops. Decreases in respiratory pump strength, increases in load, or a combination of the two, can result in carbon dioxide retention. Respiratory pump failure can occur because of depressed central drive, abnormal neuromuscular transmission, or respiratory muscle dysfunction. A higher load can be caused by increased ventilatory demand, augmented airway flow resistance, and stiffness of the lungs or chest wall. In most cases, causes of the various determinants of carbon dioxide retention, and thus respiratory acidosis, are categorized into acute and chronic subgroups, taking into consideration their usual mode of onset and duration [2].

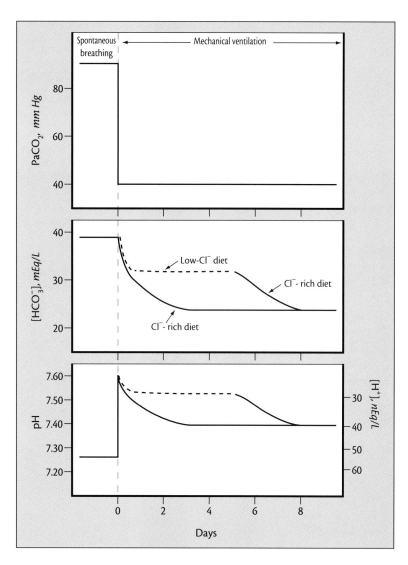

FIGURE 6-6

Posthypercapnic metabolic alkalosis. Development of posthypercapnic metabolic alkalosis is shown after abrupt normalization of the arterial carbon dioxide tension ($PaCO_2$) by way of mechanical ventilation in a 70-year-old man with respiratory decompensation who has chronic obstructive pulmonary disease and chronic hypercapnia. The acute decrease in plasma bicarbonate concentration ($[HCO_3^-]$) over the first few minutes after the decrease in $PaCO_2$ originates from alkaline titration of the nonbicarbonate buffers of the body. When a diet rich in chloride (Cl^-) is provided, the excess bicarbonate is excreted by the kidneys over the next 2 to 3 days, and acid-base equilibrium is normalized. In contrast, a low-chloride diet sustains the hyperbicarbonatemia and perpetuates the posthypercapnic metabolic alkalosis. Abrupt correction of severe hypercapnia by way of mechanical ventilation generally is not recommended. Rather, gradual return toward the patient's baseline $PaCO_2$ level should be pursued [1,2]. [H^+]—hydrogen ion concentration.

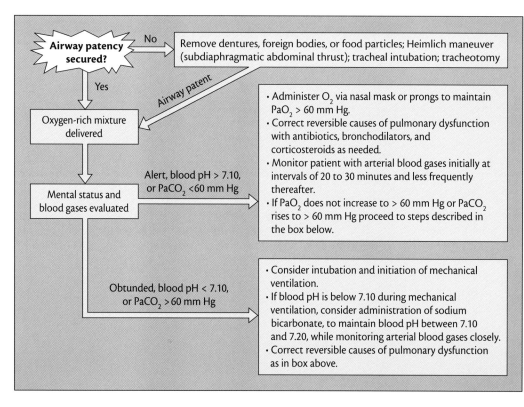

FIGURE 6-7

Acute respiratory acidosis management. Securing airway patency and delivering an oxygen-rich mixture are critical initial steps in management. Subsequent measures must be directed at identifying and correcting the underlying cause, whenever possible [1,9]. $PaCO_2$—arterial carbon dioxide tension.

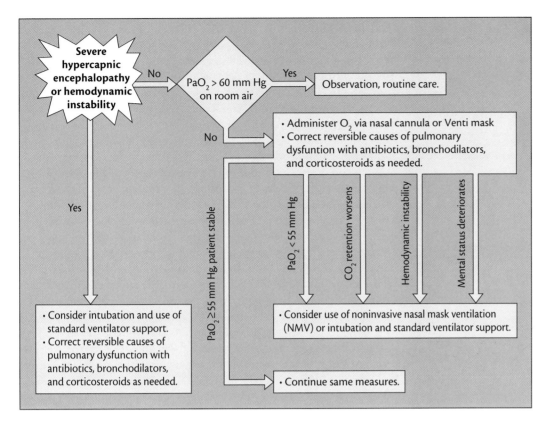

FIGURE 6-8

Chronic respiratory acidosis management. Therapeutic measures are guided by the presence or absence of severe hypercapnic encephalopathy or hemodynamic instability. An aggressive approach that favors the early use of ventilator assistance is most appropriate for patients with acute respiratory acidosis. In contrast, a more conservative approach is advisable in patients with chronic hypercapnia because of the great difficulty often encountered in weaning these patients from ventilators. As a rule, the lowest possible inspired fraction of oxygen that achieves adequate oxygenation (PaO_2 on the order of 60 mm Hg) is used. Contrary to acute respiratory acidosis, the underlying cause of chronic respiratory acidosis only rarely can be resolved [1,9].

Respiratory Alkalosis

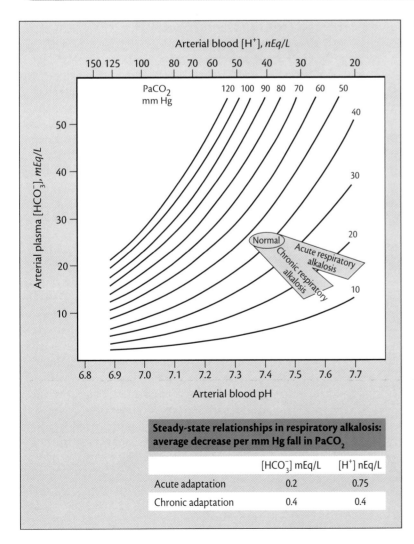

Steady-state relationships in respiratory alkalosis: average decrease per mm Hg fall in $PaCO_2$		
	$[HCO_3^-]$ mEq/L	$[H^+]$ nEq/L
Acute adaptation	0.2	0.75
Chronic adaptation	0.4	0.4

FIGURE 6-9

Adaptation to respiratory alkalosis. Respiratory alkalosis, or primary hypocapnia, is the acid-base disturbance initiated by a decrease in arterial carbon dioxide tension ($PaCO_2$) and entails alkalinization of body fluids. Hypocapnia elicits adaptive decrements in plasma bicarbonate concentration that should be viewed as an integral part of respiratory alkalosis. An immediate decrement in plasma bicarbonate occurs in response to hypocapnia. This acute adaptation is complete within 5 to 10 minutes from the onset of hypocapnia and is accounted for principally by alkaline titration of the nonbicarbonate buffers of the body. To a lesser extent, this acute adaptation reflects increased production of organic acids, notably lactic acid. When hypocapnia is sustained, renal adjustments cause an additional decrease in plasma bicarbonate, further ameliorating the resulting alkalemia. This chronic adaptation requires 2 to 3 days for completion and reflects retention of hydrogen ions by the kidneys as a result of downregulation of renal acidification [2,10]. Shown are the average decreases in plasma bicarbonate and hydrogen ion concentrations per mm Hg decrease in $PaCO_2$ after completion of the acute or chronic adaptation to respiratory alkalosis. Empiric observations on these adaptations have been used for constructing 95% confidence intervals for graded degrees of acute or chronic respiratory alkalosis, which are represented by the areas in color in the acid-base template. The black ellipse near the center of the figure indicates the normal range for the acid-base parameters. Note that for the same level of $PaCO_2$, the degree of alkalemia is considerably lower in chronic than it is in acute respiratory alkalosis. Assuming that a steady state is present, values falling within the areas in color are consistent with but not diagnostic of the corresponding simple disorders. Acid-base values falling outside the areas in color denote the presence of a mixed acid-base disturbance [4].

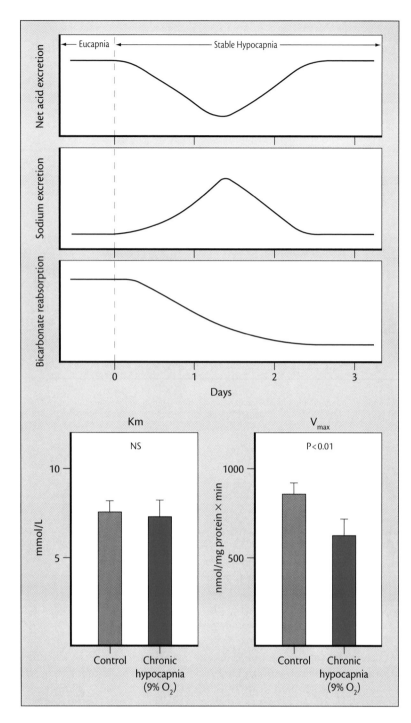

FIGURE 6-10

Renal acidification response to chronic hypocapnia. **A,** Sustained hypocapnia entails a persistent decrease in the renal tubular secretory rate of hydrogen ions and a persistent increase in the chloride reabsorption rate. As a result, transient suppression of net acid excretion occurs. This suppression is largely manifested by a decrease in ammonium excretion and, early on, by an increase in bicarbonate excretion. The transient discrepancy between net acid excretion and endogenous acid production, in turn, leads to positive hydrogen ion balance and a reduction in the bicarbonate stores of the body. Maintenance of the resulting hypobicarbonatemia is ensured by the gradual suppression in the rate of renal bicarbonate reabsorption. This suppression itself is a reflection of the hypocapnia-induced decrease in the hydrogen ion secretory rate. A new steady state emerges when two things occur: the reduced filtered load of bicarbonate is precisely balanced by the dampened rate of bicarbonate reabsorption and net acid excretion returns to the level required to offset daily endogenous acid production. The transient retention of acid during sustained hypocapnia is normally accompanied by a loss of sodium in the urine (and *not* by a retention of chloride as analogy with chronic respiratory acidosis would dictate). The resulting extracellular fluid loss is responsible for the hyperchloremia that typically accompanies chronic respiratory alkalosis. Hyperchloremia is sustained by the persistently enhanced chloride reabsorption rate. If dietary sodium is restricted, acid retention is achieved in the company of increased potassium excretion. The specific cellular mechanisms mediating the renal acidification response to chronic hypocapnia are under investigation. Available evidence indicates a parallel decrease in the rates of the luminal sodium ion–hydrogen ion (Na^+-H^+) exchanger and the basolateral sodium ion–3 bicarbonate ion (Na^+-$3HCO_3^-$) cotransporter in the proximal tubule. This parallel decrease reflects a decrease in the maximum velocity (V_{max}) of each transporter but no change in the substrate concentration at half-maximal velocity (K_m) for sodium (as shown in **B** for the Na^+-H^+ exchanger in rabbit renal cortical brush-border membrane vesicles) [11]. Moreover, hypocapnia induces endocytotic retrieval of H^+-adenosine triphosphatase (ATPase) pumps from the luminal membrane of the proximal tubule cells as well as type A intercalated cells of the cortical and medullary collecting ducts. It remains unknown whether chronic hypocapnia alters the quantity of the H^+-ATPase pumps as well as the kinetics or quantity of other acidification transporters in the renal cortex or medulla [6]. NS—not significant. (**B,** *From* Hilden and coworkers [11]; with permission.)

SIGNS AND SYMPTOMS OF RESPIRATORY ALKALOSIS

Central Nervous System	Cardiovascular System	Neuromuscular System
Cerebral vasoconstriction	Chest oppression	Numbness and paresthesias of the extremities
Reduction in intracranial pressure	Angina pectoris	
Light-headedness	Ischemic electrocardiographic changes	Circumoral numbness
Confusion	Normal or decreased blood pressure	Laryngeal spasm
Increased deep tendon reflexes	Cardiac arrhythmias	Manifestations of tetany
Generalized seizures	Peripheral vasoconstriction	Muscle cramps
		Carpopedal spasm
		Trousseau's sign
		Chvostek's sign

FIGURE 6-11

Signs and symptoms of respiratory alkalosis. The manifestations of primary hypocapnia frequently occur in the acute phase, but seldom are evident in chronic respiratory alkalosis. Several mechanisms mediate these clinical manifestations, including cerebral hypoperfusion, alkalemia, hypocalcemia, hypokalemia, and decreased release of oxygen to the tissues by hemoglobin. The cardiovascular effects of respiratory alkalosis are more prominent in patients undergoing mechanical ventilation and those with ischemic heart disease [2].

CAUSES OF RESPIRATORY ALKALOSIS

Hypoxemia or Tissue Hypoxia	Central Nervous System Stimulation	Drugs or Hormones	Stimulation of Chest Receptors	Miscellaneous
Decreased inspired oxygen tension	Voluntary	Nikethamide, ethamivan	Pneumonia	Pregnancy
High altitude	Pain	Doxapram	Asthma	Gram-positive septicemia
Bacterial or viral pneumonia	Anxiety syndrome-hyperventilation syndrome	Xanthines	Pneumothorax	Gram-negative septicemia
Aspiration of food, foreign object, or vomitus	Psychosis	Salicylates	Hemothorax	Hepatic failure
Laryngospasm	Fever	Catecholamines	Flail chest	Mechanical hyperventilation
Drowning	Subarachnoid hemorrhage	Angiotensin II	Acute respiratory distress syndrome	Heat exposure
Cyanotic heart disease	Cerebrovascular accident	Vasopressor agents	Cardiogenic and noncardiogenic pulmonary edema	Recovery from metabolic acidosis
Severe anemia	Meningoencephalitis	Progesterone	Pulmonary embolism	
Left shift deviation of oxyhemoglobin curve	Tumor	Medroxyprogesterone	Pulmonary fibrosis	
Hypotension	Trauma	Dinitrophenol		
Severe circulatory failure		Nicotine		
Pulmonary edema				

FIGURE 6-12

Respiratory alkalosis is the most frequent acid-base disorder encountered because it occurs in normal pregnancy and high-altitude residence. Pathologic causes of respiratory alkalosis include various hypoxemic conditions, pulmonary disorders, central nervous system diseases, pharmacologic or hormonal stimulation of ventilation, hepatic failure, sepsis, the anxiety-hyperventilation syndrome, and other entities. Most of these causes are associated with the abrupt occurrence of hypocapnia; however, in many instances, the process might be sufficiently prolonged to permit full chronic adaptation to occur. Consequently, no attempt has been made to separate these conditions into acute and chronic categories. Some of the major causes of respiratory alkalosis are benign, whereas others are life-threatening. Primary hypocapnia is particularly common among the critically ill, occurring either as the simple disorder or as a component of mixed disturbances. Its presence constitutes an ominous prognostic sign, with mortality increasing in direct proportion to the severity of the hypocapnia [2].

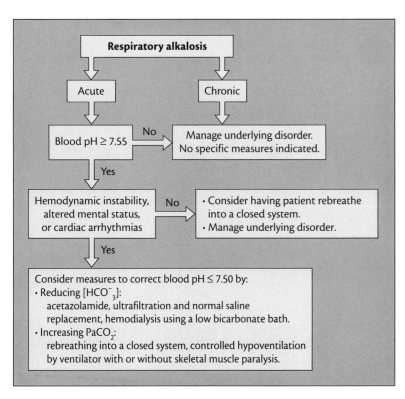

FIGURE 6-13

Respiratory alkalosis management. Because chronic respiratory alkalosis poses a low risk to health and produces few or no symptoms, measures for treating the acid-base disorder itself are not required. In contrast, severe alkalemia caused by acute primary hypocapnia requires corrective measures that depend on whether serious clinical manifestations are present. Such measures can be directed at reducing plasma bicarbonate concentration ($[HCO_3^-]$), increasing the arterial carbon dioxide tension ($PaCO_2$), or both. Even if the baseline plasma bicarbonate is moderately decreased, reducing it further can be particularly rewarding in this setting. In addition, this maneuver combines effectiveness with relatively little risk [1,2].

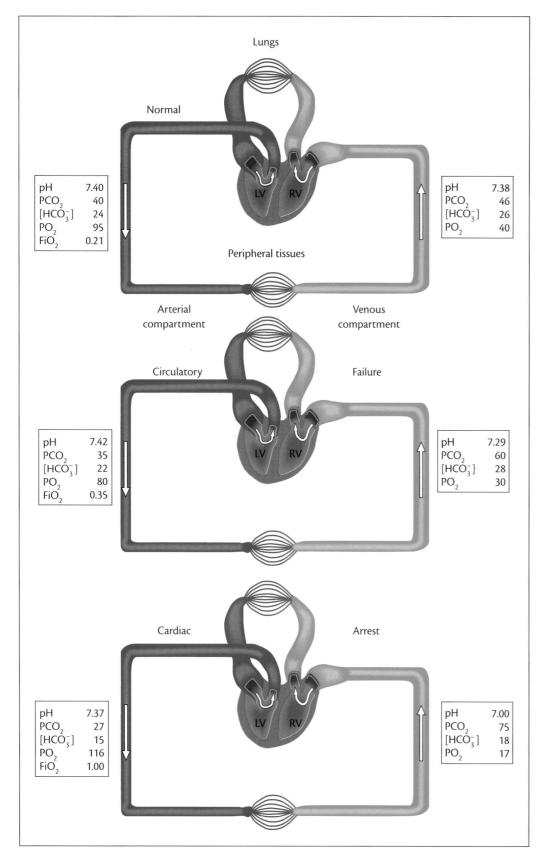

Normal		
pH	7.40
PCO$_2$	40
[HCO$_3^-$]	24
PO$_2$	95
FiO$_2$	0.21

pH	7.38
PCO$_2$	46
[HCO$_3^-$]	26
PO$_2$	40

Lungs

Peripheral tissues

Arterial compartment

Venous compartment

Circulatory		
pH	7.42
PCO$_2$	35
[HCO$_3^-$]	22
PO$_2$	80
FiO$_2$	0.35

Failure		
pH	7.29
PCO$_2$	60
[HCO$_3^-$]	28
PO$_2$	30

Cardiac		
pH	7.37
PCO$_2$	27
[HCO$_3^-$]	15
PO$_2$	116
FiO$_2$	1.00

Arrest		
pH	7.00
PCO$_2$	75
[HCO$_3^-$]	18
PO$_2$	17

FIGURE 6-14

Pseudorespiratory alkalosis. This entity develops in patients with profound depression of cardiac function and pulmonary perfusion but relative preservation of alveolar ventilation. Patients include those with advanced circulatory failure and those undergoing cardiopulmonary resuscitation. The severely reduced pulmonary blood flow limits the amount of carbon dioxide delivered to the lungs for excretion, thereby increasing the venous carbon dioxide tension (PCO$_2$). In contrast, the increased ventilation-to-perfusion ratio causes a larger than normal removal of carbon dioxide per unit of blood traversing the pulmonary circulation, thereby giving rise to arterial hypocapnia [12,13]. Note a progressive widening of the arteriovenous difference in pH and PCO$_2$ in the two settings of cardiac dysfunction. The hypobicarbonatemia in the setting of cardiac arrest represents a complicating element of lactic acidosis. Despite the presence of arterial hypocapnia, pseudorespiratory alkalosis represents a special case of respiratory acidosis, as absolute carbon dioxide excretion is decreased and body carbon dioxide balance is positive. Furthermore, the extreme oxygen deprivation prevailing in the tissues might be completely disguised by the reasonably preserved arterial oxygen values. Appropriate monitoring of acid-base composition and oxygenation in patients with advanced cardiac dysfunction requires mixed (or central) venous blood sampling in addition to arterial blood sampling. Management of pseudorespiratory alkalosis must be directed at optimizing systemic hemodynamics [1,13].

Metabolic Acidosis

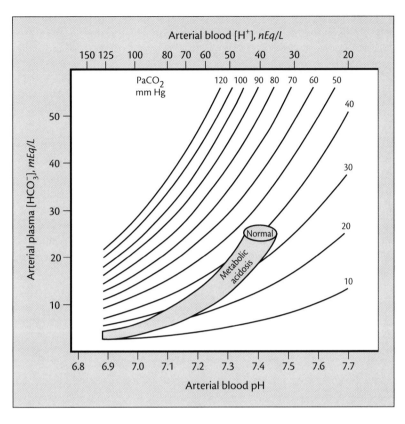

FIGURE 6-15

Ninety-five percent confidence intervals for metabolic acidosis. Metabolic acidosis is the acid-base disturbance initiated by a decrease in plasma bicarbonate concentration ($[HCO_3^-]$). The resultant acidemia stimulates alveolar ventilation and leads to the secondary hypocapnia characteristic of the disorder. Extensive observations in humans encompassing a wide range of stable metabolic acidosis indicate a roughly linear relationship between the steady-state decrease in plasma bicarbonate concentration and the associated decrement in arterial carbon dioxide tension ($PaCO_2$). The slope of the steady state $\Delta PaCO_2$ versus $\Delta[HCO_3^-]$ relationship has been estimated as approximately 1.2 mm Hg per mEq/L decrease in plasma bicarbonate concentration. Such empiric observations have been used for construction of 95% confidence intervals for graded degrees of metabolic acidosis, represented by the area in color in the acid-base template. The black ellipse near the center of the figure indicates the normal range for the acid-base parameters [3]. Assuming a steady state is present, values falling within the area in color are consistent with but not diagnostic of simple metabolic acidosis. Acid-base values falling outside the area in color denote the presence of a mixed acid-base disturbance [4]. [H^+]—hydrogen ion concentration.

SIGNS AND SYMPTOMS OF METABOLIC ACIDOSIS

Respiratory System	Cardiovascular System	Metabolism	Central Nervous System	Skeleton
Hyperventilation	Impairment of cardiac contractility, arteriolar dilation, venoconstriction, and centralization of blood volume	Increased metabolic demands	Impaired metabolism	Osteomalacia
Respiratory distress and dyspnea		Insulin resistance	Inhibition of cell volume regulation	Fractures
Decreased strength of respiratory muscles and promotion of muscle fatigue	Reductions in cardiac output, arterial blood pressure, and hepatic and renal blood flow	Inhibition of anaerobic glycolysis	Progressive obtundation	
		Reduction in adenosine triphosphate synthesis	Coma	
	Sensitization to reentrant arrhythmias and reduction in threshold for ventricular fibrillation	Hyperkalemia		
	Increased sympathetic discharge but attenuation of cardiovascular responsiveness to catecholamines	Increased protein degradation		

FIGURE 6-16

Signs and symptoms of metabolic acidosis. Among the various clinical manifestations, particularly pernicious are the effects of severe acidemia (blood pH < 7.20) on the cardiovascular system. Reductions in cardiac output, arterial blood pressure, and hepatic and renal blood flow can occur and life-threatening arrhythmias can develop. Chronic acidemia, as it occurs in untreated renal tubular acidosis and uremic acidosis, can cause calcium dissolution from the bone mineral and consequent skeletal abnormalities.

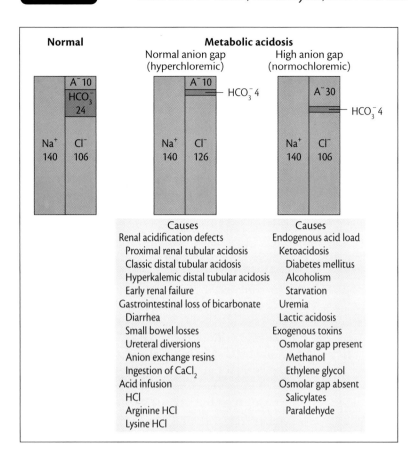

Normal	Metabolic acidosis	
	Normal anion gap (hyperchloremic)	High anion gap (normochloremic)

FIGURE 6-17

Causes of metabolic acidosis tabulated according to the prevailing pattern of plasma electrolyte composition. Assessment of the plasma unmeasured anion concentration (anion gap) is a very useful first step in approaching the differential diagnosis of unexplained metabolic acidosis. The plasma anion gap is calculated as the difference between the sodium concentration and the sum of chloride and bicarbonate concentrations. Under normal circumstances, the plasma anion gap is primarily composed of the net negative charges of plasma proteins, predominantly albumin, with a smaller contribution from many other organic and inorganic anions. The normal value of the plasma anion gap is 12 ± 4 (mean $\pm$ 2 SD) mEq/L, where SD is the standard deviation. However, recent introduction of ion-specific electrodes has shifted the normal anion gap to the range of about 6 ± 3 mEq/L. In one pattern of metabolic acidosis, the decrease in bicarbonate concentration is offset by an increase in the concentration of chloride, with the plasma anion gap remaining normal. In the other pattern, the decrease in bicarbonate is balanced by an increase in the concentration of unmeasured anions (*ie*, anions not measured routinely), with the plasma chloride concentration remaining normal.

Causes

Renal acidification defects
  Proximal renal tubular acidosis
  Classic distal tubular acidosis
  Hyperkalemic distal tubular acidosis
  Early renal failure
Gastrointestinal loss of bicarbonate
  Diarrhea
  Small bowel losses
  Ureteral diversions
  Anion exchange resins
  Ingestion of CaCl₂
Acid infusion
  HCl
  Arginine HCl
  Lysine HCl

Causes

Endogenous acid load
  Ketoacidosis
    Diabetes mellitus
    Alcoholism
    Starvation
  Uremia
  Lactic acidosis
Exogenous toxins
  Osmolar gap present
    Methanol
    Ethylene glycol
  Osmolar gap absent
    Salicylates
    Paraldehyde

Lactic acidosis

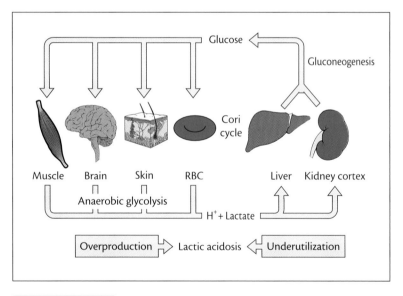

FIGURE 6-18

Lactate-producing and lactate-consuming tissues under basal conditions and pathogenesis of lactic acidosis. Although all tissues pro-

duce lactate during the course of glycolysis, those listed contribute substantial quantities of lactate to the extracellular fluid under normal aerobic conditions. In turn, lactate is extracted by the liver and to a lesser degree by the renal cortex and primarily is reconverted to glucose by way of gluconeogenesis (a smaller portion of lactate is oxidized to carbon dioxide and water). This cyclical relationship between glucose and lactate is known as the *Cori cycle*. The basal turnover rate of lactate in humans is enormous, on the order of 15 to 25 mEq/kg/d. Precise equivalence between lactate production and its use ensures the stability of plasma lactate concentration, normally ranging from 1 to 2 mEq/L. Hydrogen ions (H+) released during lactate generation are quantitatively consumed during the use of lactate such that acid-base balance remains undisturbed. Accumulation of lactate in the circulation, and consequent lactic acidosis, is generated whenever the rate of production of lactate is higher than the rate of utilization. The pathogenesis of this imbalance reflects overproduction of lactate, underutilization, or both. Most cases of persistent lactic acidosis actually involve both overproduction and underutilization of lactate. During hypoxia, almost all tissues can release lactate into the circulation; indeed, even the liver can be converted from the premier consumer of lactate to a net producer [1,14].

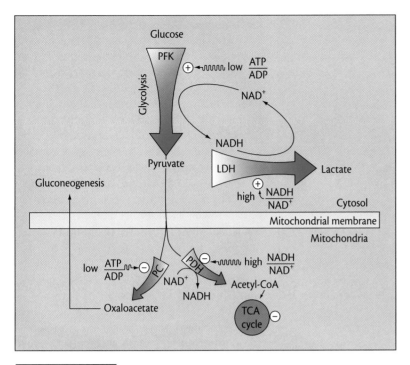

FIGURE 6-19

Hypoxia-induced lactic acidosis. Accumulation of lactate during hypoxia, by far the most common clinical setting of the disorder, originates from impaired mitochondrial oxidative function that reduces the availability of adenosine triphosphate (ATP) and NAD+ (oxidized nicotinamide adenine dinucleotide) within the cytosol. In turn, these changes cause cytosolic accumulation of pyruvate as a consequence of both increased production and decreased utilization. Increased production of pyruvate occurs because the reduced cytosolic supply of ATP stimulates the activity of 6-phosphofructokinase (PFK), thereby accelerating glycolysis. Decreased utilization of pyruvate reflects the fact that both pathways of its consumption depend on mitochondrial oxidative reactions: oxidative decarboxylation to acetyl coenzyme A (acetyl-CoA), a reaction catalyzed by pyruvate dehydrogenase (PDH), requires a continuous supply of NAD+; and carboxylation of pyruvate to oxaloacetate, a reaction catalyzed by pyruvate carboxylase (PC), requires ATP. The increased [NADH]/[NAD+] ratio (NADH refers to the reduced form of the dinucleotide) shifts the equilibrium of the lactate dehydrogenase (LDH) reaction (that catalyzes the interconversion of pyruvate and lactate) to the right. In turn, this change coupled with the accumulation of pyruvate in the cytosol results in increased accumulation of lactate. Despite the prevailing mitochondrial dysfunction, continuation of glycolysis is assured by the cytosolic regeneration of NAD+ during the conversion of pyruvate to lactate. Provision of NAD+ is required for the oxidation of glyceraldehyde 3-phosphate, a key step in glycolysis. Thus, lactate accumulation can be viewed as the toll paid by the organism to maintain energy production during anaerobiosis (hypoxia) [14]. ADP—adenosine diphosphate; TCA cycle—tricarboxylic acid cycle.

CAUSES OF LACTIC ACIDOSIS

Type A: Impaired Tissue Oxygenation	Type B: Preserved Tissue Oxygenation	
	Diseases and conditions	Drugs and toxins
Shock	Diabetes mellitus	Epinephrine, norepinephrine, vasoconstrictor agents
Severe hypoxemia	Hypoglycemia	
Generalized convulsions	Renal failure	
Vigorous exercise	Hepatic failure	Salicylates
Exertional heat stroke	Severe infections	Ethanol
Hypothermic shivering	Alkaloses	Methanol
Massive pulmonary emboli	Malignancies (lymphoma, leukemia, sarcoma)	Ethylene glycol
Severe heart failure		Biguanides
Profound anemia	Thiamine deficiency	Acetaminophen
Mesenteric ischemia	Acquired immunodeficiency syndrome	Zidovudine
Carbon monoxide poisoning		Fructose, sorbitol, and xylitol
Cyanide poisoning	Pheochromocytoma	Streptozotocin
	Iron deficiency	Isoniazid
	D-Lactic acidosis	Nitroprusside
	Congenital enzymatic defects	Papaverine
		Nalidixic acid

FIGURE 6-20

Conventionally, two broad types of lactic acidosis are recognized. In type A, clinical evidence exists of impaired tissue oxygenation. In type B, no such evidence is apparent. Occasionally, the distinction between the two types may be less than obvious. Thus, inadequate tissue oxygenation can at times defy clinical detection, and tissue hypoxia can be a part of the pathogenesis of certain causes of type B lactic acidosis. Most cases of lactic acidosis are caused by tissue hypoxia arising from circulatory failure [14,15].

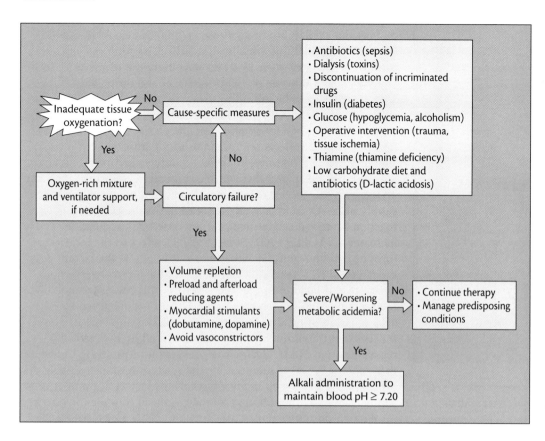

FIGURE 6-21

Lactic acidosis management. Management of lactic acidosis should focus primarily on securing adequate tissue oxygenation and on aggressively identifying and treating the underlying cause or predisposing condition. Monitoring of the patient's hemodynamics, oxygenation, and acid-base status should be used to guide therapy. In the presence of severe or worsening metabolic acidemia, these measures should be supplemented by judicious administration of sodium bicarbonate, given as an infusion rather than a bolus. Alkali administration should be regarded as a temporizing maneuver adjunctive to cause-specific measures. Given the ominous prognosis of lactic acidosis, clinicians should strive to prevent its development by maintaining adequate fluid balance, optimizing cardiorespiratory function, managing infection, and using drugs that predispose to the disorder cautiously. Preventing the development of lactic acidosis is all the more important in patients at special risk for developing it, such as those with diabetes mellitus or advanced cardiac, respiratory, renal, or hepatic disease [1,14–16].

Diabetic ketoacidosis and nonketotic hyperglycemia

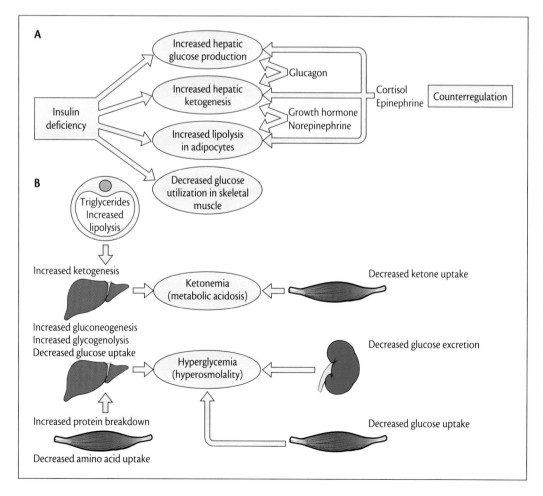

FIGURE 6-22

Role of insulin deficiency and the counterregulatory hormones, and their respective sites of action, in the pathogenesis of hyperglycemia and ketosis in diabetic ketoacidosis (DKA). **A,** Metabolic processes affected by insulin deficiency, on the one hand, and excess of glucagon, cortisol, epinephrine, norepinephrine, and growth hormone, on the other. **B,** The roles of the adipose tissue, liver, skeletal muscle, and kidney in the pathogenesis of hyperglycemia and ketonemia. Impairment of glucose oxidation in most tissues and excessive hepatic production of glucose are the main determinants of hyperglycemia. Excessive counterregulation and the prevailing hypertonicity, metabolic acidosis, and electrolyte imbalance superimpose a state of insulin resistance. Prerenal azotemia caused by volume depletion can contribute significantly to severe hyperglycemia. Increased hepatic production of ketones and their reduced utilization by peripheral tissues account for the ketonemia typically observed in DKA.

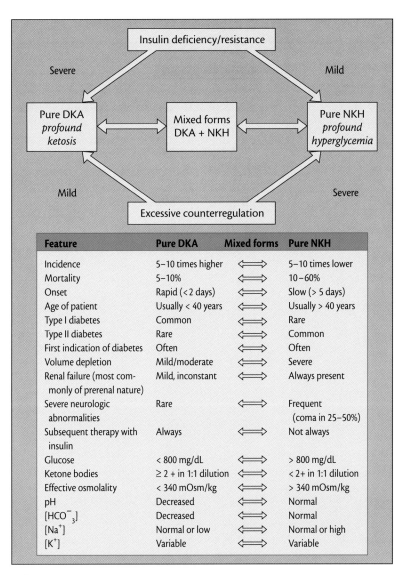

Feature	Pure DKA	Mixed forms	Pure NKH
Incidence	5–10 times higher	⟺	5–10 times lower
Mortality	5–10%	⟺	10–60%
Onset	Rapid (< 2 days)	⟺	Slow (> 5 days)
Age of patient	Usually < 40 years	⟺	Usually > 40 years
Type I diabetes	Common	⟺	Rare
Type II diabetes	Rare	⟺	Common
First indication of diabetes	Often	⟺	Often
Volume depletion	Mild/moderate	⟺	Severe
Renal failure (most commonly of prerenal nature)	Mild, inconstant	⟺	Always present
Severe neurologic abnormalities	Rare	⟺	Frequent (coma in 25–50%)
Subsequent therapy with insulin	Always	⟺	Not always
Glucose	< 800 mg/dL	⟺	> 800 mg/dL
Ketone bodies	≥ 2 + in 1:1 dilution	⟺	< 2+ in 1:1 dilution
Effective osmolality	< 340 mOsm/kg	⟺	> 340 mOsm/kg
pH	Decreased	⟺	Normal
$[HCO_3^-]$	Decreased	⟺	Normal
$[Na^+]$	Normal or low	⟺	Normal or high
$[K^+]$	Variable	⟺	Variable

FIGURE 6-23

Clinical features of diabetic ketoacidosis (DKA) and nonketotic hyperglycemia (NKH). DKA and NKH are the most important acute metabolic complications of patients with uncontrolled diabetes mellitus. These disorders share the same overall pathogenesis that includes insulin deficiency and resistance and excessive counterregulation; however, the importance of each of these endocrine abnormalities differs significantly in DKA and NKH. As depicted here, pure NKH is characterized by profound hyperglycemia, the result of mild insulin deficiency and severe counterregulation (eg, high glucagon levels). In contrast, pure DKA is characterized by profound ketosis that largely is due to severe insulin deficiency, with counterregulation being generally of lesser importance. These pure forms define a continuum that includes mixed forms incorporating clinical and biochemical features of both DKA and NKH. Dyspnea and Kussmaul's respiration result from the metabolic acidosis of DKA, which is generally absent in NKH. Sodium and water deficits and secondary renal dysfunction are more severe in NKH than in DKA. These deficits also play a pathogenetic role in the profound hypertonicity characteristic of NKH. The severe hyperglycemia of NKH, often coupled with hypernatremia, increases serum osmolality, thereby causing the characteristic functional abnormalities of the central nervous system. Depression of the sensorium, somnolence, obtundation, and coma, are prominent manifestations of NKH. The degree of obtundation correlates with the severity of serum hypertonicity [17].

MANAGEMENT OF DIABETIC KETOACIDOSIS AND NONKETOTIC HYPERGLYCEMIA

Insulin	Fluid Administration	Potassium repletion	Alkali
1. Give initial IV bolus of 0.2 U/kg actual body weight. 2. Add 100 U of regular insulin to 1 L of normal saline (0.1 U/mL), and follow with continuous IV drip of 0.1 U/kg actual body weight per h until correction of ketosis. 3. Give double rate of infusion if the blood glucose level does not decrease in a 2-h interval (expected decrease is 40–80 mg/dL/h or 10% of the initial value.) 4. Give SQ dose (10–30 U) of regular insulin when ketosis is corrected and the blood glucose level decreases to 300 mg/dL, and continue with SQ insulin injection every 4 h on a sliding scale (ie, 5 U if below 150, 10 U if 150–200, 15 U if 200–250, and 20 U if 250–300 mg/dL).	Shock absent: Normal saline (0.9% NaCl) at 7 mL/kg/h for 4 h, and half this rate thereafter Shock present: Normal saline and plasma expanders (ie, albumin, low molecular weight dextran) at maximal possible rate Start a glucose-containing solution (eg, 5% dextrose in water) when blood glucose level decreases to 250 mg/dL.	Potassium chloride should be added to the third liter of IV infusion and subsequently if urinary output is at least 30–60 mL/h and plasma $[K^+]$ < 5 mEq/L. Add K^+ to the initial 2 L of IV fluids if initial plasma $[K^+]$ < 4 mEq/L and adequate diuresis is secured.	Half-normal saline (0.45% NaCl) plus 1–2 ampules (44-88 mEq) $NaHCO_3$ per liter when blood pH < 7.0 or total CO_2 < 5 mmol/L; in hyperchloremic acidosis, add $NaHCO_3$ when pH < 7.20; discontinue $NaHCO_3$ in IV infusion when total CO_2 > 8–10 mmol/L.

CO_2—carbon dioxide; IV—intravenous; K^+—potassium ion; NaCl—sodium chloride; $NaHCO_3$—sodium bicarbonate; SQ—subcutaneous.

FIGURE 6-24

Diabetic ketoacidosis (DKA) and nonketotic hyperglycemia (NKH) management. Administration of insulin is the cornerstone of management for both DKA and NKH. Replacement of the prevailing water, sodium, and potassium deficits is also required. Alkali are administered only under certain circumstances in DKA and virtually never in NKH, in which ketoacidosis is generally absent. Because the fluid deficit is generally severe in patients with NKH, many of whom have preexisting heart disease and are relatively old, safe fluid replacement may require monitoring of central venous pressure, pulmonary capillary wedge pressure, or both [1,17,18].

Renal tubular acidosis

FEATURES OF THE RENAL TUBULAR ACIDOSIS (RTA) SYNDROMES

Feature	Proximal RTA	Classic Distal RTA	Hyperkalemic Distal RTA
Plasma bicarbonate ion concentration	14–18 mEq/L	Variable, may be < 10 mEq/L	15–20 mEq/L
Plasma chloride ion concentration	Increased	Increased	Increased
Plasma potassium ion concentration	Mildly decreased	Mildly to severely decreased	Mildly to severely increased
Plasma anion gap	Normal	Normal	Normal
Glomerular filtration rate	Normal or slightly decreased	Normal or slightly decreased	Normal to moderately decreased
Urine pH during acidosis	≤ 5.5	>6.0	≤ 5.5
Urine pH after acid loading	≤ 5.5	>6.0	≤ 5.5
U-B PCO_2 in alkaline urine	Normal	Decreased	Decreased
Fractional excretion of HCO_3^- at normal $[HCO_3^-]_p$	>15%	<5%	<5%
Tm HCO_3^-	Decreased	Normal	Normal
Nephrolithiasis	Absent	Present	Absent
Nephrocalcinosis	Absent	Present	Absent
Osteomalacia	Present	Present	Absent
Fanconi's syndrome*	Usually present	Absent	Absent
Alkali therapy	High dose	Low dose	Low dose

Tm HCO_3^-—maximum reabsorption of bicarbonate; U-B PCO_2—difference between partial pressure of carbon dioxide values in urine and arterial blood.

*This syndrome signifies generalized proximal tubule dysfunction and is characterized by impaired reabsorption of glucose, amino acids, phosphate, and urate.

FIGURE 6-25

Renal tubular acidosis (RTA) defines a group of disorders in which tubular hydrogen ion secretion is impaired out of proportion to any reduction in the glomerular filtration rate. These disorders are characterized by normal anion gap (hyperchloremic) metabolic acidosis. The defects responsible for impaired acidification give rise to three distinct syndromes known as proximal RTA (type 2), classic distal RTA (type 1), and hyperkalemic distal RTA (type 4).

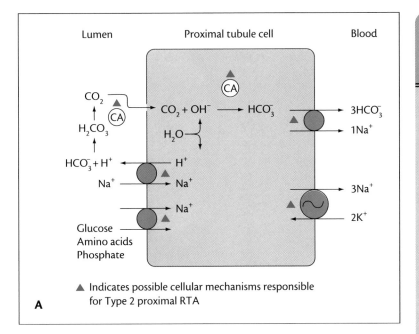

Lumen Proximal tubule cell Blood

▲ Indicates possible cellular mechanisms responsible for Type 2 proximal RTA

A

FIGURE 6-26

A and B, Potential defects and causes of proximal renal tubular acidosis (RTA) (type 2). Excluding the case of carbonic anhydrase inhibitors, the nature of the acidification defect responsible for bicarbonate (HCO_3) wastage remains unknown. It might represent defects in the luminal sodium ion– hydrogen ion (Na^+-H^+) exchanger, basolateral Na^+-$3HCO_3^-$ cotransporter, or carbonic anhydrase activity. Most patients with proximal RTA have additional defects in proximal tubule function (Fanconi's syndrome); this generalized proximal tubule dysfunction might reflect a defect in the basolateral Na^+-K^+ adenosine triphosphatase. K^+—potassium ion; CA—carbonic anhydrase. Causes of proximal renal tubular acidosis (RTA) (type 2). An idiopathic form and cystinosis are the most common causes of proximal RTA in children. In adults, multiple myeloma and carbonic anhydrase inhibitors (eg, acetazolamide) are the major causes. Ifosfamide is an increasingly common cause of the disorder in both age groups.

B. CAUSES OF PROXIMAL RENAL TUBULAR ACIDOSIS

Selective defect (isolated bicarbonate wasting)
  Primary (no obvious associated disease)
    Genetically transmitted
    Transient (infants)
  Due to altered carbonic anhydrase activity
    Acetazolamide
    Sulfanilamide
    Mafenide acetate
    Genetically transmitted
    Idiopathic
    Osteopetrosis with carbonic
      anhydrase II deficiency
    York-Yendt syndrome

Generalized defect (associated with multiple
    dysfunctions of the proximal tubule)
  Primary (no obvious associated disease)
    Sporadic
    Genetically transmitted
  Genetically transmitted systemic disease
    Tyrosinemia
    Wilson's disease
    Lowe syndrome
    Hereditary fructose intolerance (during
      administration of fructose)
    Cystinosis
    Pyruvate carboxylate deficiency
    Metachromatic leukodystrophy
    Methylmalonic acidemia

Conditions associated with chronic hypocalcemia
    and secondary hyperparathyroidism
  Vitamin D deficiency or resistance
  Vitamin D dependence

Dysproteinemic states
  Multiple myeloma
  Monoclonal gammopathy

Drug- or toxin-induced
  Outdated tetracycline
  3-Methylchromone
  Streptozotocin
  Lead
  Mercury
  Arginine
  Valproic acid
  Gentamicin
  Ifosfamide

Tubulointerstitial diseases
  Renal transplantation
  Sjögren's syndrome
  Medullary cystic disease

Other renal diseases
  Nephrotic syndrome
  Amyloidosis

Miscellaneous
  Paroxysmal
    nocturnal hemoglobinuria
  Hyperparathyroidism

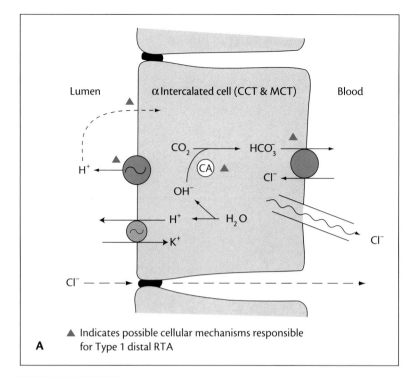

▲ Indicates possible cellular mechanisms responsible
for Type 1 distal RTA

A

FIGURE 6-27

A and B, Potential defects and causes of classic distal renal tubular acidosis (RTA) (type 1). Potential cellular defects underlying classic distal RTA include a faulty luminal hydrogen ion–adenosine triphosphatase (H^+ pump failure or secretory defect), an abnormality in the basolateral bicarbonate ion–chloride ion exchanger, inadequacy of carbonic anhydrase activity, or an increase in the luminal membrane permeability for hydrogen ions (backleak of protons or permeability defect). Most of the causes of classic distal RTA likely reflect a secretory defect, whereas amphotericin B is the only established cause of a permeability defect. The hereditary form is the most common cause of this disorder in children. Major causes in adults include autoimmune disorders (*eg*, Sjögren's syndrome) and hypercalciuria [19]. CA—carbonic anhydrase.

B. CAUSES OF CLASSIC DISTAL RENAL TUBULAR ACIDOSIS

Primary (no obvious associated disease)
  Sporadic
  Genetically transmitted

Autoimmune disorders
  Hypergammaglobulinemia
  Hyperglobulinemic purpura
  Cryoglobulinemia
  Familial
  Sjögren's syndrome
  Thyroiditis
  Pulmonary fibrosis
  Chronic active hepatitis
  Primary biliary cirrhosis
  Systemic lupus erythematosus
  Vasculitis

Genetically transmitted systemic disease
  Ehlers-Danlos syndrome
  Hereditary elliptocytosis
  Sickle cell anemia
  Marfan syndrome
  Carbonic anhydrase I deficiency
    or alteration
  Osteopetrosis with carbonic
    anhydrase II deficiency
  Medullary cystic disease
  Neuroaxonal dystrophy

Disorders associated
    with nephrocalcinosis
  Primary or familial hyperparathyroidism
  Vitamin D intoxication
  Milk-alkali syndrome
  Hyperthyroidism
  Idiopathic hypercalciuria
    Genetically transmitted
    Sporadic
  Hereditary fructose intolerance
    (after chronic fructose ingestion)
  Medullary sponge kidney
  Fabry's disease
  Wilson's disease

Drug- or toxin-induced
  Amphotericin B
  Toluene
  Analgesics
  Lithium
  Cyclamate
  Balkan nephropathy

Tubulointerstitial diseases
  Chronic pyelonephritis
  Obstructive uropathy
  Renal transplantation
  Leprosy
  Hyperoxaluria

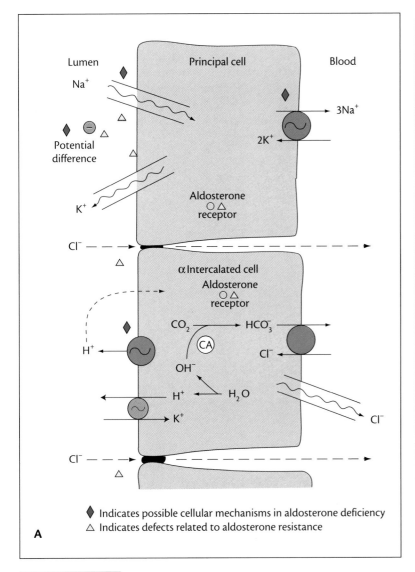

Indicates possible cellular mechanisms in aldosterone deficiency

△ Indicates defects related to aldosterone resistance

A

B. CAUSES OF HYPERKALEMIC DISTAL RENAL TUBULAR ACIDOSIS

Deficiency of aldosterone
  Associated with glucocorticoid deficiency
    Addison's disease
    Bilateral adrenalectomy
    Enzymatic defects
      21-Hydroxylase deficiency
      3-β-ol-Dehydrogenase deficiency
      Desmolase deficiency
    Acquired immunodeficiency syndrome
  Isolated aldosterone deficiency
    Genetically transmitted
      Corticosterone methyl
        oxidase deficiency
    Transient (infants)
    Sporadic
    Heparin
    Deficient renin secretion
      Diabetic nephropathy
      Tubulointerstitial renal disease
      Nonsteroidal antiinflammatory drugs
      β-adrenergic blockers
      Acquired immunodeficiency syndrome
      Renal transplantation
  Angiotensin I-converting enzyme inhibition
    Endogenous
    Captopril and related drugs
  Angiotensin AT, receptor blockers

Resistance to aldosterone action
  Pseudohypoaldosteronism type I
    (with salt wasting)
    Childhood forms with
      obstructive uropathy
    Adult forms with
      renal insufficiency
  Spironolactone
  Pseudohypoaldosteronism type II
    (without salt wasting)
  Combined aldosterone deficiency
    and resistance
    Deficient renin secretion
    Cyclosporine nephrotoxicity
    Uncertain renin status
  Voltage-mediated defects
    Obstructive uropathy
    Sickle cell anemia
    Lithium
    Triamterene
    Amiloride
    Trimethoprim, pentamidine
  Renal transplantation

FIGURE 6-28

A and **B**, Potential defects and causes of hyperkalemic distal renal tubular acidosis (RTA) (type 4). This syndrome represents the most common type of RTA encountered in adults. The characteristic hyperchloremic metabolic acidosis in the company of hyperkalemia emerges as a consequence of generalized dysfunction of the collecting tubule, including diminished sodium reabsorption and impaired hydrogen ion and potassium secretion. The resultant hyperkalemia causes impaired ammonium excretion that is an important contribution to the generation of the metabolic acidosis. The causes of this syndrome are broadly classified into disorders resulting in aldosterone deficiency and those that impose resistance to the action of aldosterone. Aldosterone deficiency can arise from

hyporeninemia, impaired conversion of angiotensin I to angiotensin II, or abnormal aldosterone synthesis. Aldosterone resistance can reflect the following: blockade of the mineralocorticoid receptor; destruction of the target cells in the collecting tubule (*tubulointerstitial nephropathies*); interference with the sodium channel of the principal cell, thereby decreasing the lumen-negative potential difference and thus the secretion of potassium and hydrogen ions (voltage-mediated defect); inhibition of the basolateral sodium ion, potassium ion–adenosine triphosphatase; and enhanced chloride ion permeability in the collecting tubule, with consequent shunting of the transepithelial potential difference. Some disorders cause combined aldosterone deficiency and resistance [20].

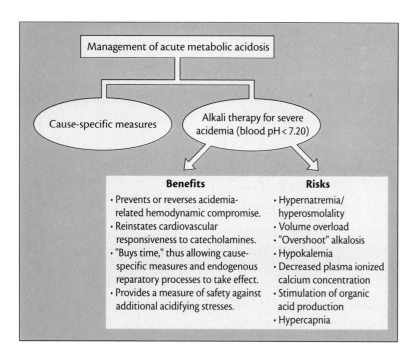

FIGURE 6-29

Treatment of acute metabolic acidosis. Whenever possible, cause-specific measures should be at the center of treatment of metabolic acidosis. In the presence of severe acidemia, such measures should be supplemented by judicious administration of sodium bicarbonate. The goal of alkali therapy is to return the blood pH to a safer level of about 7.20. Anticipated benefits and potential risks of alkali therapy are depicted here [1].

Metabolic Alkalosis

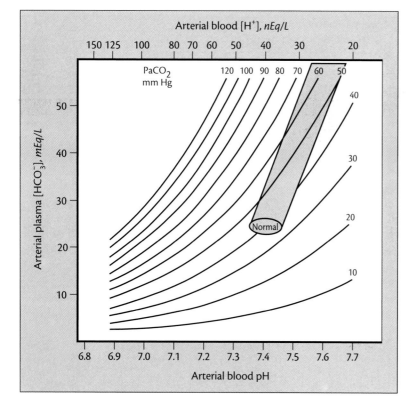

FIGURE 6-30

Ninety-five percent confidence intervals for metabolic alkalosis. Metabolic alkalosis is the acid-base disturbance initiated by an increase in plasma bicarbonate concentration ($[HCO_3^-]$). The resultant alkalemia dampens alveolar ventilation and leads to the secondary hypercapnia characteristic of the disorder. Available observations in humans suggest a roughly linear relationship between the steady-state increase in bicarbonate concentration and the associated increment in the arterial carbon dioxide tension ($PaCO_2$). Although data are limited, the slope of the steady-state $\Delta PaCO_2$ versus $\Delta[HCO_3^-]$ relationship has been estimated as about a 0.7 mm Hg per mEq/L increase in plasma bicarbonate concentration. The value of this slope is virtually identical to that in dogs that has been derived from rigorously controlled observations [21]. Empiric observations in humans have been used for construction of 95% confidence intervals for graded degrees of metabolic alkalosis represented by the area in color in the acid-base template. The black ellipse near the center of the figure indicates the normal range for the acid-base parameters [3]. Assuming a steady state is present, values falling within the area in color are consistent with but not diagnostic of simple metabolic alkalosis. Acid-base values falling outside the area in color denote the presence of a mixed acid-base disturbance [4]. [H^+]—hydrogen ion concentration.

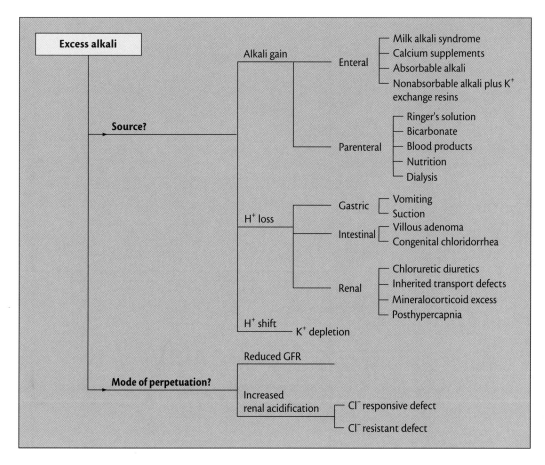

FIGURE 6-31

Pathogenesis of metabolic alkalosis. Two crucial questions must be answered when evaluating the pathogenesis of a case of metabolic alkalosis. 1) What is the source of the excess alkali? Answering this question addresses the primary event responsible for *generating* the hyperbicarbonatemia. 2) What factors perpetuate the hyperbicarbonatemia? Answering this question addresses the pathophysiologic events that *maintain* the metabolic alkalosis.

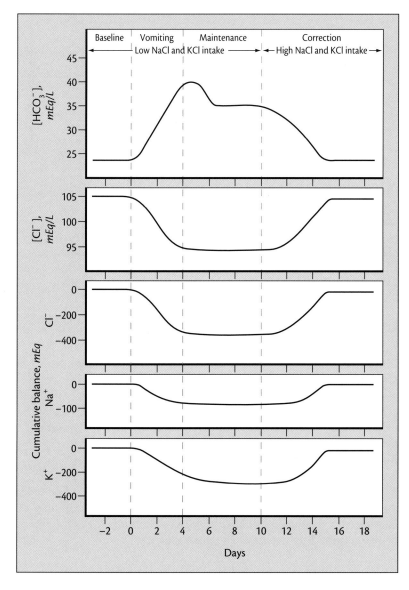

FIGURE 6-32

Changes in plasma anionic pattern and body electrolyte balance during development, maintenance, and correction of metabolic alkalosis induced by vomiting. Loss of hydrochloric acid from the stomach as a result of vomiting (or gastric drainage) generates the hypochloremic hyperbicarbonatemia characteristic of this disorder. During the generation phase, renal sodium and potassium excretion increases, yielding the deficits depicted here. Renal potassium losses continue in the early days of the maintenance phase. Subsequently, and as long as the low-chloride diet is continued, a new steady state is achieved in which plasma bicarbonate concentration ($[HCO_3^-]$) stabilizes at an elevated level, and renal excretion of electrolytes matches intake. Addition of sodium chloride (NaCl) and potassium chloride (KCl) in the correction phase repairs the electrolyte deficits incurred and normalizes the plasma bicarbonate and chloride concentration ($[Cl^-]$) levels [22,23].

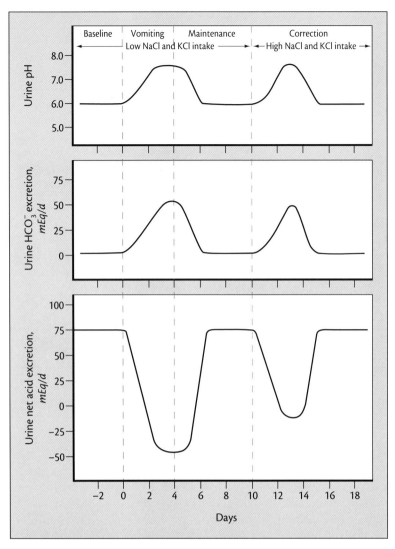

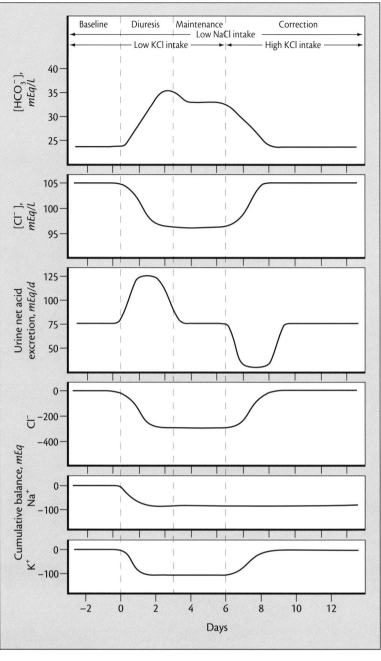

FIGURE 6-33

Changes in urine acid-base composition during development, maintenance, and correction of vomiting-induced metabolic alkalosis. During acid removal from the stomach as well as early in the phase after vomiting (maintenance), an alkaline urine is excreted as acid excretion is suppressed, and bicarbonate excretion (in the company of sodium and, especially potassium; *see* Fig. 6-32) is increased, with the net acid excretion being negative (net alkali excretion). This acid-base profile moderates the steady-state level of the resulting alkalosis. In the steady state (late maintenance phase), as all filtered bicarbonate is reclaimed the pH of urine becomes acidic, and the net acid excretion returns to baseline. Provision of sodium chloride (NaCl) and potassium chloride (KCl) in the correction phase alkalinizes the urine and suppresses the net acid excretion, as bicarbonaturia in the company of exogenous cations (sodium and potassium) supervenes [22,23]. HCO_3^-—bicarbonate ion.

FIGURE 6-34

Changes in plasma anionic pattern, net acid excretion, and body electrolyte balance during development, maintenance, and correction of diuretic-induced metabolic alkalosis. Administration of a loop diuretic, such as furosemide, increases urine net acid excretion (largely in the form of ammonium) as well as the renal losses of chloride (Cl^-), sodium (Na^+), and potassium (K^+). The resulting hyperbicarbonatemia reflects both loss of excess ammonium chloride in the urine and an element of contraction (consequent to diuretic-induced sodium chloride [NaCl] losses) that limits the space of distribution of bicarbonate. During the phase after diuresis (maintenance), and as long as the low-chloride diet is continued, a new steady state is attained in which the plasma bicarbonate concentration ([HCO_3^-]) remains elevated, urine net acid excretion returns to baseline, and renal excretion of electrolytes matches intake. Addition of potassium chloride (KCl) in the correction phase repairs the chloride and potassium deficits, suppresses net acid excretion, and normalizes the plasma bicarbonate and chloride concentration ([Cl^-]) levels [23,24]. If extracellular fluid volume has become subnormal folllowing diuresis, administration of NaCl is also required for repair of the metabolic alkalosis.

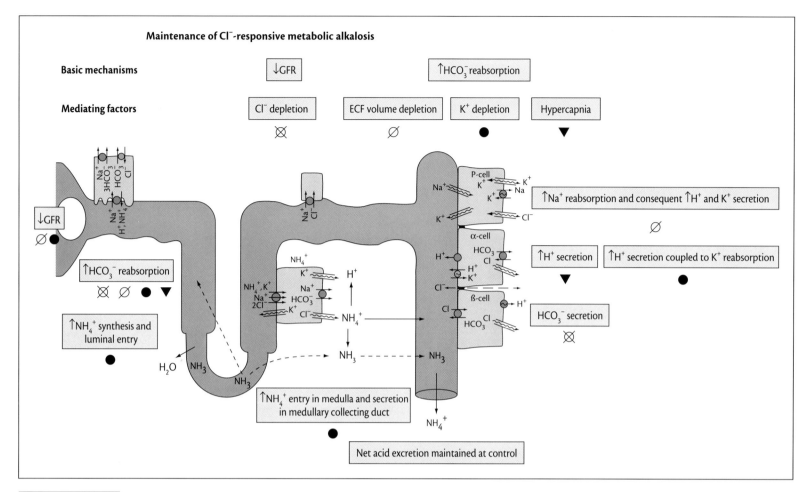

FIGURE 6-35

Maintenance of chloride-responsive metabolic alkalosis. Increased renal bicarbonate reabsorption frequently coupled with a reduced glomerular filtration rate are the basic mechanisms that maintain chloride-responsive metabolic alkalosis. These mechanisms have been ascribed to three mediating factors: chloride depletion itself, extracellular fluid (ECF) volume depletion, and potassium depletion. Assigning particular roles to each of these factors is a vexing task. Notwithstanding, here depicted is our current understanding of the participation of each of these factors in the nephronal processes that maintain chloride-responsive metabolic alkalosis [22–24]. In addition to these factors, the secondary hypercapnia of metabolic alkalosis contributes importantly to the maintenance of the prevailing hyperbicarbonatemia [25].

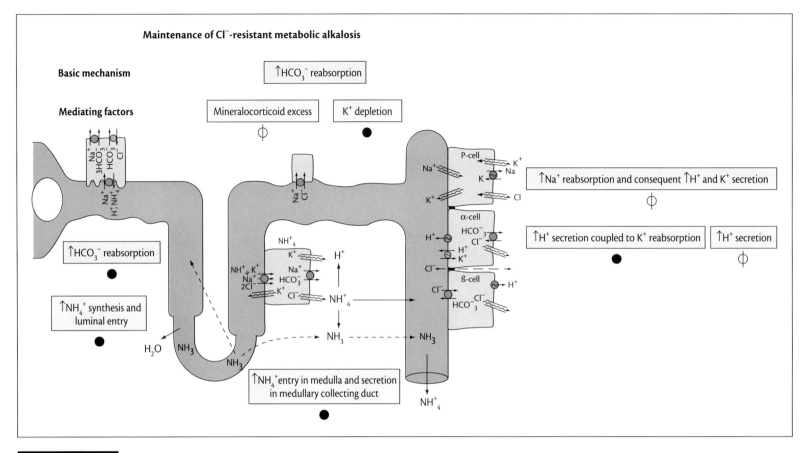

FIGURE 6-36

Maintenance of chloride-resistant metabolic alkalosis. Increased renal bicarbonate reabsorption is the sole basic mechanism that maintains chloride-resistant metabolic alkalosis. As its name implies, factors independent of chloride intake mediate the height-ened bicarbonate reabsorption and include mineralocorticoid excess and potassium depletion. The participation of these factors in the nephronal processes that maintain chloride-resistant meta-bolic alkalosis is depicted [22–24, 26].

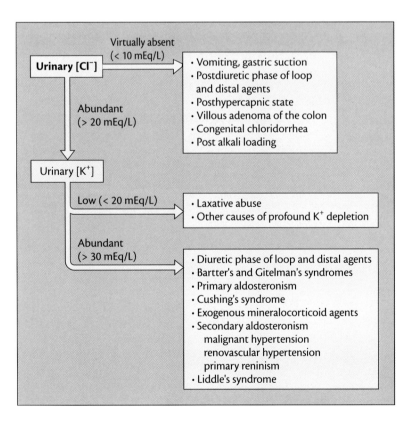

FIGURE 6-37

Urinary composition in the diagnostic evaluation of metabolic alka-losis. Assessing the urinary composition can be an important aid in the diagnostic evaluation of metabolic alkalosis. Measurement of uri-nary chloride ion concentration ($[Cl^-]$) can help distinguish between chloride-responsive and chloride-resistant metabolic alkalosis. The virtual absence of chloride (urine $[Cl^-]$ < 10 mEq/L) indicates signifi-cant chloride depletion. Note, however, that this test loses its diag-nostic significance if performed within several hours of administra-tion of chloruretic diuretics, because these agents promote urinary chloride excretion. Measurement of urinary potassium ion concen-tration ($[K^+]$) provides further diagnostic differentiation. With the exception of the diuretic phase of chloruretic agents, abundance of both urinary chloride and potassium signifies a state of mineralocor-ticoid excess [22].

SIGNS AND SYMPTOMS OF METABOLIC ALKALOSIS

Central Nervous System	Cardiovascular System	Respiratory System	Neuromuscular System	Metabolic Effects	Renal (Associated Potassium Depletion)
Headache	Supraventricular and ventricular arrhythmias	Hypoventilation with attendant hypercapnia and hypoxemia	Chvostek's sign	Increased organic acid and ammonia production	Polyuria
Lethargy	Potentiation of digitalis toxicity		Trousseau's sign	Hypokalemia	Polydipsia
Stupor			Weakness (severity depends on degree of potassium depletion)	Hypocalcemia	Urinary concentration defect
Delirium	Positive inotropic ventricular effect			Hypomagnesemia	Cortical and medullary renal cysts
Tetany				Hypophosphatemia	
Seizures					
Potentiation of hepatic encephalopathy					

FIGURE 6-38

Signs and symptoms of metabolic alkalosis. Mild to moderate metabolic alkalosis usually is accompanied by few if any symptoms, unless potassium depletion is substantial. In contrast, severe metabolic alkalosis ($[HCO_3^-] > 40$ mEq/L) is usually a symptomatic disorder. Alkalemia, hypokalemia, hypoxemia, hypercapnia, and decreased plasma ionized calcium concentration all contribute to these clinical manifestations. The arrhythmogenic potential of alkalemia is more pronounced in patients with underlying heart disease and is heightened by the almost constant presence of hypokalemia, especially in those patients taking digitalis. Even mild alkalemia can frustrate efforts to wean patients from mechanical ventilation [23,24].

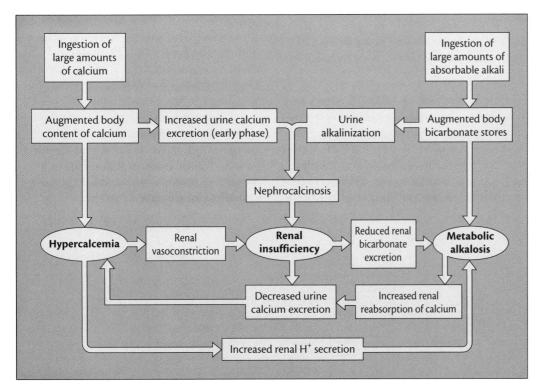

FIGURE 6-39

Pathophysiology of the milk-alkali syndrome. The milk-alkali syndrome comprises the triad of hypercalcemia, renal insufficiency, and metabolic alkalosis and is caused by the ingestion of large amounts of calcium and absorbable alkali. Although large amounts of milk and absorbable alkali were the culprits in the classic form of the syndrome, its modern version is usually the result of large doses of calcium carbonate alone. Because of recent emphasis on prevention and treatment of osteoporosis with calcium carbonate and the availability of this preparation over the counter, milk-alkali syndrome is currently the third leading cause of hypercalcemia after primary hyperparathyroidism and malignancy. Another common presentation of the syndrome originates from the current use of calcium carbonate in preference to aluminum as a phosphate binder in patients with chronic renal insufficiency. The critical element in the pathogenesis of the syndrome is the development of hypercalcemia that, in turn, results in renal dysfunction. Generation and maintenance of metabolic alkalosis reflect the combined effects of the large bicarbonate load, renal insufficiency, and hypercalcemia. Metabolic alkalosis contributes to the maintenance of hypercalcemia by increasing tubular calcium reabsorption. Superimposition of an element of volume contraction caused by vomiting, diuretics, or hypercalcemia-induced natriuresis can worsen each one of the three main components of the syndrome. Discontinuation of calcium carbonate coupled with a diet high in sodium chloride or the use of normal saline and furosemide therapy (depending on the severity of the syndrome) results in rapid resolution of hypercalcemia and metabolic alkalosis. Although renal function also improves, in a considerable fraction of patients with the chronic form of the syndrome serum creatinine fails to return to baseline as a result of irreversible structural changes in the kidneys [27].

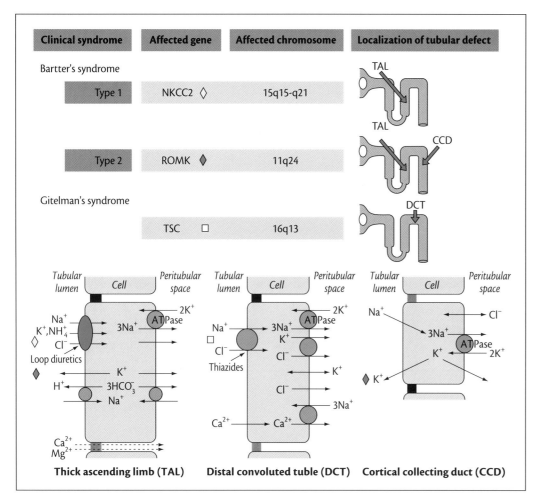

FIGURE 6-40

Clinical features and molecular basis of tubular defects of Bartter's and Gitelman's syndromes. These rare disorders are characterized by chloride-resistant metabolic alkalosis, renal potassium wasting and hypokalemia, hyperreninemia and hyperplasia of the juxtaglomerular apparatus, hyperaldosteronism, and normotension. Regarding differentiating features, Bartter's syndrome presents early in life, frequently in association with growth and mental retardation. In this syndrome, urinary concentrating ability is usually decreased, polyuria and polydipsia are present, the serum magnesium level is normal,

and hypercalciuria and nephrocalcinosis are present. In contrast, Gitelman's syndrome is a milder disease presenting later in life. Patients often are asymptomatic, or they might have intermittent muscle spasms, cramps, or tetany. Urinary concentrating ability is maintained; hypocalciuria, renal magnesium wasting, and hypomagnesemia are almost constant features. On the basis of certain of these clinical features, it had been hypothesized that the primary tubular defects in Bartter's and Gitelman's syndromes reflect impairment in sodium reabsorption in the thick ascending limb (TAL) of the loop of Henle and the distal tubule, respectively. This hypothesis has been validated by recent genetic studies [28-31]. As illustrated here, Bartter's syndrome now has been shown to be caused by loss-of-function mutations in the loop diuretic–sensitive sodium-potassium-2chloride cotransporter (NKCC2) of the TAL (type 1 Bartter's syndrome) [28] or the apical potassium channel ROMK of the TAL (where it recycles reabsorbed potassium into the lumen for continued operation of the NKCC2 cotransporter) and the cortical collecting duct (where it mediates secretion of potassium by the principal cell) (type 2 Bartter's syndrome) [29,30]. On the other hand, Gitelman's syndrome is caused by mutations in the thiazide-sensitive Na-Cl cotransporter (TSC) of the distal tubule [31]. Note that the distal tubule is the major site of active calcium reabsorption. Stimulation of calcium reabsorption at this site is responsible for the hypocalciuric effect of thiazide diuretics.

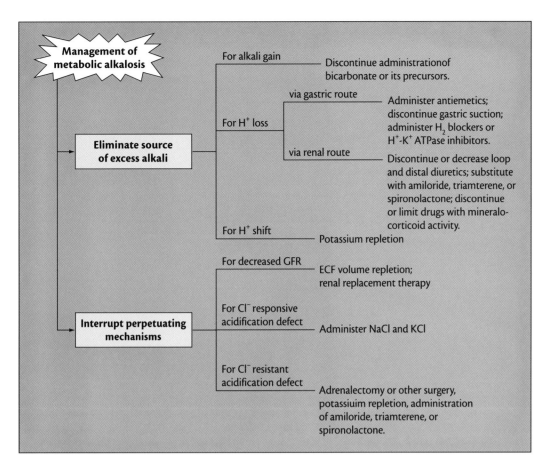

Metabolic alkalosis management. Effective management of metabolic alkalosis requires sound understanding of the underlying pathophysiology. Therapeutic efforts should focus on eliminating or moderating the processes that generate the alkali excess and on interrupting the mechanisms that perpetuate the hyperbicarbonatemia. Rarely, when the pace of correction of metabolic alkalosis must be accelerated, acetazolamide or an infusion of hydrochloric acid can be used. Treatment of severe metabolic alkalosis can be particularly challenging in patients with advanced cardiac or renal dysfunction. In such patients, hemodialysis or continuous hemofiltration might be required [1].

References

1. Adrogué HJ, Madias NE: Management of life-threatening acid-base disorders. *N Engl J Med*, 1998, 338:26–34, 107–111.

2. Madias NE, Adrogué HJ: Acid-base disturbances in pulmonary medicine. In *Fluid, Electrolyte, and Acid-Base Disorders.* Edited by Arieff Al, DeFronzo RA. New York: Churchill Livingstone; 1995:223–253.

3. Madias NE, Adrogué HJ, Horowitz GL, *et al.*: A redefinition of normal acid-base equilibrium in man: carbon dioxide tension as a key determinant of plasma bicarbonate concentration. *Kidney Int* 1979, 16:612–618.

4. Adrogué HJ, Madias NE: Mixed acid-base disorders. In *The Principles and Practice of Nephrology.* Edited by Jacobson HR, Striker GE, Klahr S. St. Louis: Mosby-Year Book; 1995:953–962.

5. Krapf R: Mechanisms of adaptation to chronic respiratory acidosis in the rabbit proximal tubule. *J Clin Invest* 1989, 83:890–896.

6. Al-Awqati Q: The cellular renal response to respiratory acid-base disorders. *Kidney Int* 1985, 28:845–855.

7. Bastani B: Immunocytochemical localization of the vacuolar H+-ATPase pump in the kidney. *Histol Histopathol* 1997, 12:769–779.

8. Teixeira da Silva JC Jr, Perrone RD, Johns CA, Madias NE: Rat kidney band 3 mRNA modulation in chronic respiratory acidosis. *Am J Physiol* 1991, 260:F204–F209.

9. Respiratory pump failure: primary hypercapnia (respiratory acidosis). In *Respiratory Failure.* Edited by Adrogué HJ, Tobin MJ. Cambridge, MA: Blackwell Science; 1997:125–134.

10. Krapf R, Beeler I, Hertner D, Hulter HN: Chronic respiratory alkalosis: the effect of sustained hyperventilation on renal regulation of acid-base equilibrium. *N Engl J Med* 1991, 324:1394–1401.

11. Hilden SA, Johns CA, Madias NE: Adaptation of rabbit renal cortical Na+-H+-exchange activity in chronic hypocapnia. *Am J Physiol* 1989, 257:F615–F622.

12. Adrogué HJ, Rashad MN, Gorin AB, *et al.*: Arteriovenous acid-base disparity in circulatory failure: studies on mechanism. *Am J Physiol* 1989, 257:F1087–F1093.

13. Adrogué HJ, Rashad MN, Gorin AB, *et al.*: Assessing acid-base status in circulatory failure: differences between arterial and central venous blood. *N Engl J Med* 1989, 320:1312–1316.

14. Madias NE: Lactic acidosis. *Kidney Int* 1986, 29:752–774.

15. Kraut JA, Madias NE: Lactic acidosis. In *Textbook of Nephrology.* Edited by Massry SG, Glassock RJ. Baltimore: Williams and Wilkins; 1995:449–457.

16. Hindman BJ: Sodium bicarbonate in the treatment of subtypes of acute lactic acidosis: physiologic considerations. *Anesthesiology* 1990, 72:1064–1076.

17. Adroguè HJ: Diabetic ketoacidosis and hyperosmolar nonketotic syndrome. In *Therapy of Renal Diseases and Related Disorders.* Edited by Suki WN, Massry SG. Boston: Kluwer Academic Publishers; 1997:233–251.

18. Adrogué HJ, Barrero J, Eknoyan G: Salutary effects of modest fluid replacement in the treatment of adults with diabetic ketoacidosis. *JAMA* 1989, 262:2108–2113.

19. Bastani B, Gluck SL: New insights into the pathogenesis of distal renal tubular acidosis. *Miner Electrolyte Metab* 1996, 22:396–409.

20. DuBose TD Jr: Hyperkalemic hyperchloremic metabolic acidosis: pathophysiologic insights. *Kidney Int* 1997, 51:591–602.

21. Madias NE, Bossert WH, Adrogué HJ: Ventilatory response to chronic metabolic acidosis and alkalosis in the dog. *J Appl Physiol* 1984, 56:1640–1646.

22. Gennari FJ: Metabolic alkalosis. In *The Principles and Practice of Nephrology.* Edited by Jacobson HR, Striker GE, Klahr S. St Louis: Mosby-Year Book; 1995:932–942.

23. Sabatini S, Kurtzman NA: Metabolic alkalosis: biochemical mechanisms, pathophysiology, and treatment. In *Therapy of Renal Diseases and Related Disorders* Edited by Suki WN, Massry SG. Boston: Kluwer Academic Publishers; 1997:189–210.

24. Galla JH, Luke RG: Metabolic alkalosis. In *Textbook of Nephrology.* Edited by Massry SG, Glassock RJ. Baltimore: Williams & Wilkins; 1995:469–477.

25. Madias NE, Adrogué HJ, Cohen JJ: Maladaptive renal response to secondary hypercapnia in chronic metabolic alkalosis. *Am J Physiol* 1980, 238:F283–289.

26. Harrington JT, Hulter HN, Cohen JJ, Madias NE: Mineralocorticoid-stimulated renal acidification in the dog: the critical role of dietary sodium. *Kidney Int* 1986, 30:43–48.

27. Beall DP, Scofield RH: Milk-alkali syndrome associated with calcium carbonate consumption. *Medicine* 1995, 74:89–96.

28. Simon DB, Karet FE, Hamdan JM, *et al.*: Bartter's syndrome, hypokalaemic alkalosis with hypercalciuria, is caused by mutations in the Na-K-2Cl cotransporter NKCC2. *Nat Genet* 1996, 13:183–188.

29. Simon DB, Karet FE, Rodriguez-Soriano J, *et al.*: Genetic heterogeneity of Bartter's syndrome revealed by mutations in the K+ channel, ROMK. *Nat Genet* 1996, 14:152–156.

30. International Collaborative Study Group for Bartter-like Syndromes. Mutations in the gene encoding the inwardly-rectifying renal potassium channel, ROMK, cause the antenatal variant of Bartter syndrome: evidence for genetic heterogeneity. *Hum Mol Genet* 1997, 6:17–26.

31. Simon DB, Nelson-Williams C, *et al.*: Gitelman's variant of Bartter's syndrome, inherited hypokalaemic alkalosis, is caused by mutations in the thiazide-sensitive Na-Cl cotransporter. *Nat Genet* 1996, 12:24–30.

Disorders of Phosphate Balance

Moshe Levi
Mordecai Popovtzer

The physiologic concentration of serum phosphorus (phosphate) in normal adults ranges from 2.5 to 4.5 mg/dL (0.80–1.44 mmol/L). A diurnal variation occurs in serum phosphorus of 0.6 to 1.0 mg/dL, the lowest concentration occurring between 8 AM and 11 AM. A seasonal variation also occurs; the highest serum phosphorus concentration is in the summer and the lowest in the winter. Serum phosphorus concentration is markedly higher in growing children and adolescents than in adults, and it is also increased during pregnancy [1,2].

Of the phosphorus in the body, 80% to 85% is found in the skeleton. The rest is widely distributed throughout the body in the form of organic phosphate compounds. In the extracellular fluid, including in serum, phosphorous is present mostly in the inorganic form. In serum, more than 85% of phosphorus is present as the free ion and less than 15% is protein-bound.

Phosphorus plays an important role in several aspects of cellular metabolism, including adenosine triphosphate synthesis, which is the source of energy for many cellular reactions, and 2,3-diphosphoglycerate concentration, which regulates the dissociation of oxygen from hemoglobin. Phosphorus also is an important component of phospholipids in cell membranes. Changes in phosphorus content, concentration, or both, modulate the activity of a number of metabolic pathways.

Major determinants of serum phosphorus concentration are dietary intake and gastrointestinal absorption of phosphorus, urinary excretion of phosphorus, and shifts between the intracellular and extracellular spaces. Abnormalities in any of these steps can result either in hypophosphatemia or hyperphosphatemia [3–7].

The kidney plays a major role in the regulation of phosphorus homeostasis. Most of the inorganic phosphorus in serum is ultrafilterable at the level of the glomerulus. At physiologic levels of serum phosphorus and during a normal dietary phosphorus intake, approximately 6 to 7 g/d of phosphorous is filtered by the kidney. Of that

CHAPTER

7

amount, 80% to 90% is reabsorbed by the renal tubules and the rest is excreted in the urine. Most of the filtered phosphorus is reabsorbed in the proximal tubule by way of a sodium gradient-dependent process (Na-P_i cotransport) located on the apical brush border membrane [8–10]. Recently two distinct Na-P_i cotransport proteins have been cloned from the kidney (type I and type II Na-P_i cotransport proteins). Most of the hormonal and metabolic factors that regulate renal tubular phosphate reabsorption, including alterations in dietary phosphate content and parathyroid hormone, have been shown to modulate the proximal tubular apical membrane expression of the type II Na-P_i cotransport protein [11–16].

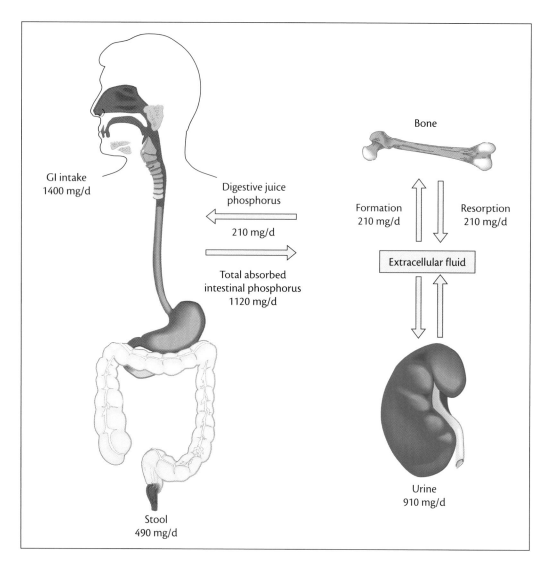

FIGURE 7-1

Summary of phosphate metabolism for a normal adult in neutral phosphate balance. Approximately 1400 mg of phosphate is ingested daily, of which 490 mg is excreted in the stool and 910 mg in the urine. The kidney, gastrointestinal (GI) tract, and bone are the major organs involved in phosphorus homeostasis.

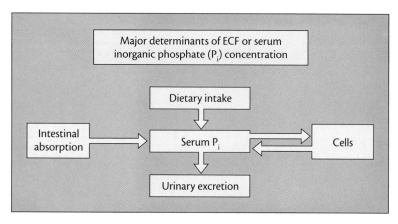

FIGURE 7-2

Major determinants of extracellular fluid or serum inorganic phosphate (P_i) concentration include dietary P_i intake, intestinal P_i absorption, urinary Pi excretion and shift into the cells.

Renal Tubular Phosphate Reabsorption

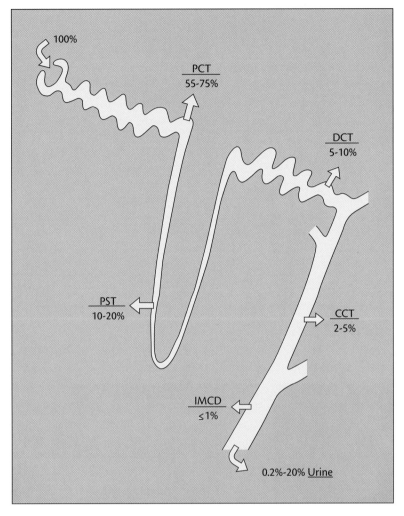

FIGURE 7-3

Renal tubular reabsorption of phosphorus. Most of the inorganic phosphorus in serum is ultrafilterable at the level of the glomerulus. At physiologic levels of serum phosphorus and during a normal dietary phosphorus intake, most of the filtered phosphorous is reabsorbed in the proximal convoluted tubule (PCT) and proximal straight tubule (PST). A significant amount of filtered phosphorus is also reabsorbed in distal segments of the nephron [7,9,10]. CCT—cortical collecting tubule; IMCD—inner medullary collecting duct or tubule; PST—proximal straight tubule.

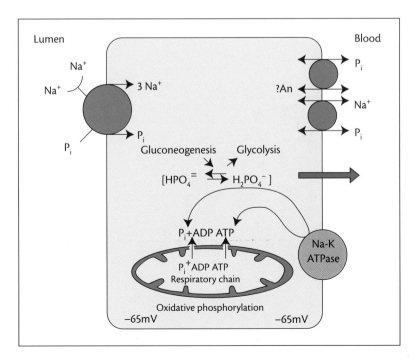

FIGURE 7-4

Cellular model for renal tubular reabsorption of phosphorus in the proximal tubule. Phosphate reabsorption from the tubular fluid is sodium gradient–dependent and is mediated by the sodium gradient–dependent phosphate transport (Na-P_i cotransport) protein located on the apical brush border membrane. The sodium gradient for phosphate reabsorption is generated by then sodium-potassium adenosine triphosphatase (Na-K ATPase) pump located on the basolateral membrane. Recent studies indicate that the Na-P_i cotransport system is electrogenic [8,11]. ADP—adenosine diphosphate; An—anion.

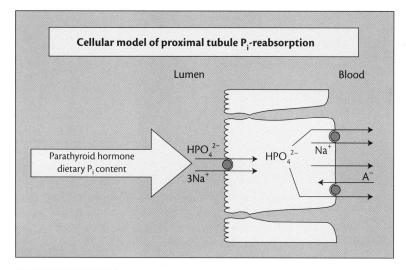

Cellular model of proximal tubule P$_i$-reabsorption

Lumen   Blood

Parathyroid hormone
dietary P$_i$ content   HPO$_4^{2-}$ HPO$_4^{2-}$ Na$^+$

                         3Na$^+$ A$^-$

FIGURE 7-5

Celluar model of proximal tubular phosphate reabsorption. Major physiologic determinants of renal tubular phosphate reabsorption are alterations in parathyroid hormone activity and alterations in dietary phosphate content. The regulation of renal tubular phosphate reabsorption occurs by way of alterations in apical membrane sodium-phosphate (Na-P$_i$) cotransport 3Na$^+$-HPO$^{2-}_4$ activity [11–14].

FACTORS REGULATING RENAL PROXIMAL TUBULAR PHOSPHATE REABSORPTION

Decreased transport	Increased transport
High phosphate diet	Low phosphate diet
Parathyroid hormone and parathyroid-hormone–related protein	Growth hormone
Glucocorticoids	Insulin
Chronic metabolic acidosis	Thyroid hormone
Acute respiratory acidosis	1,25-dihydroxy-vitamin D$_3$
Aging	Chronic metabolic alkalosis
Calcitonin	High calcium diet
Atrial natriuretic peptide	High potassium diet
Fasting	Stanniocalcin
Hypokalemia	
Hypercalcemia	
Diuretics	
Phosphatonin	

FIGURE 7-6

Factors regulating renal proximal tubular phosphate reabsorption.

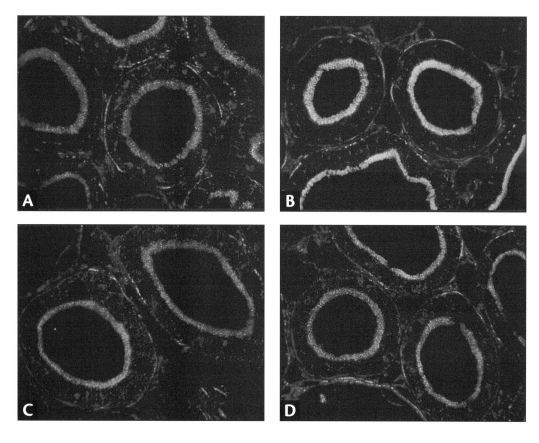

FIGURE 7-7 (*see* Color Plate)

Effects of a diet low in phosphate on renal tubular phosphate reabsorption in rats. **A,** Chronic high P$_i$ diet. **B,** Acute low P$_i$ diet. **C,** Colchicine and high P$_i$ diet. **D,** Colchicine and low P$_i$ diet. In response to a low phosphate diet, a rapid adaptive increase occurs in the sodium-phosphate (Na-P$_i$) cotransport activity of the proximal tubular apical membrane (**A, B**). The increase in Na-P$_i$ cotransport activity is mediated by rapid upregulation of the type II Na-P$_i$ cotransport protein, in the absence of changes in Na-P$_i$ messenger RNA (mRNA) levels. This rapid upregulation is dependent on an intact microtubular network because pretreatment with colchicine prevents the upregulation of Na-P$_i$ cotransport activity and Na-P$_i$ protein expression (**C, D**). In this immunofluorescence micrograph, the Na-P$_i$ protein is stained green (fluorescein) and the actin cytoskeleton is stained red (rhodamine). Colocalization of green and red at the level of the apical membrane results in yellow color [14].

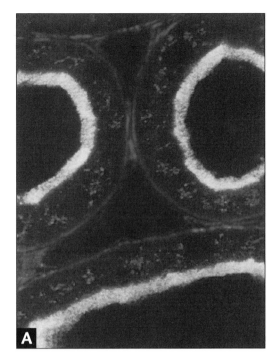
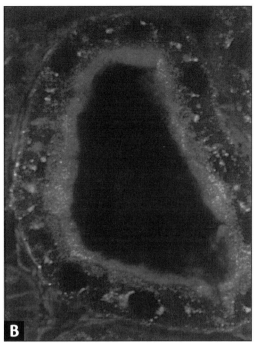

FIGURE 7-8 (*see* Color Plate)

Effects of parathyroid hormone (PTH) on renal tubular phosphate reabsorption in rats. In response to PTH administration to parathyroidectomized rats, a rapid decrease occurs in the sodium-phosphate (Na-P$_i$) cotransport activity of the proximal tubular apical membrane. The decrease in Na-P$_i$ cotransport activity is mediated by rapid downregulation of the type II Na-P$_i$ cotransport protein. In this immunofluorescence micrograph, the Na-P$_i$ protein is stained green (fluorescein) and the actin cytoskeleton is stained red (rhodamine). Colocalization of green and red at the level of the apical membrane results in yellow color [13]. **A,** parathyroidectomized (PTX) effects. **B,** effects of PTX and PTH.

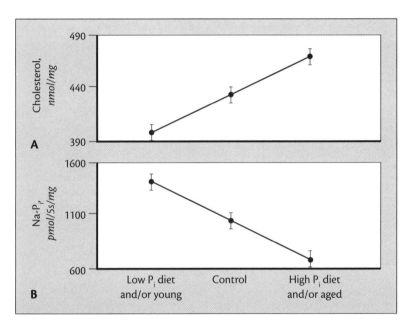

FIGURE 7-9

Renal cholesterol content modulates renal tubular phosphate reabsorption. In aged rats versus young rats and rats fed a diet high in phosphate versus a diet low in phosphate, an inverse correlation exists between the brush border membrane (BBM) cholesterol content (**A**) and Na-P$_i$ cotransport activity (**B**). Studies in isolated BBM vesicles and recent studies in opossum kidney cells grown in culture indicate that direct alterations in cholesterol content *per se* modulate Na-P$_i$ cotransport activity [15]. CON—controls.

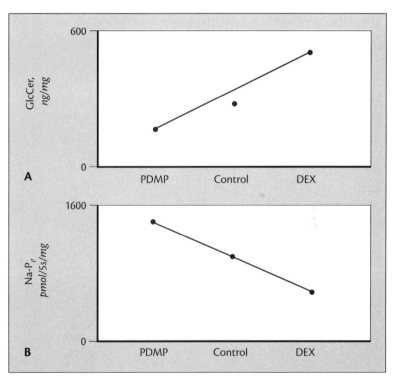

FIGURE 7-10

Renal glycosphingolipid content modulates renal tubular phosphate reabsorption. In rats treated with dexamethasone (DEX) and in rats fed a potassium-deficient diet, an inverse correlation exists between brush border membrane (BBM) glucosylceramide (GluCer)—and ganglioside GM$_3$, content and Na-P$_i$ cotransport activity. Treatment of rats with a glucosylceramide synthase inhibitor PDMP lowers BBM glucosylceramide content (**A**) and increases Na-P$_i$ cotransport activity (**B**) [16].

Hypophosphatemia/Hyperphosphatemia

MAJOR CAUSES OF HYPOPHOSPHATEMIA

Internal redistribution	Decreased intestinal absorption	Increased urinary excretion
Increased insulin, particularly during refeeding	Inadequate intake	Primary and secondary hyperparathyroidism
Acute respiratory alkalosis	Antacids containing aluminum or magnesium	Vitamin D deficiency or resistance
Hungry bone syndrome	Steatorrhea and chronic diarrhea	Fanconi's syndrome
		Miscellaneous: osmotic diuresis, proximally acting diuretics, acute volume expansion

FIGURE 7-11

Major causes of hypophosphatemia. (*From* Angus [1]; with permission.)

CAUSES OF MODERATE HYPOPHOSPHATEMIA

Pseudohypophosphatemia
  Mannitol
  Bilirubin
  Acute leukemia
Decreased dietary intake
Decreased intestinal absorption
  Vitamin D deficiency
  Malabsorption
  Steatorrhea
  Secretory diarrhea
  Vomiting
  PO_4^3-binding antacids
Shift from serum into cells
  Respiratory alkalosis
    Sepsis
    Heat stroke
    Neuroleptic malignant syndrome
    Hepatic coma
    Salicylate poisoning
    Gout
    Panic attacks
    Psychiatric depression

Hormonal effects
  Insulin
  Glucagon
  Epinephrine
  Androgens
  Cortisol
  Anovulatory hormones
Nutrient effects
  Glucose
  Fructose
  Glycerol
  Lactate
  Amino acids
  Xylitol

Cellular uptake syndromes
  Recovery from hypothermia
  Burkitt's lymphoma
  Histiocytic lymphoma
  Acute myelomonocytic leukemia
  Acute myelogenous leukemia
  Chronic myelogenous leukemia
    in blast crisis
  Treatment of pernicious anemia
  Erythropoietin therapy
  Erythrodermic psoriasis
  Hungry bone syndrome
  After parathyroidectomy
  Acute leukemia

Increased excretion into urine
  Hyperparathyroidism
  Renal tubule defects
    Fanconi's syndrome
    X-linked hypophosphatemic rickets
    Hereditary hypophosphatemic rickets
      with hypercalciuria
    Polyostotic fibrous dysphasia
    Panostotic fibrous dysphasia
    Neurofibromatosis
    Kidney transplantation
    Oncogenic osteomalacia
    Recovery from hemolytic-uremic
      syndrome
  Aldosteronism
  Licorice ingestion
  Volume expansion
  Inappropriate secretion of antidiuretic
  hormone
  Mineralocorticoid administration
  Corticosteroid therapy
  Diuretics
  Aminophylline therapy

FIGURE 7-12

Causes of moderate hypophosphatemia. (*From* Popovtzer, *et al.* [6]; with permission.)

CAUSES OF SEVERE HYPOPHOSPHATEMIA

Acute renal failure: excessive P binders

Chronic alcoholism and alcohol withdrawal

Dietary deficiency and PO_4^3-binding antacids

Hyperalimentation

Neuroleptic malignant syndrome

Recovery from diabetic ketoacidosis

Recovery from exhaustive exercise

Kidney transplantation

Respiratory alkalosis

Severe thermal burns

Therapeutic hypothermia

Reye's syndrome

After major surgery

Periodic paralysis

Acute malaria

Drug therapy

　Ifosfamide

　Cisplatin

Acetaminophen intoxication

Cytokine infusions

　Tumor necrosis factor

　Interleukin-2

FIGURE 7-13

Causes of severe hypophosphatemia. (*From* Popovtzer, *et al.* [6]; with permission.)

CAUSES OF HYPOPHOSPHATEMIA IN PATIENTS WITH NONKETOTIC HYPERGLYCEMIA OR DIABETIC KETOACIDOSIS

Decreased net intestinal phosphate absorption	Increased urinary phosphate excretion	Acute movement of extracellular phosphate into the cells
Decreased phosphate intake	Glucosuria-induced osmotic diuresis	Insulin therapy
	Acidosis	

FIGURE 7-14

Causes of hypophosphatemia in patients with nonketotic hyperglycemia or diabetic ketoacidosis.

CAUSES OF HYPOPHOSPHATEMIA IN PATIENTS WITH ALCOHOLISM

Decreased net intestinal phosphate absorption	Increased urinary phosphate excretion	Acute movement of extracellular phosphate into the cells
Poor dietary intake of phosphate and vitamin D	Alcohol-induced reversible proximal tubular defect	Insulin release induced by intravenous solutions containing dextrose
Use of phosphate binders to treat recurring gastritis	Secondary hyperparathyroidism induced by vitamin D deficiency	Acute respiratory alkalosis caused by alcohol withdrawal, sepsis, or hepatic cirrhosis
Chronic diarrhea		Refeeding of the patient who is malnourished

FIGURE 7-15

Causes of hypophosphatemia in patients with alcoholism.

CAUSES OF HYPOPHOSPHATEMIA IN PATIENTS WITH RENAL TRANSPLANTATION

Increased urinary phosphate excretion
Persistent hyperparathyroidism (hyperplasia or adenoma)
Proximal tubular defect (possibly induced by glucocorticoids, cyclosporine, or both)

FIGURE 7-16

Causes of hypophosphatemia in patients with renal transplantation.

MAJOR CONSEQUENCES OF HYPOPHOSPHATEMIA

Decreased erythrocyte 2,3-diphosphoglycerate levels, which result in increased affinity of hemoglobin for oxygen and reduced oxygen release at the tissue level

Decreased intracellular adenosine triphosphate levels, which result in impairment of cell functions dependent on energy-rich phosphate compounds

FIGURE 7-17

Major consequences of hypophosphatemia.

SIGNS AND SYMPTOMS OF HYPOPHOSPHATEMIA

Central nervous system dysfunction	Cardiac dysfunction	Pulmonary dysfunction	Skeletal and smooth muscle dysfunction	Hematologic dysfunction	Bone disease	Renal effects	Metabolic effects
Metabolic encephalopathy owing to tissue ischemia	Impaired myocardial contractility	Weakness of the diaphragm	Proximal myopathy	Erythrocytes	Increased bone resorption	Decreased glomerular filtration rate	Low parathyroid hormone levels
Irritability	Congestive heart failure	Respiratory failure	Dysphagia and ileus	Increased erythrocyte rigidity	Rickets and osteo-malacia caused by decreased bone mineralization	Decreased tubular transport maximum for bicarbonate	Increased 1,25-dihy-droxy-vitamin D_3 levels
Paresthesias			Rhabdomyolysis	Hemolysis			Increased creatinine phosphokinase levels
Confusion				Leukocytes		Decreased renal gluconeogenesis	Increased aldolase levels
Delirium				Impaired phagocytosis		Decreased titratable acid excretion	
Coma				Decreased granulocyte chemotaxis		Hypercalciuria	
				Platelets		Hypermagnesuria	
				Defective clot retraction			
				Thrombocytopenia			

FIGURE 7-18

Signs and symptoms of hypophosphatemia. (*Adapted from* Hruska and Slatopolsky [2] *and* Hruska and Gupta [7].)

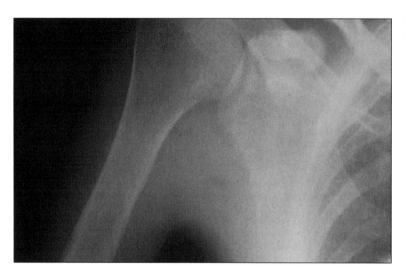

FIGURE 7-19

Pseudofractures (Looser's transformation zones) at the margins of the scapula in a patient with oncogenic osteomalacia. Similar to the genetic X-linked hypophosphatemic rickets, a circulating phospha-turic factor is believed to be released by the tumor, causing phosphate wasting and reduced calcitriol formation by the kidney. Note the radiolucent ribbonlike decalcification extending into bone at a right angle to its axillary margin. Pseudofractures are pathognomonic of osteomalacia with a low remodeling rate.

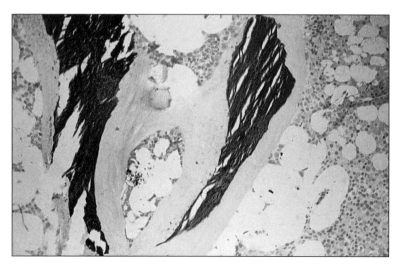

FIGURE 7-20 (*see* Color Plate)

Histologic appearance of trabecular bone from a patient with oncogenic osteomalacia. Undecalcified bone section with impaired mineralization and a wide osteoid (organic matrix) seam stained with von Kossa's stain is illustrated. Note the wide bands of osteoid around the mineralized bone. Absence of osteoblasts on the circumference of the trabecular bone portion indicates a low remodeling rate.

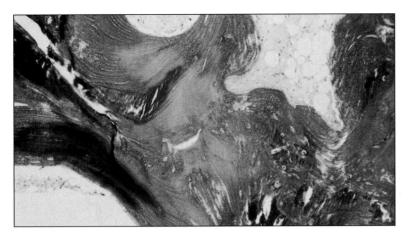

FIGURE 7-21(*see* Color Plate)

Microscopic appearance of bone section from a patient with vitamin D deficiency caused by malabsorption. The bone section was stained with Masson trichrome stain. Hypophosphatemia and hypocalcemia were present. Note the trabecular bone consisting of very wide osteoid areas (red) characteristic of osteomalacia.

USUAL DOSAGES FOR PHOSPHORUS REPLETION

Severe symptomatic hypophosphatemia (plasma phosphate concentration < 1 mg/dL)	Phosphate depletion	Hypophosphatemic rickets
10 mg/kg/d, intravenously, until the plasma phosphate concentration reaches 2 mg/dL	2–4 g/d (64 to 128 mmol/d), orally, in 3 to 4 divided doses	1–4 g/d (32 to 128 mmol/d), orally, in 3 to 4 divided doses

FIGURE 7-22

Usual dosages for phosphorus repletion.

PHOSPHATE PREPARATIONS FOR ORAL USE

Preparation	Phosphate, *mg*	Sodium, *mEq*	Potassium, *mEq*
K-Phos Neutral®, tablet (Beach Pharmaceuticals, Conestee, SC)	250	13	1.1
Neutra-Phos®, capsule or 75-mL solution (Baker Norton Pharmaceuticals, Miami, FL)	250	7.1	7.1
Neutra-Phos K®, capsule or 75-mL solution (Baker Norton Pharmaceuticals, Miami, FL)	250	0	14.2

FIGURE 7-23

Phosphate preparations for oral use.

PHOSPHATE PREPARATIONS FOR INTRAVENOUS USE

Phosphate preparation	Composition, *mg/mL*	Phosphate, *mmol/mL*	Sodium, *mEq/mL*	Potassium, *mEq/mL*
Potassium	236 mg K_2HPO_4 224 mg KH_2PO_4	3.0	0	4.4
Sodium	142 mg Na_2HPO_4 276 mg $NaH_2PO_4.H_2O$	3.0	4.0	0
Neutral sodium	10.0 mg Na_2HPO 2.7 mg $NaH_2PO_4.H_2O$	0.09	0.2	0
Neutral sodium, potassium	11.5 mg Na_2HPO_4 2.6 mg KH_2PO_4	1.10	0.2	0.02

3 mmol/mL of phosphate corresponds to 93 mg of phosphorus.

FIGURE 7-24

Phosphate preparations for intravenous use. (*From* Popovtzer, *et al.* [6]; with permission.)

CAUSES OF HYPERPHOSPHATEMIA

Pseudohyperphosphatemia
Multiple myeloma
Extreme hypertriglyceridemia
In vitro hemolysis

Increased exogenous phosphorus load or absorption
Phosphorus-rich cow's milk in premature neonates
Vitamin D intoxication
PO^3_4-containing enemas
Intravenous phosphorus supplements
White phosphorus burns
Acute phosphorus poisoning

Increased endogenous loads
Tumor lysis syndrome
Rhabdomyolysis
Bowel infarction
Malignant hyperthermia
Heat stroke
Acid-base disorders
Organic acidosis
Lactic acidosis
Ketoacidosis
Respiratory acidosis
Chronic respiratory alkalosis

Reduced urinary excretion
Renal failure
Hypoparathyroidism
Hereditary
Acquired
Pseudohypoparathyroidism
Vitamin D intoxication
Growth hormone
Insulin-like growth factor-1
Glucocorticoid withdrawal
Mg^{2+} deficiency
Tumoral calcinosis
Diphosphonate therapy
Hyopophosphatasia

Miscellaneous
Fluoride poisoning
β-Blocker therapy
Verapamil
Hemorrhagic shock
Sleep deprivation

FIGURE 7-25

Causes of hyperphosphatemia. (*From* Knochel and Agarwal [5]; with permission.)

CLINICAL MANIFESTATIONS OF HYPERPHOSPHATEMIA

Consequences of secondary changes in calcium, parathyroid hormone, vitamin D metabolism and hypocalcemia:	Consequences of ectopic calcification:
Neuromuscular irritability	Periarticular and soft tissue calcification
Tetany	Vascular calcification
Hypotension	Ocular calcification
Increased QT interval	Conduction abnormalities
	Pruritus

FIGURE 7-26

Clinical manifestations of hyperphosphatemia.

TREATMENT OF HYPERPHOSPHATEMIA

Acute hyperphosphatemia in patients with adequate renal function	Chronic hyperphosphatemia in patients with end-stage renal disease
Saline diuresis that causes phosphaturia	Dietary phosphate restriction
	Phosphate binders to decrease gastrointestinal phosphate reabsorption

FIGURE 7-27

Treatment of hyperphosphatemia.

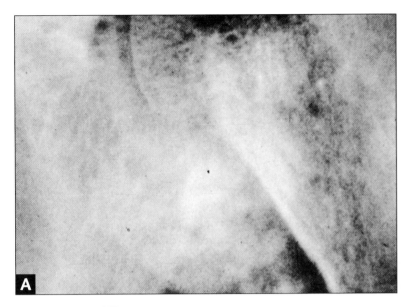

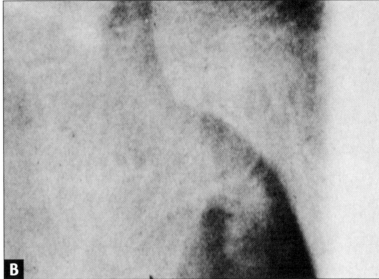

FIGURE 7-28

Periarticular calcium phosphate deposits in a patient with end-stage renal disease who has severe hyperphosphatemia and a high level of the product of calcium and phosphorus. Note the partial resolution of calcific masses after dietary phosphate restriction and oral phosphate binders. Left shoulder joint before (**A**) and after (**B**) treatment. (*From* Pinggera and Popovtzer [17]; with permission.)

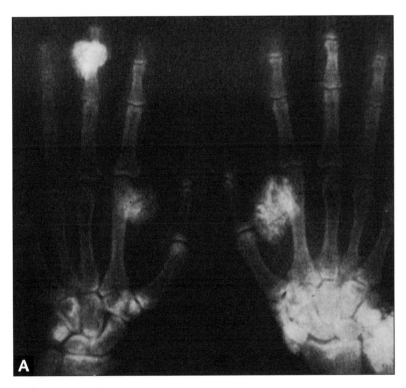

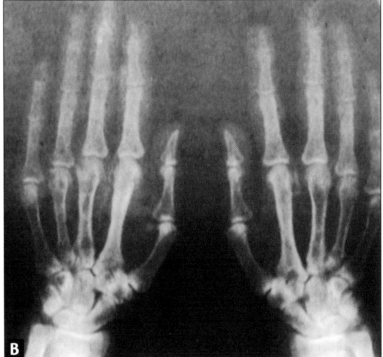

FIGURE 7-29

Resolution of soft tissue calcifications. The palms of the hands of the patient in Figure 7-28 with end-stage renal disease are shown before (**A**) and after (**B**) treatment of hyperphosphatemia. The patient has a high level of the product of calcium and phosphorus. (*From* Pinggera and Popovtzer [17]; with permission.)

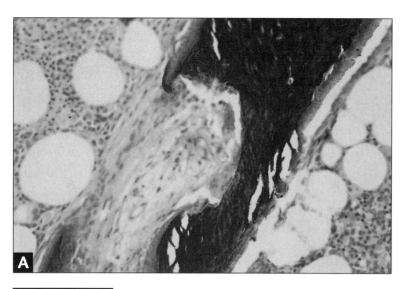
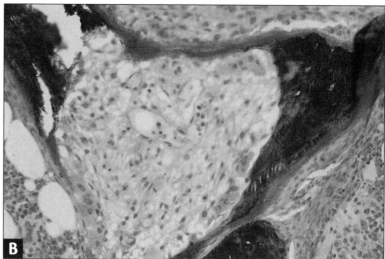

FIGURE 7-30

A, B, Bone sections from the same patient as in Figures 7-28 and 7-29, illustrating osteitis fibrosa cystica caused by renal secondary hyperparathyroidism with hyperphosphatemia.

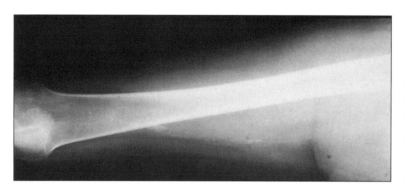

FIGURE 7-31

Roentgenographic appearance of femoral arterial vascular calcification in a patient on dialysis who has severe hyperphosphatemia. The patient has a high level of the product of calcium and phosphorus.

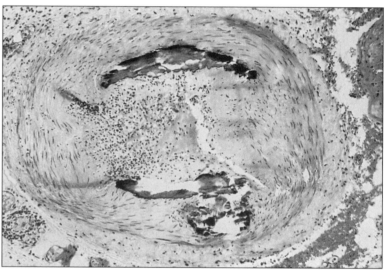

FIGURE 7-32 (*see* Color Plate)

Microscopic appearance of a cross section of a calcified artery in a patient with end-stage renal disease undergoing chronic dialysis. The patient has severe hyperphosphatemia and a high level of the product of calcium and phosphorus. Note the intimal calcium phosphate deposit with a secondary occlusion of the arterial lumen.

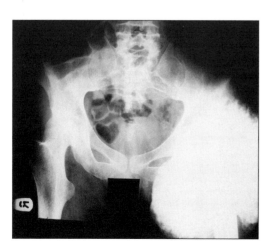

FIGURE 7-33

Massive periarticular calcium phosphate deposit (around the hip joint) in a patient with genetic tumoral calcinosis. The patient exhibits hyperphosphatemia and increased renal tubular phosphate reabsorption. Normal parathyroid hormone levels and elevated calcitriol levels are present. The same disease affects two of the patient's brothers.

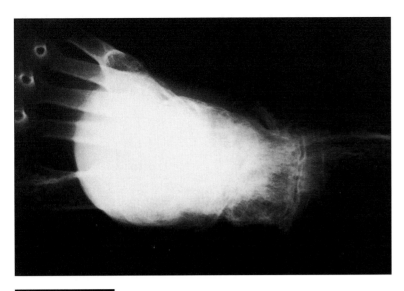

FIGURE 7-34

Massive periarticular calcium phosphate deposit in the plantar joints in the same patient in Figure 7-33 who has genetic tumoral calcinosis.

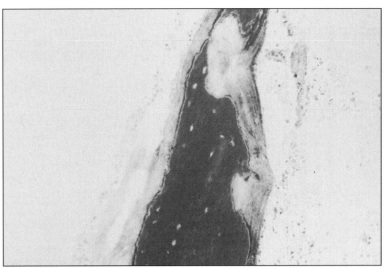

FIGURE 7-35 (*see* Color Plate)

Complications of the use of aluminum-based phosphate binders to control hyperphosphatemia. Appearance of bone section from a patient with end-stage renal disease who was treated with oral aluminum gels to control severe hyperphosphatemia. A bone biopsy was obtained 6 months after a parathyroidectomy was performed. Note the wide areas of osteoid filling previously resorbed bone.

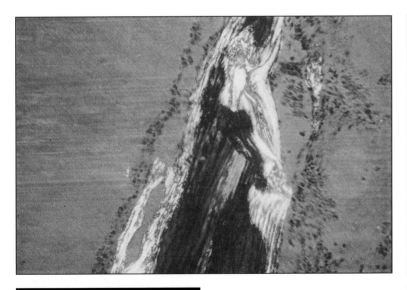

FIGURE 7-36 (*see* Color Plate)

The same bone section as in Figure 7-35 but under polarizing lenses, illustrating the partially woven appearance of osteoid typical of chronic renal failure.

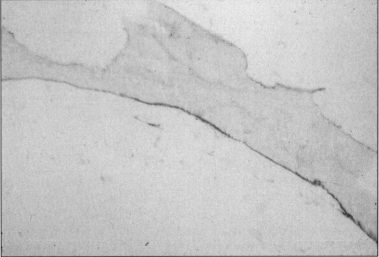

FIGURE 7-37 (*see* Color Plate)

The same bone section as in Figure 7-35 with positive aluminum stain of the trabecular surface. These findings are consistent with aluminum-related osteomalacia.

Acknowledgments

The authors thank Sandra Nickerson and Teresa Autrey for secretarial assistance and the Medical Media Department at the Dallas VA Medical Center for the illustrations.

References

1. Agus ZS: Phosphate metabolism. In *UpToDate, Inc.*. Edited by Burton D. Rose, 1998.

2. Hruska KA, Slatopolsky E: Disorders of phosphorus, calcium, and magnesium metabolism. In *Diseases of the Kidney*, edn 6. Edited by Schrier RW, Gottschalk CW. Boston: Little and Brown; 1997.

3. Levi M, Knochel JP: The management of disorders of phosphate metabolism. In *Therapy of Renal Diseases and Related Disorders*. Edited by Massry SG, Suki WN. Boston, Martinus Nijhoff; 1990.

4. Levi M, Cronin RE, Knochel JP: Disorders of phosphate and magnesium metabolism. In *Disorders of Bone and Mineral Metabolism*. Edited by Coe FL, Favus MJ. New York: Raven Press; 1992.

5. Knochel JP, Agarwal R: Hypophosphatemia and hyperphosphatemia. In *The Kidney*, edn 5. Edited by Brenner BM. Philadelphia: WB Saunders; 1996.

6. Popovtzer M, Knochel JP, Kumar R: Disorders of calcium, phosphorus, vitamin D, and parathyroid hormone activity. In *Renal Electrolyte Disorders*, edn 5. Edited by Schrier RW. Philadelphia: Lippincott-Raven; 1997.

7. Hruska K, Gupta A: Disorders of phosphate homeostasis. In *Metabolic Bone Disease*, edn 3. Edited by Avioli LV, SM Krane. New York: Academic Press; 1998.

8. Murer H, Biber J: Renal tubular phosphate transport: cellular mechanisms. In *The Kidney: Physiology and Pathophysiology*, edn 2. Edited by Seldin DW, Giebisch G. New York: Raven Press; 1997.

9. Berndt TJ, Knox FG: Renal regulation of phosphate excretion. In *The Kidney: Physiology and Pathophysiology*, edn 2. Edited by Seldin DW, Giebisch G. New York: Raven Press; 1992.

10. Suki WN, Rouse D: Renal Transport of calcium, magnesium, and phosphate. In *The Kidney*, edn 5. Edited by Brenner BM. Philadelphia: WB Saunders; 1996.

11. Levi M, Kempson, SA, Lötscher M, *et al.*: Molecular regulation of renal phosphate transport. *J Membrane Biol* 1996, 154:1–9.

12. Levi M, Lötscher M, Sorribas V, *et al.*: Cellular mechanisms of acute and chronic adaptation of rat renal phosphate transporter to alterations in dietary phosphate. *Am J Physiol* 1994, 267:F900–F908.

13. Kempson SA, Lötscher M, Kaissling B, *et al.*: Effect of parathyroid hormone on phosphate transporter mRNA and protein in rat renal proximal tubules. *Am J Physiol* 1995, 268:F784–F791.

14. Lötscher M, Biber J, Murer H, *et al.*: Role of microtubules in the rapid upregulation of rat renal proximal tubular Na-Pi cotransport following dietary P restriction. *J Clin Invest* 1997, 99:1302–1312.

15. Levi M, Baird B, Wilson P: Cholesterol modulates rat renal brush border membrane phosphate transport. *J Clin Invest* 1990, 85:231–237.

16. Levi M, Shayman J, Abe A, *et al.*: Dexamethasone modulates rat renal brush border membrane phosphate transporter mRNA and protein abundance and glycosphingolipid composition. *J Clin Invest* 1995, 96:207–216.

17. Pinggera WF, Popovtzer MM: Uremic osteodystrophy: the therapeutic consequences of effective control of serum phosphorus. *JAMA* 1972, 222:1640–1642.

Acute Renal Failure

Introduction
Joseph V. Bonventre

Acute renal failure (ARF) is a clinical syndrome characterized by a deterioration of renal function over hours to days, resulting in the failure of the kidney to excrete nitrogenous waste products and to maintain fluid and electrolyte homeostasis. ARF was established by Bywaters as a clinical entity in victims buried under collapsed buildings during World War II. In these victims, Bywaters described the histologic hallmarks of hypotensive- and pigment-induced damage to the kidney: tubular cell necrosis and intratubular pigmented casts. In the past five decades we have come to appreciate other important causes of ARF and the pathophysiologic mechanisms that underlie renal dysfunction.

Despite many developments in the treatment of critically ill patients, the introduction of various renal replacement therapies, and a more profound understanding leading to early diagnosis and prevention of many complications, ARF remains the most costly kidney or urologic condition requiring hospitalization when cost is measured by mortality as well as when measured by financial parameters. The mortality rate remains at approximately 40%, and this rate has not changed significantly over the last 40 years. While a great deal of attention has been devoted to understanding the mechanisms involved in the pathogenesis of acute renal failure, the processes responsible for cell death and organ dysfunction remain poorly understood. Various pathophysiological mechanisms have been proposed, although there is no general consensus even on issues as basic as the primary site of injury or the relative contributions of vascular and tubular components to the pathophysiology.

The kidney, in contrast to the heart or brain, has the ability to completely restore its structure and function after an ischemic or toxic insult. The repair process has been analyzed using the tools and insight of basic cellular, molecular, and developmental biology. Repair has been found to recapitulate many aspects of renal development. A number of therapeutic agents have been tried based upon animal studies and our current understanding of pathophysiology and repair. Unfortunately the results of these therapeutic trials have been disappointing. Thus, a better understanding of the disease, with better insight into pathophysiology and repair mechanisms, is critical to arrive at effective therapies.

This section presents the concepts underlying the epidemiology, etiology, diagnosis, prognosis, complications, pathophysiology, and repair mechanisms associated with acute renal failure in the form of tables and figures with minimal text. This format rivets the reader's attention to the schematics and data just as they might be in a well-presented lecture by each of the distinguished authors. The format serves as an ideal tool for the teacher who can utilize the figures and tables to effectively transmit the latest in the field. The section is useful for medical students, residents, fellows, practicing physicians, and investigators. In no other volume on ARF is so much graphical information presented in so concise a fashion.

Acute Renal Failure: Causes and Prognosis

Fernando Liaño
Julio Pascual

There are many causes—more than fifty are given within this present chapter—that can trigger pathophysiological mechanisms leading to acute renal failure (ARF). This syndrome is characterized by a sudden decrease in kidney function, with a consequence of loss of the hemostatic equilibrium of the internal medium. The primary marker is an increase in the concentration of the nitrogenous components of blood. A second marker, oliguria, is seen in 50% to 70% of cases.

In general, the causes of ARF have a dynamic behavior as they change as a function of the economical and medical development of the community. Economic differences justify the different spectrum in the causes of ARF in developed and developing countries. The setting where ARF appears (community versus hospital), or the place where ARF is treated (intensive care units [ICU] versus other hospital areas) also show differences in the causes of ARF.

While functional outcome after ARF is usually good among the surviving patients, mortality rate is high: around 45% in general series and close to 70% in ICU series. Although it is unfortunate that these mortality rates have remained fairly constant over the past decades, it should be noted that today's patients are generally much older and display a generally much more severe condition than was true in the past. These age and severity factors, together with the more aggressive therapeutical possibilities presently available, could account for this apparent paradox.

As is true for any severe clinical condition, a prognostic estimation of ARF is of great utility for both the patients and their families, the medical specialists (for analysis of therapeutical maneuvers and options), and for society in general (demonstrating the monetary costs of treatment). This chapter also contains a brief review of the prognostic tools available for application to ARF.

CHAPTER

8

Causes of Acute Renal Failure

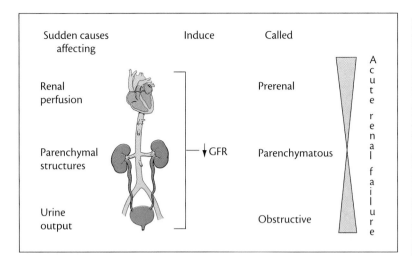

FIGURE 8-1

Characteristics of acute renal failure. Acute renal failure is a syndrome characterized by a sudden decrease of the glomerular filtration rate (GFR) and consequently an increase in blood nitrogen products (blood urea nitrogen and creatinine). It is associated with oliguria in about two thirds of cases. Depending on the localization or the nature of the renal insult, ARF is classified as prerenal, parenchymatous, or obstructive (postrenal).

CAUSES OF PRERENAL ACUTE RENAL FAILURE

Decreased effective extracellular volume

Renal losses: hemorrhage, vomiting, diarrhea, burns, diuretics

Redistribution: hepatopathy, nephrotic syndrome, intestinal obstruction, pancreatitis, peritonitis, malnutrition

Decreased cardiac output: cardiogenic shock, valvulopathy, myocarditis, myocardial infarction, arrhythmia, congestive heart failure, pulmonary emboli, cardiac tamponade

Peripheral vasodilation: hypotension, sepsis, hypoxemia, anaphylactic shock, treatment with interleukin L2 or interferons, ovarian hyperstimulation syndrome

Renal vasoconstriction: prostaglandin synthesis inhibition, α-adrenergics, sepsis, hepatorenal syndrome, hypercalcemia

Efferent arteriole vasodilation: converting-enzyme inhibitors

FIGURE 8-2

Causes of prerenal acute renal failure (ARF). *Prerenal* ARF, also known as prerenal uremia, supervenes when glomerular filtration rate falls as a consequence of decreased effective renal blood supply. The condition is reversible if the underlying disease is resolved.

CAUSES OF PARENCHYMATOUS ACUTE RENAL FAILURE

Acute tubular necrosis

Hemodynamic: cardiovascular surgery,* sepsis,* prerenal causes*

Toxic: antimicrobials,* iodide contrast agents,* anesthesics, immunosuppressive or antineoplastic agents,* Chinese herbs, Opiaceous, Extasis, mercurials, organic solvents, venoms, heavy metals, mannitol, radiation

Intratubular deposits: acute uric acid nephropathy, myeloma, severe hypercalcemia, primary oxalosis, sulfadiazine, fluoride anesthesics

Organic pigments (endogenous nephrotoxins):

Myoglobin rhabdomyolisis: muscle trauma; infections; dermatopolymyositis; metabolic alterations; hyperosmolar coma; diabetic ketoacidosis; severe hypokalemia; hyper- or hyponatremia; hypophosphatemia; severe hypothyroidism; malignant hyperthermia; toxins such as ethylene glycol, carbon monoxide, mercurial chloride, stings; drugs such as fibrates, statins, opioids and amphetamines; hereditary diseases such as muscular dystrophy, metabolopathies, McArdle disease and carnitine deficit

Hemoglobinuria: malaria; mechanical destruction of erythrocytes with extracorporeal circulation or metallic prosthesis, transfusion reactions, or other hemolysis; heat stroke; burns; glucose-6-phosphate dehydrogenase; nocturnal paroxystic hemoglobinuria; chemicals such as aniline, quinine, glycerol, benzene, phenol, hydralazine; insect venoms

Acute tubulointerstitial nephritis (*see* Fig. 8-4)

Vascular occlusion

Principal vessels: bilateral (unilateral in solitary functioning kidney) renal artery thrombosis or embolism, bilateral renal vein thrombosis

Small vessels: atheroembolic disease, thrombotic microangiopathy, hemolytic-uremic syndrome or thrombotic thrombocytopenic purpura, postpartum acute renal failure, antiphospholipid syndrome, disseminated intravascular coagulation, scleroderma, malignant arterial hypertension, radiation nephritis, vasculitis

Acute glomerulonephritis

Postinfectious: streptococcal or other pathogen associated with visceral abscess, endocarditis, or shunt

Henoch-Schonlein purpura

Essential mixed cryoglobulinemia

Systemic lupus erythematosus

ImmunoglobulinA nephropathy

Mesangiocapillary

With antiglomerular basement membrane antibodies with lung disease (Goodpasture is syndrome) or without it

Idiopathic, rapidly progressive, without immune deposits

Cortical necrosis, abruptio placentae, septic abortion, disseminated intravascular coagulation

FIGURE 8-3

Causes of parenchymal acute renal failure (ARF). When the sudden decrease in glomerular filtration rate that characterizes ARF is secondary to intrinsic renal damage mainly affecting tubules, interstitium, glomeruli and/or vessels, we are facing a *parenchymatous ARF*. Multiple causes have been described, some of them constituting the most frequent ones are marked with an asterisk.

MOST FREQUENT CAUSES OF ACUTE TUBULOINTERSTITIAL NEPHRITIS

Antimicrobials
  Penicillin
  Ampicillin
  Rifampicin
  Sulfonamides
Analgesics, anti-inflammatories
  Fenoprofen
  Ibuprofen
  Naproxen
  Amidopyrine
  Glafenine
Other drugs
  Cimetidine
  Allopurinol

Immunological
  Systemic lupus erythematosus
  Rejection
  Infections (at present quite rare)
Neoplasia
  Myeloma
  Lymphoma
  Acute leukemia
Idiopathic
  Isolated
  Associated with uveitis

FIGURE 8-4

Most common causes of tubulointerstitial nephritis. During the last years, acute tubulointerstitial nephritis is increasing in importance as a cause of acute renal failure. For decades infections were the most important cause. At present, antimicrobials and other drugs are the most common causes.

CAUSES OF OBSTRUCTIVE ACUTE RENAL FAILURE

Congenital anomalies
  Ureterocele
  Bladder diverticula
  Posterior urethral valves
  Neurogenic bladder
Acquired uropathies
  Benign prostatic hypertrophy
  Urolithiasis
  Papillary necrosis
  Iatrogenic ureteral ligation
Malignant diseases
  Prostate
  Bladder
  Urethra
  Cervix
  Colon
  Breast (metastasis)

Retroperitoneal fibrosis
  Idiopathic
  Associated with
    aortic aneurysm
  Trauma
  Iatrogenic
  Drug-induced
Gynecologic non-neoplastic
  Pregnancy-related
  Uterine prolapse
  Endometriosis
Acute uric acid nephropathy
Drugs
  ε-Aminocaproic acid
  Sulfonamides

Infections
  Schistosomiasis
  Tuberculosis
  Candidiasis
  Aspergillosis
  Actinomycosis
Other
  Accidental urethral
  catheter occlusion

FIGURE 8-5

Causes of obstructive acute renal failure. Obstruction at any level of the urinary tract frequently leads to acute renal failure. These are the most frequent causes.

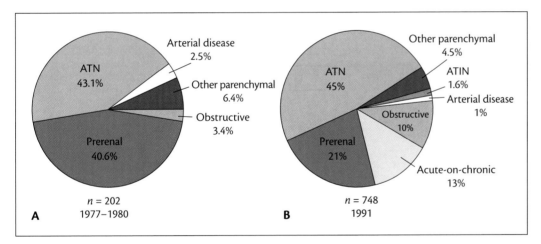

A *n* = 202 1977–1980

B *n* = 748 1991

FIGURE 8-6

This figure shows a comparison of the percentages of the different types of acute renal failure (ARF) in a western European country in 1977–1980 and 1991: **A**, distribution in a typical Madrid hospital; **B**, the Madrid ARF Study [1]. There are two main differences: 1) the appearance of a new group in 1991, "acute on chronic ARF," in which only mild forms (serum creatinine concentrations between 1.5 and 3.0 mg/dL) were considered, for methodological reasons; 2) the decrease in prerenal ARF suggests improved medical care. This low rate of prerenal ARF has been observed by other workers in an intensive care setting [2]. The other types of ARF remain unchanged.

FIGURE 8-7

Incidences of different forms of acute renal failure (ARF) in the Madrid ARF Study [1]. Figures express cases per million persons per year with 95% confidence intervals (CI).

FINDINGS OF THE MADRID STUDY

Condition	Incidence (per million persons per year)	95% CI
Acute tubular necrosis	88	79–97
Prerenal acute renal failure	46	40–52
Acute on chronic renal failure	29	24–34
Obstructive acute renal failure	23	19–27
Glomerulonephritis (primary or secondary)	6.3	4.8–8.3
Acute tubulointerstitial nephritis	3.5	1.7–5.3
Vasculitis	3.5	1.7–5.3
Other vascular acute renal failure	2.1	0.8–3.4
Total	209	195–223

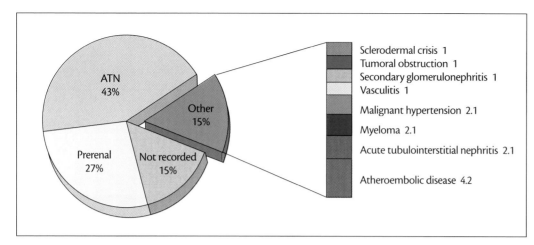

FIGURE 8-8

The most frequent causes of acute renal failure (ARF) in patients with preexisting chronic renal failure are acute tubular necrosis (ATN) and prerenal failure. The distribution of causes of ARF in these patients is similar to that observed in patients without previous kidney diseases. (*Data from* Liaño *et al.* [1])

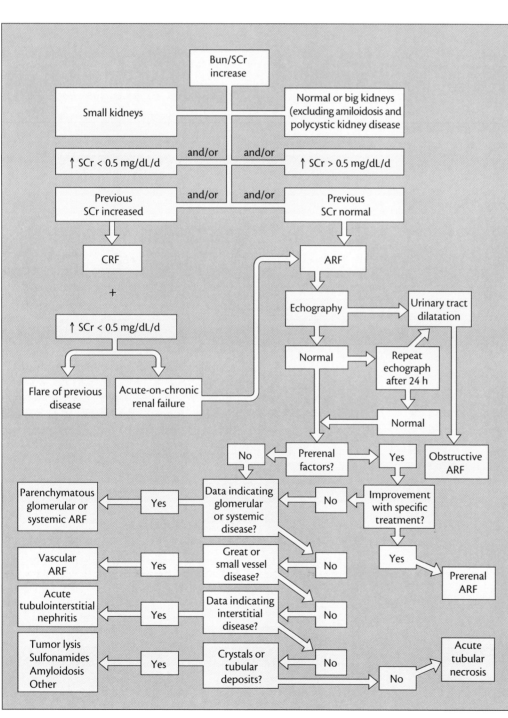

FIGURE 8-9

Discovering the cause of acute renal failure (ARF). This is a great challenge for clinicians. This algorithm could help to determine the cause of the increase in blood urea nitrogen (BUN) or serum creatinine (SCr) in a given patient.

BIOPSY RESULTS IN THE MADRID STUDY

Disease	Patients, n
Primary GN	12
Extracapillary	6
Acute proliferative	3
Endocapillary and extracapillary	2
Focal sclerosing	1
Secondary GN	6
Antiglomerular basement membrane	3
Acute postinfectious	2
Diffuse proliferative (systemic lupus erythematosus)	1*
Vasculitis	10
Necrotizing	5*
Wegener's granulomatosis	3
Not specified	2
Acute tubular necrosis	4*
Acute tubulointerstitial nephritis	4
Atheroembolic disease	2
Kidney myeloma	2*
Cortical necrosis	1
Malignant hypertension	1
ImmunoglobulinA GN + ATN	1
Hemolytic-uremic syndrome	1
Not recorded	2

* One patient with acute-on-chronic renal failure.

FIGURE 8-10

Biopsy results in the Madrid acute renal failure (ARF) study. Kidney biopsy has had fluctuating roles in the diagnostic work-up of ARF. After extrarenal causes of ARF are excluded, the most common cause is acute tubular necrosis (ATN). Patients with well-established clinical and laboratory features of ATN receive no benefit from renal biopsy. This histologic tool should be reserved for parenchymatous ARF cases when there is no improvement of renal function after 3 weeks' evolution of ARF. By that time, most cases of ATN have resolved, so other causes could be influencing the poor evolution. Biopsy is mandatory when a potentially treatable cause is suspected, such as vasculitis, systemic disease, or glomerulonephritis (GN) in adults. Some types of parenchymatous non-ATN ARF might have histologic confirmation; however kidney biopsy is not strictly necessary in cases with an adequate clinical diagnosis such as myeloma, uric acid nephropathy, or some types of acute tubulointerstitial nephritis . Other parenchymatous forms of ARF can be accurately diagnosed without a kidney biopsy. This is true of acute post-streptococcal GN and of hemolytic-uremic syndrome in children. Kidney biopsy was performed in only one of every 16 ARF cases in the Madrid ARF Study [1]. All patients with primary GN, 90% with vasculitis and 50% with secondary GN were diagnosed by biopsy at the time of ARF. As many as 15 patients were diagnosed as having acute tubulointerstitial nephritis, but only four (27%) were biopsied. Only four of 337 patients with ATN (1.2%) underwent biopsy. (*Data from* Liaño *et al.* [1].)

Predisposing Factors for Acute Renal Failure

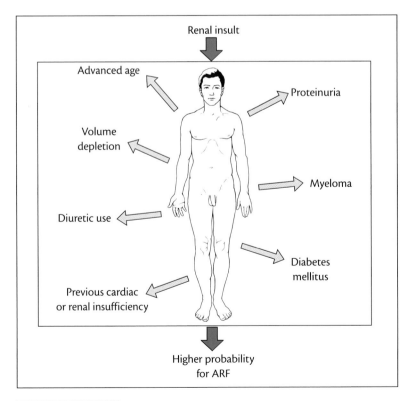

FIGURE 8-11

Factors that predispose to acute renal failure (ARF). Some of them act synergistically when they occur in the same patient. Advanced age and volume depletion are particularly important.

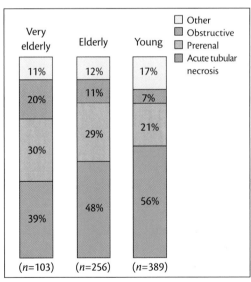

FIGURE 8-12

Causes of acute renal failure (ARF) relative to age. Although the cause of ARF is usually multifactorial, one can define the cause of each case as the most likely contributor to impairment of renal function. One interesting approach is to distribute the causes of ARF according to age. This figure shows the main causes of ARF, dividing a population diagnosed with ARF into the very elderly (at least 80 years), elderly (65 to 79), and young (younger than 65). Essentially, acute tubular necrosis (ATN) is less frequent (*P*=0.004) and obstructive ARF more frequent (*P*<0.001) in the very old than in the youngest patients. Prerenal diseases appear with similar frequency in the three age groups. (*Data from* Pascual *et al.* [3].)

Epidemiology of Acute Renal Failure

EPIDEMIOLOGY OF ACUTE RENAL FAILURE

Investigator, Year	Country (City)	Study Period (Study Length)	Study Population (millions)	Incidence (pmp/y)
Eliahou et al., 1973 [4]	Israel	1965–1966 (2 yrs)	2.2	52
Abraham et al., 1989 [5]	Kuwait	1984–1986 (2 yrs)	0.4	95
McGregor et al., 1992 [6]	United Kingdom (Glasgow)	1986–1988 (2 yrs)	0.94	185
Sanchez et al., 1992 [7]	Spain (Cuenca)	1988–1989 (2 yrs)	0.21	254
Feest et al., 1993 [8]	United Kingdom (Bristol and Devon)	1986–1987 (2 yrs)	0.44	175
Madrid ARF Study Group, 1996 [1]	Spain (Madrid)	1991–1992 (9 mo)	4.23	209

FIGURE 8-13

Prospective studies. Prospective epidemiologic studies of acute renal failure (ARF) in large populations have not often been published . The first study reported by Eliahou and colleagues [4] was developed in Israel in the 1960s and included only Jewish patients. This summary of available data suggests a progressive increase in ARF incidence that at present seems to have stabilized around 200 cases per million population per year (pmp/y). No data about ARF incidence are available from undeveloped countries.

EPIDEMIOLOGY OF ACUTE RENAL FAILURE: NEED OF DIALYSIS

Investigator, Year	Country	Cases (pmp/y)
Lunding et al., 1964 [9]	Scandinavia	28
Eliahou et al., 1973 [4]	Israel	17*
Lachhein et al., 1978 [10]	West Germany	30
Wing et al., 1983 [11]	European Dialysis and Transplant Association	29
Wing et al., 1983 [11]	Spain	59
Abraham et al., 1989 [5]	Kuwait	31
Sanchez et al., 1992 [7]	Spain	21†
McGregor et al., 1992 [6]	United Kingdom	31
Gerrard et al., 1992 [12]	United Kingdom	71
Feest et al., 1993 [8]	United Kingdom	22†
Madrid ARF Study Group [1]	Spain	57

* Very restrictive criteria.
† Only secondary care facilities.

FIGURE 8-14

Number of patients needing dialysis for acute renal failure (ARF), expressed as cases per million population per year (pmp/y). This has been another way of assessing the incidence of the most severe cases of ARF. Local situations, mainly economics, have an effect on dialysis facilities for ARF management. In 1973 Israeli figures showed a lower rate of dialysis than other countries at the same time. The very limited access to dialysis in developing countries supports this hypothesis. At present, the need for dialysis in a given area depends on the level of health care offered there. In two different countries (eg, the United Kingdom and Spain) the need for dialysis for ARF was very much lower when only secondary care facilities were available. At this level of health care, both countries had the same rate of dialysis. The Spanish data of the EDTA-ERA Registry in 1982 gave a rate of dialysis for ARF of 59 pmp/y. This rate was similar to that found in the Madrid ARF Study 10 years later. These data suggest that, when a certain economical level is achieved, the need of ARF patients for dialysis tends to stabilize.

HISTORICAL PATTERNS OF ACUTE RENAL FAILURE

	Proportion of Cases, %				
	France 1973	India 1965–1974	France 1981–1986	India 1981–1986	South Africa 1986–1988
Surgical	46	11	30	30	8
Medical	30	67	70	61	77
Obstetric	24	22	2	9	15

FIGURE 8-15

Historical perspective of acute renal failure (ARF) patterns in France, India, and South Africa. In the 1960s and 1970s, obstetrical causes were a great problem in both France and India and overall incidences of ARF were similar. Surgical cases were almost negligible in India at that time, probably because of the relative unavailability of hospital facilities. During the 1980s surgical and medical causes were similar in both countries. In India, the increase in surgical cases may be explained by advances in health care, so that more surgical procedures could be done. The decrease in surgical cases in France, despite the fact that surgery had become very sophisticated, could be explained by better management of surgical patients.

(Legend continued on next page)

FIGURE 8-15 *(Continued)*

Changes in classification criteria—inclusion of a larger percentage of medical cases than a decade before—could be an alternative explanation. In addition, obstetric cases had almost disappeared in France in the 1980s, but they were still an important cause of ARF in India. In a South African study that excluded the white population the distribution of ARF causes was almost identical to that observed in India 20 years earlier. In conclusion, 1) the economic level of a country determines the spectrum of ARF causes observed; 2) when a developing country improves its economic situation, the spectrum moves toward that observed in developed countries; and 3) great differences can be detected in ARF causes among developing countries, depending on their individual economic power. (*Data from* Kleinknecht [13]; Chugh *et al*. [14]; Seedat *et al*. [15].)

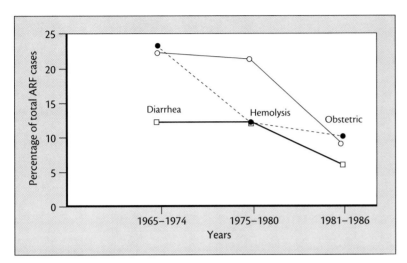

FIGURE 8-16

Changing trends in the causes of acute renal failure (ARF) in the Third-World countries. Trends can be identified from the analysis of medical and obstetric causes by the Chandigarh Study [14]. Chugh and colleagues showed how obstetric (septic abortion) and hemolytic (mainly herbicide toxicity) causes tended to decrease as economic power and availability of hospitalization improved with time. These causes of ARF, however, did not completely disappear. By contrast, diarrheal causes of ARF, such as cholera and other gastrointestinal diseases, remained constant. In conclusion, gastrointestinal causes of ARF will remain important in ARF until structural and sanitary measures (*eg*, water treatment) are implemented. Educational programs and changes in gynecological attention, focused on controlled medical abortion and contraceptive measures, should be promoted to eradicate other forms of ARF that constitute a plague in Third World countries.

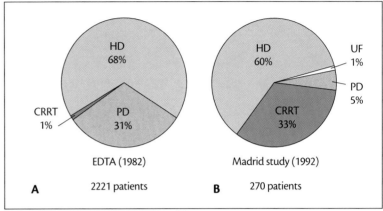

FIGURE 8-17

Evolution of dialysis techniques for acute renal failure (ARF) in Spain. **A,** The percentages of different modalities of dialysis performed in Spain in the early 1980s. **B,** The same information obtained a decade. At this latter time, 90% of conventional hemodialysis (HD) was performed using bicarbonate as a buffer. These rates are those of a developed country. In developing countries, dialysis should be performed according to the available facilities and each individual doctor's experience in the different techniques. PD—peritoneal dialysis; CRRT—continuous renal replacement technique; UF—isolated ultrafiltration. (**A,** *Data from* the EDTA-ERA Registry [11]; **B** *data from* the Madrid ARF Study [1].)

Hospital-Related Epidemiologic Data

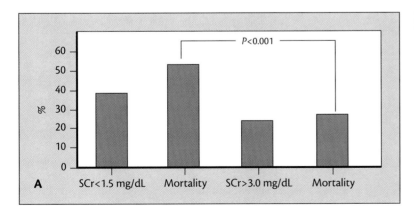

FIGURE 8-18

Serum creatinine (SCr) at hospital admission has diagnostic and prognostic implications for acute renal failure (ARF). **A,** Of the patients included in an ARF epidemiologic study 39% had a normal SCr concentration (less than 1.5 mg/dL) at hospital admission. It is worth noting that only 22% of the patients had clearly established ARF (SCr greater than 3 mg/dL) when admitted (no acute-on-chronic case was included). Mortality was significantly higher in patients with normal SCr at admission.

(Continued on next page)

ARF	Community-acquired (SCr at admission>3 mg/dL)	Hospital-acquired (SCr at admission<1.5 mg/dL)
ATN	41.8	58.2
Prerenal	47.5	52.5
Obstructive	77.3	22.7
Total	49.7	50.3

B

FIGURE 8-18 (*Continued*)

B, With the same two groups, acute tubular necrosis (ATN) predominated among the hospital-induced ARF group, whereas the obstructive form was the main cause of community-acquired ARF. In conclusion, the hospital could be considered an ARF generator, particularly of the most severe forms. Nonetheless, these iatrogenic ARF cases are usually "innocent," and are an unavoidable consequence of diagnostic and therapeutic maneuvers. (*Data from* Liaño et al. [1].)

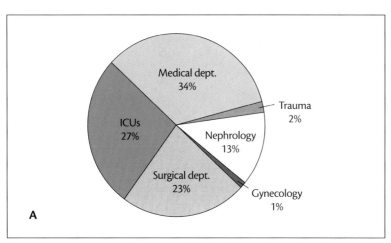

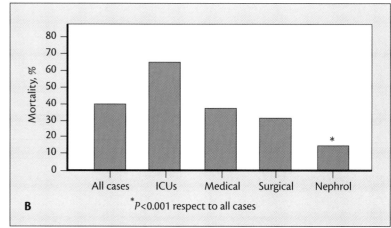

FIGURE 8-19

Acute renal failure: initial hospital location and mortality. **A**, Initial departmental location of ARF patients in a hospital in a Western country. The majority of the cases initially were seen in medical, surgical, and intensive care units (ICUs). The cases initially treated in nephrology departments were community acquired, whereas the ARF patients in the other settings generally acquired ARF in those settings. Obstetric-gynecologic ARF cases have almost disappeared. ARF of traumatic origin is also rare, for two reasons: 1) polytrauma patients are now treated in the ICU and 2) early and effective treatments applied today to trauma patients at the accident scene, and quick transfer to hospital, have decreased this cause of ARF. **B**, Mortality was greater for patients initially treated in the ICU and lower in the nephrology setting than rates observed in other departments. These figures were obtained from 748 ARF patients admitted to 13 different adult hospitals. (*Data from* Liaño et al. [1].)

EPIDEMIOLOGIC VARIABLES

Investigator, Year	Acute Renal Failure in Hospitalized Patients (per 1000 admissions)
Hou et al., 1983*	49.0
Shusterman et al., 1987*	19.0
Lauzurica et al., 1989*	
First period	16.0
Second period	6.5
Abraham et al., 1989	1.3
Madrid Study, 1992	1.5

* Case-control studies.

FIGURE 8-20

Epidemiologic variable. The incidence of hospital-acquired acute renal failure (ARF) depends on what epidemiologic method is used. In case-control studies the incidence varied between 49 and 19 per thousand. When the real occurrence was measured in large populations over longer intervals, the incidence of hospital-acquired ARF decreased to 1.5 per thousand admissions. (*Data from* [1,5,16,17,18].)

Prognosis

HISTORICAL PERSPECTIVE OF MEDICAL PROGNOSIS APPLIED IN ACUTE RENAL FAILURE

Criteria	Derivation	Applications	Advantages	Drawbacks
Classical	Doctor's experience	Individual prognosis	Easy	Doctor's inexperience Unmeasurable
Traditional	Univariate statistical analysis	Risk stratification	Easy	Only one determinant of prognosis is considered
Present	Multivariate statistical analysis Computing facilities	Risk stratification Individual prognosis?	Measurable Theoretically, "all" factors influencing outcome are considered	Complexity (variable, depending on model)
Future	Multivariate analysis Computing facilities	Risk stratification Individual prognosis Patient's quality of life evaluation Functional prediction	Measurable "All" factors considered	Ideally, none

FIGURE 8-21

Estimating prognosis. The criteria for estimating prognosis in acute renal failure can be classified into four periods. The *Classical* or heuristic way is similar to that used since the Hippocratic aphorisms. The *Traditional* one based on simple statistical procedures, is not useful for individual prognosis. The *Present* form is more or less complex, depending on what method is used, and it is possible, thanks to computing facilities and the development of multivariable analysis. Theoretically, few of these methods can give an individual prognosis [19]. They have not been used for triage. The next step will need a great deal of work to design and implement adequate tools to stratify risks and individual prognosis. In addition, the estimate of residual renal function and survivors' quality of life, mainly for older people, are future challenges.

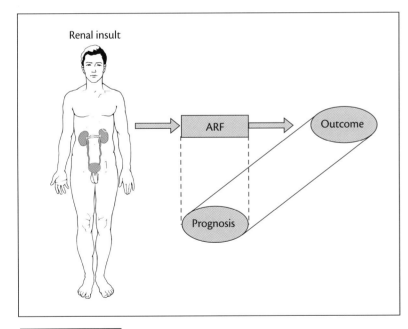

FIGURE 8-22

Ideally, prognosis should be established as the problem, the episode of acute renal failure (ARF), starts. Correct prognostic estimation gives the real outcome for a patient or group of patients as precisely as possible. In this ideal scenario, this fact is illustrated by giving the same surface area for the concepts of outcome and prognosis.

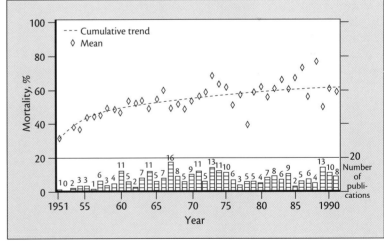

FIGURE 8-23

Mortality trends in acute renal failure (ARF). This figure shows the evolution of mortality during a 40-year period, starting in 1951. The graphic was elaborated after reviewing the outcome of 32,996 ARF patients reported in 258 published papers. As can be appreciated, mortality rate increases slowly but constantly during this follow-up, despite theoretically better availability of therapeutic armamentarium (mainly antibiotics and vasoactive drugs), deeper knowledge of dialysis techniques, and wider access to intensive care facilities. This improvement in supporting measures allows the physician to keep alive, for longer periods of time patients who otherwise would have died. A complementary explanation could be that the patients treated now are usually older, sicker, and more likely to be treated more aggressively. (*From* Kierdorf *et al.* [20]; with permission.)

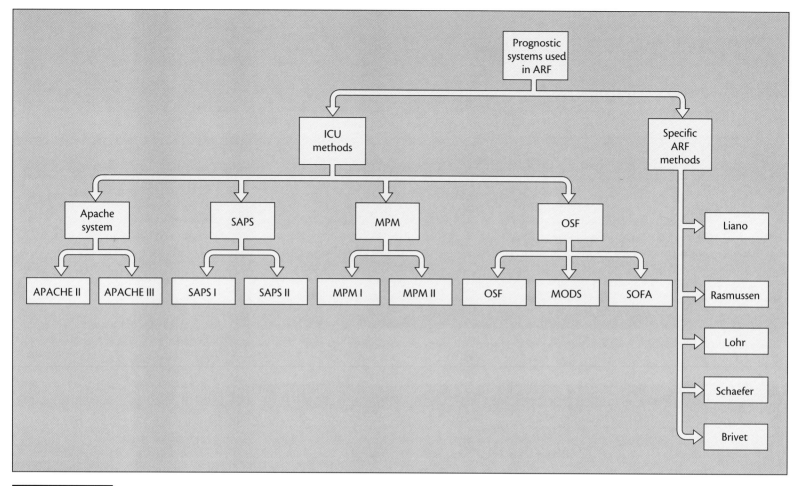

FIGURE 8-24

Ways of estimating prognosis in acute renal failure (ARF). This can be done using either general intensive care unit (ICU) score systems or methods developed specifically for ARF patients. ICU systems include Acute Physiological and Chronic Health Evaluation (APACHE) [21,22], Simplified Physiologic Score (SAPS)[23,24], Mortality Prediction Model (MPM) [25,26], and Organ System Failure scores (OSF) [27]. Multiple Organ Dysfunction Score (MODS) [28] and

Sepsis-Related Organ Failure Assessment Score (SOFA) [29] are those that seem most suitable for this purpose. APACHE II used to be most used. Other systems (white boxes) have been used in ARF.
On the other hand, at least 17 specific ARF prognostic methods have been developed [20,30]. The figure shows only those that have been used after their publication [31], plus one recently published system which is not yet in general use [2].

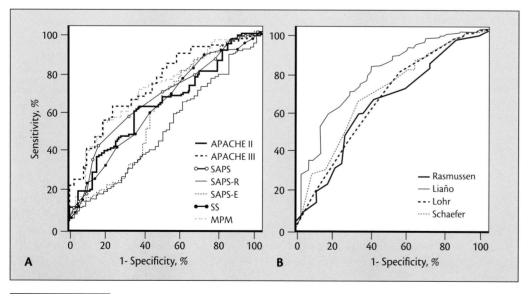

FIGURE 8-25

Comparison of prognostic methods for acute renal failure (ARF) by ROC curve analysis [31]. A method is better when its ROC-curve moves to the upper left square determined by the sensitivity and the reciprocal of the specificity. **A,** ROC curves of seven

prognostic methods usually employed in the ICU setting. The best curve comes from the APACHE III method, which has an area under the ROC curve of 0.74 ± 0.04 (SE). **B,** Four ROC curves corresponding to prognostic methods specifically developed for ARF patients are depicted. The best curve in this panel comes from the Liaño method for ARF prognosis. Its area under the curve is 0.78 ± 0.03 (SE). APACHE—Acute Physiology and Chronic Health Evaluation, (II second version [21]; III third version [22]); SAPS—Simplified Acute Physiology Score [23]; SAPS-R— SAPS-reduced [33]; SAPS-E—SAPS- Extended [32]; SS—Sickness Score [33]; MPM—Mortality Prediction Model [25]; ROC curve—Receiving Operating Characteristic curve; SE—Standard Error. (*From* Douma [31]; with permission.)

ACUTE RENAL FAILURE: VARIABLES STUDIED WITH UNIVARIATE ANALYSIS

Age	Hypotension
Jaundice	Catabolism
Sepsis	Hemolysis
Burns	Hepatic disease
Trauma	Kind of surgery
NSAIDs	Hyperkalemia
BUN increments	Need for dialysis
Coma	Assisted respiration
Oliguria	Site of war injuries
Obstetric origin	Disseminated intravascular coagulopathy
Malignancies	Pancreatitis
Cardiovascular disease	Antibiotics
X-ray contrast agents	Timing of treatment
Acidosis	

FIGURE 8-26

Individual factors that have been associated with acute renal failure (ARF) outcome. Most of these innumerable variables have been related to an adverse outcome, whereas few (nephrotoxicity as a cause of ARF and early treatment) have been associated with more favorable prognosis. For a deep review of variables studied with univariate statistical analysis [34, 35]. NSAID—nonsteroidal anti-inflammatory drugs; BUN—blood urea nitrogen.

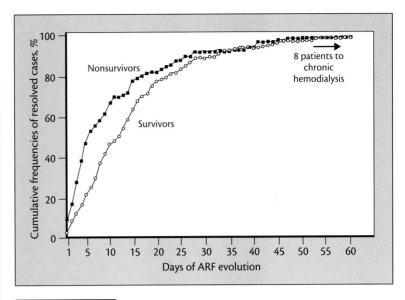

FIGURE 8-27

Duration and resolution of acute renal failure (ARF). Most of the episodes of ARF resolved in the first month of evolution. Mean duration of ARF was 14 days. Seventy-eight percent of the patients with ARF who died did so within 2 weeks after the renal insult. Similarly, 60% of survivors had recovered renal function at that time. After 30 days, 90% of the patients had had a final resolution of the ARF episode, one way or the other. Patients who finally lost renal function and needed to be included in a chronic periodic dialysis program usually had severe forms of glomerulonephritis, vasculitis, or systemic disease. (*From* Liaño *et al.* [1]; with permission.)

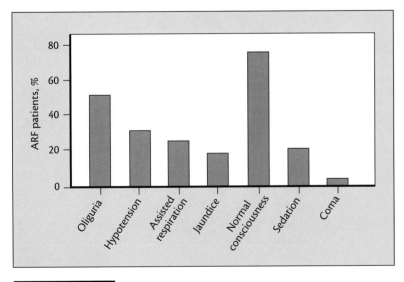

FIGURE 8-28

Precipitating condition of acute renal failure (ARF). The initial clinical condition observed in ARF patients is shown. *Oliguria*: urine output of less than 400 mL per day; *hypotension*: systolic blood pressure lower than 100 mm Hg for at least 10 hours per day independent of the use of vasoactive drugs; *jaundice*: serum bilirubin level higher than 2 mg/dL; *coma*: Glasgow coma score of 5 or less. The presence of these factors is associated with poorer outcome (*see* Fig. 8-29). (*Data from* Liaño *et al.* [1].)

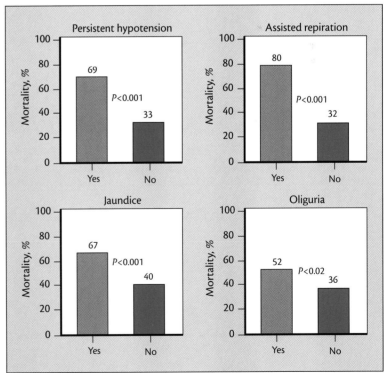

FIGURE 8-29

Mortality associated with the presence or absence of oliguria, persistent hypotension, assisted respiration and jaundice (as defined in Fig. 8-28). The presence of an unfavorable factor was significantly associated with higher mortality. (*Data from* Liaño *et al.* [1].)

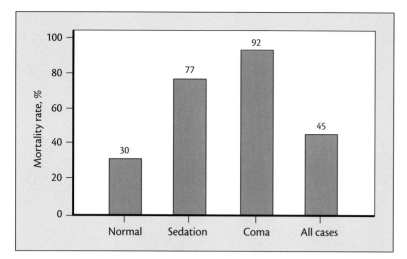

FIGURE 8-30

Consciousness level and mortality. Coma patients had a Glasgow coma score of 5 or lower. *Sedation* refers to the use of this kind of treatment, primarily in patients with assisted respiration. Both situations are associated with significantly higher mortality ($P<0.001$) than that observed in either patients with a normal consciousness level or the total population. (*Data from* Liaño *et al.* [1].)

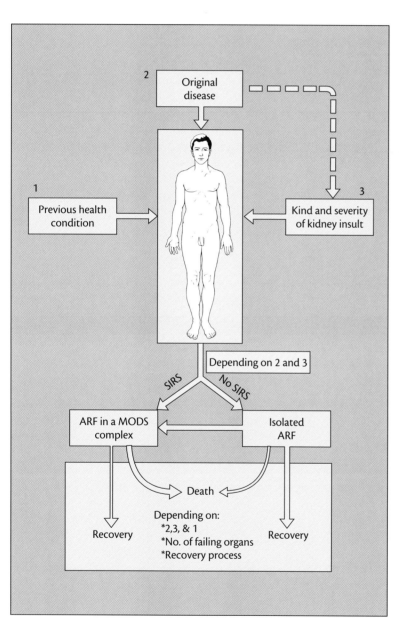

FIGURE 8-31

Outcome of acute renal failure (ARF). Two groups of factors play a role on ARF outcome. The first includes factors that affect the patient: 1) previous health condition; 2) initial disease—usually, the direct or indirect (*eg*, treatments) cause of kidney failure; 3) the kind and severity of kidney injury. While 1 is a conditioning element, 2 and 3 trigger the second group of factors: the response of the patient to the insult. If this response includes a systemic inflammatory response syndrome (SIRS) like that usually seen in intensive care patients (*eg*, sepsis, pancreatitis, burns), a multiple organ dysfunction syndrome (MODS) frequently appears and consequently outcome is associated with a higher fatality rate (*thick line*). On the contrary, if SIRS does not develop and isolated ARF predominates, death (*thin line, right*) is less frequent than survival (*thick line*).

INDIVIDUAL SEVERITY INDEX

ISI=0.032 (age-decade) − 0.086 (male) − 0.109 (nephrotoxic) + 0.109 (oliguria) + 0.116 (hypotension) + 0.122 (jaundice) + 0.150 (coma) − 0.154 (consciousness) + 0.182 (assisted respiration) + 0.210

Case example

A 55-year-old man was seen because of oliguria following pancreatic surgery. At that moment he was hypotensive and connected to a respirator, and jaundice was evident. He was diagnosed with acute tubular necrosis. His ISI was calculated as follows:

ISI=0.032(6) − 0.086 + 0.109 + 0.116 + 0.122 + 0.182 + 0.210 = 0.845

FIGURE 8-32

Individual severity index (ISI). The ISI was published in its second version in 1993 [36]. The ISI estimates the probability of death. *Nephrotoxic* indicates an ARF of that origin; the other variables have been defined in preceding figures. The numbers preceding these keys denote the contribution of each one to the prognosis and are the factor for multiplying the clinical variables; 0.210 is the equation constant. Each clinical variable takes a value of 1 or 0, depending, respectively, on its presence or absence (with the exception of the age, which takes the value of the patient's decade). The parameters are recorded when the nephrologist sees the patient the first time. Calculation is easy: only a card with the equation values, a pen, and paper are necessary. A real example is given.

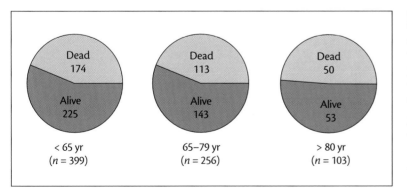

FIGURE 8-33

Outcome of acute renal failure (ARF). Long-term outcome of ARF has been studied only in some series of intrinsic or parenchymatous ARF. The figure shows the different long-term prognoses for intrinsic ARF of various causes. *Left*, The percentages of recovery rate of renal function 1 year after the acute episode of renal failure. *Right*, The situation of renal function 5 years after the ARF episode. Acute tubulointerstitial nephritis (TIN) carries the better prognosis: the vast majority of patients had recovered renal function after 1 and 5 years. Two thirds of the patients with acute tubule necrosis (ATN) recovered normal renal function, 31% showed partial recovery, and 6% experienced no functional recovery. Some patients with ATN lost renal function over the years. Patients with ARF due to glomerular lesions have a poorer prognosis; 24% at 1 year and 47% at 5 years show terminal renal failure. The poorest evolution is observed with severe forms of acute cortical necrosis or hemolytic-uremic syndrome. GN—glomerulonephritis; HUS—hemolytic-uremic syndrome; ACN—acute cortical necrosis. (*Data from* Bonomini *et al.* [37].)

FIGURE 8-34

Age as a prognostic factor in acute renal failure (ARF). There is a tendency to treat elders with ARF less aggressively because of the presumed worse outcomes; however, prognosis may be similar to that found in the younger population. In the multicenter prospective longitudinal study in Madrid, relative risk for mortality in patients older than 80 years was not significantly different (1.09 as compared with 1 for the group younger than 65 years). Age probably is not a poor prognostic sign, and outcome seems to be within acceptable limits for elderly patients with ARF. Dialysis should not be withheld from patients purely because of their age.

VARIABLES ASSOCIATED WITH PROGNOSIS: MULTIVARIATE ANALYSIS (16 STUDIES)

Assisted respiration	11
Hypotension or inotropic support	10
Age	8
Cardiac failure/complications	6
Jaundice	6
Diuresis volume	5
Coma	5
Male sex	4
Sepsis	3
Chronic disease	3
Neoplastic disease	2
Other organ failures	2
Serum creatinine	2
Other conditions	12
Summary	
Clinical variables	20
Laboratory variables	6

FIGURE 8-35

Outcome of acute renal failure (ARF). A great number of variables have been associated with outcome in ARF by multivariate analysis. This figure gives the frequency with which these variables appear in 16 ARF studies performed with multivariable analysis (all cited in [30]).

PROGNOSIS IN ACUTE RENAL FAILURE

	1960–1969	P	1980–1989
No.	119		124
Mortality (%)	51	NS	63
Mean age (y)	50.9	< 0.0001	63
Median APACHE II score	32	< 0.0001	35
Range	(22–45)		(25–49)

FIGURE 8-36

Prognosis in acute renal failure (ARF). This figure shows the utility of a prognostic system for evaluating the severity of ARF over time, using the experience of Turney [38]. He compared the age, mortality, and APACHE II score of ARF patients treated at one hospital between 1960 and 1969 and 1980 and 1989. In the latter period there were significant increases in both the severity of the illness as measured by APACHE II and age. Although there was a tendency to a higher mortality rate in the second period, this tendency was not great enough to be statistically significant.

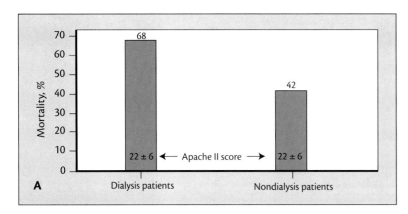

Time	Nonsurvivors	Survivors
Admission in ICU	24	22
Before dialysis	22	22
24 h after dialysis	25	22
48 h after dialysis	24	22

B

FIGURE 8-37

APACHE score. The APACHE II score is not a good method for estimating prognosis in acute renal failure (ARF) patients. **A,** Data from Verde and coworkers show how mortality was higher in their ICU patients with ARF needing dialysis than in those without need of dialysis, despite the fact that the APACHE II score before dialysis was equal in both groups [39]. **B,** Similar data were observed by Schaefer's group [40], who found that the median APACHE II score was similar in both the surviving or nonsurviving ARF patients treated in an intensive care unit. Recently Brivet and associates have found that APACHE II score influences ARF prognosis when included as a factor in a more complex logistic equation [2]. Although not useful for prognostic estimations, APACHE II score has been used in ARF for risk stratification.

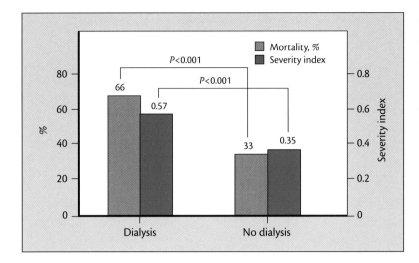

FIGURE 8-38

Analysis of the severity and mortality in acute renal failure (ARF) patients needing dialysis. This figure is an example of the uses of a severity index for analyzing the effect of treatment on the outcome of ARF. Looking at the mortality rate, it is clear that it is higher in patients who need dialysis than in those who do not. It could lead to the sophism that dialysis is not a good treatment; however, it is also clear that the severity index score for ARF was higher in patients who needed dialysis. Severity index is the mean of the individual severity index of each of the patients in each group [36]. (*Data from* Liaño *et al.* [1].)

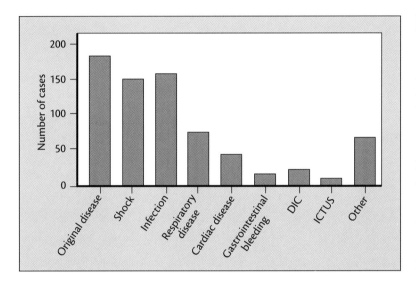

FIGURE 8-39

Causes of death. The causes of death from acute renal failure (ARF) were analyzed in 337 patients in the Madrid ARF Study [1]. In this work all the potential causes of death were recorded; thus, more than one cause could be present in a given patient. In fact, each dead patient averaged two causes, suggesting multifactorial origin. This could be the expression of a high presence of multiple organ dysfunction syndrome (MODS) among the nonsurviving patients. The main cause of death was the original disease, which was present in 55% of nonsurviving patients. Infection and shock were the next most common causes of death, usually concurrent in septic patients. It is worth noting that, if we exclude from the mortality analysis patients who died as a result of the original disease, the corrected mortality due to the ARF episode itself and its complications, drops to 27%. GI—gastrointestinal; DIC—disseminated intravascular coagulation.

References

1. Liaño F, Pascual J the Madrid ARF Study Group: Epidemiology of acute renal failure: A prospective, multicenter, community-based study. *Kidney Int* 1996, 50:811–818.

2. Brivet FG, Kleinknecht DJ, Loirat P, *et al.*: Acute renal failure in intensive care units—causes, outcome and prognostic factors of hospital mortality: A prospective, multicenter study. *Crit Care Med* 1995, 24:192–197.

3. Pascual J, Liaño F, the Madrid ARF Study Group: Causes and prognosis of acute renal failure in the very old. *J Am Geriatr Soc* 1998, 46:1–5.

4. Eliahou HE, Modan B, Leslau V, *et al.*: Acute renal failure in the community: An epidemiological study. Acute Renal Failure Conference, Proceedings. New York 1973.

5. Abraham G, Gupta RK, Senthilselvan A, *et al.*: Cause and prognosis of acute renal failure in Kuwait: A 2-year prospective study. *J Trop Med Hyg* 1989, 92:325–329.

6. McGregor E, Brown I, Campbell H, *et al.*: Acute renal failure. A prospective study on incidence and outcome (Abstract). XXIX Congress of EDTA-ERA, Paris, 1992, p 54.

7. Sanchez Rodrìguez L, Martìn Escobar E, Lozano L, *et al.*: Aspectos epidemiolûgicos del fracaso renal agudo en el ·rea sanitaria de Cuenca. *Nefrologìa* 1992, 12(Suppl 4):87–91.

8. Feest TG, Round A, Hamad S: Incidence of severe acute renal failure in adults: Results of a community based study. *Br Med J* 1993, 306:481–483.

9. Lunding M, Steiness I, Thaysen JH: Acute renal failure due to tubular necrosis. Immediate prognosis and complications. *Acta Med Scand* 1964, 176:103–119.

10. Lachhein L, Kielstein R, Sauer K, *et al.*: Evaluation of 433 cases of acute renal failure. *Proc EDTA* 1978, 14:628–629.

11. Wing AJ, Broyer M, Brunner FP, *et al.*: Combined report on regular dialysis and transplantation in Europe XIII-1982. *Proc EDTA* 1983, 20:5–78.

12. Gerrard JM, Catto GRD, Jones MC: Acute renal failure: An iceberg revisited (Abstract). *Nephrol Dial Transplant* 1992, 7:458.

13. Kleinknecht D: Epidemiology of acute renal failure in France today. In *Acute Renal Failure in the Intensive Therapy Unit*. Edited by Bihari D, Neild G. London:Springer-Verlag; 1990:13–21.

14. Chugh S, Sakhuja V, Malhotra HS, Pereira BJG: Changing trends in acute renal failure in Third-World countries—Chandigarh study. *Q J Med* 1989, 272:1117–1123.

15. Seedat YK, Nathoo BC: Acute renal failure in blacks and Indians in South Africa—Comparison after 10 years. *Nephron* 1993, 64:198–201.

16. Hou SH, Bushinsky DA, Wish JB, *et al.*: Hospital-acquired renal insufficiency: A prospective study. *Am J Med* 1983, 74:243–248.

17. Shusterman N, Strom BL, Murray TG, *et al.*: Risk factors and outcome of hospital-acquired acute renal failure. *Am J Med* 1987, 83:65–71.

18. Lauzurica R, Caralps A: Insuficiencia renal aguda producida en el hospital: Estudio prospectivo y prevenciûn de la misma. *Med Clìn (Barc)* 1989, 92:331–334.

19. Liaño F, Solez K, Kleinknecht D: Scoring the patient with ARF. In *Critical Care Nephrology*. Edited by Ronco C, Bellomo R. Dordrecht:Kluwer Academic; 1998; Section 23.1: 1535–1545.

20. Kierdorf H, Sieberth HG: Continuous treatment modalities in acute renal failure. *Nephrol Dial Transplant* 1995; 10:2001–2008.

21. Knaus WA, Draper EA, Wagner DP, Zimmerman JE: APACHE II: A severity of disease classification system. *Crit Care Med* 1985, 13:818–829.

22. Knaus WA, Wagner DP, Draper EA, *et al.*: The APACHE III prognostic system: Risk prediction of hospital mortality for critically ill hospitalized adults. *Chest* 1991, 100:1619–1636.

23. Le Gall JR, Loirat P, Alperovitch A, *et al.*: A simplified acute physiology score for ICU patients. *Crit Care Med* 1984, 12:975–977.

24. Le Gall, Lemeshow S, Saulnier F: A new Simplified Acute Phisiology Score (SAPS II) based on a European/North American multicenter study. *JAMA* 1993, 270:2957–2963.

25. Lemeshow S, Teres D, Pastides H, *et al.*: A method for predicting survival and mortality of ICU patients using objectively derived weights. *Crit Care Med* 1985, 13:519–525.

26. Lemeshow S, Teres D, Klar J, *et al.*: Mortality probability models (MPM II) based on an international cohort of intensive care unit patients. *JAMA* 1993, 270:2478–2486.

27. Knaus WA, Draper EA, Wagner DP, Zimmerman JE: Prognosis in acute organ-system failure. *Ann Surg* 1985, 202:685–693.

28. Marshall JC, Cook DJ, Christou NV, *et al.*: Multiple organ dysfunction score: A reliable descriptor of a complex clinical outcome. *Crit Care Med* 1995, 23:1638–1652.

29. Vincent JL, Moreno R, Takala J, *et al.*: The SOFA (sepsis-related organ failure assessment) score to describe organ dysfunction/failure. *Intensive Care Med* 1996, 22:707–710.

30. Liaño F, Pascual J: Acute renal failure, critical illness and the artificial kidney: Can we predict outcome? *Blood Purif* 1997, 15:346–353.

31. Douma CE, Redekop WK, Van der Meulen JHP, *et al.*: Predicting mortality in intensive care patients with acute renal failure treated with dialysis. *J Am Soc Nephrol* 1997, 8:111–117.

32. Viviand X, Gouvernet J, Granthil C, Francois G: Simplification of the SAPS by selecting independent variables. *Intensive Care Med* 1991, 17:164–168.

33. Bion JF, Aitchison TC, Edlin SA, Ledingham IM: Sickness scoring and response to treatment as predictors of outcome from critical illness. *Intensive Care Med* 1988, 14:167–172.

34. Chew SL, Lins RL, Daelemans R, De Broe ME: Outcome in acute renal failure. *Nephrol Dial Transplant* 1993, 8:101–107.

35. Liaño F: Severity of acute renal failure: The need of measurement. *Nephrol Dial Transplant* 1994, 9(Suppl. 4):229–238.

36. Liaño F, Gallego A, Pascual J, *et al.*: Prognosis of acute tubular necrosis: An extended prospectively contrasted study. *Nephron* 1993, 63:21–23.

37. Bonomini V, Stefoni S, Vangelista A: Long-term patient and renal prognosis in acute renal failure. *Nephron* 1984, 36:169–172.

38. Turney JH: Why is mortality persistently high in acute renal failure? *Lancet* 1990, 335:971.

39. Verde E, Ruiz F, Vozmediano MC, *et al.*: Valor predictivo del APACHE II en el fracaso renal agudo de las unidades de cuidados intensivos (Abstract). *Nefrologìa* 1996, 16(Suppl. 19):32.

40. Schaefer JH, Jochimsen F, Keller F, *et al.*: Outcome prediction of acute renal failure in medical intensive care. *Intensive Care Med* 1991, 17:19–24.

Renal Histopathology, Urine Cytology, and Cytopathology of Acute Renal Failure

Lorraine C. Racusen
Cynthia C. Nast

Causes of acute renal failure can be divided into three categories: 1) prerenal, due to inadequate perfusion; 2) postrenal, due to obstruction of outflow; and 3) intrinsic, due to injury to renal parenchyma. Among the latter, diseases of, or injury to, glomeruli, vessels, interstitium, or tubules may lead to a decrease in glomerular filtration rate (GFR).

Glomerular diseases that lead to acute renal failure are the proliferative glomerulonephritides, including postinfectious and membranoproliferative glomerulonephritis secondary to glomerular deposition of immune complexes. If glomerular injury is severe enough to damage the glomerular basement membrane, leakage of fibrin and other plasma proteins stimulates formation of cellular extracapillary "crescents" composed of epithelial cells and monocytes and macrophages. Crescents may form as a result of an inflammatory reaction to immune complexes formed to nonglomerular antigens; antibody reaction to intrinsic glomerular antigens, as in anti–glomerular basement membrane disease; and, in the absence of immune complexes, the pauci-immune processes, which include the small vessel vasculitides, including Wegener's granulomatosis and microscopic polyarteritis. Immunohistologic examination and electron microscopy play important roles in the diagnosis of these processes. Extensive crescent formation is accompanied by rapidly progressive acute renal failure. The urine sediment in these diseases often contains red blood cells and red cell casts.

Vascular diseases (involving veins, arteries, or arterioles and capillaries) can lead to hypoperfusion and acute renal failure. Venous thrombosis, most often due to trauma or a nephrotic state, and arterial thrombosis due to trauma or vasculitis, cause parenchymal ischemia and

CHAPTER

9

infarction. Small vessel vasculitides involve small arteries, arterioles, and glomerular capillaries, causing injury and necrosis in the glomerular tuft, which may result in crescent formation. Thrombotic microangiopathies result from endothelial injury damage in small arteries and arterioles, producing thrombosis, obstruction to blood flow, and glomerular hypoperfusion. Urine sediment in these diseases often shows hematuria or cellular casts, reflecting ischemia.

Interstitial inflammatory processes lead to acute renal failure via compression of peritubular capillaries or injury to tubules. Causes of acute interstitial nephritis include infection, and immune-mediated reactions. With infection, polymorphonuclear leukocytes may be seen in tubules as well as in interstitium. Inflammatory infiltrates in hypersensitivity reactions, often due to drug exposure, feature eosinophils. Immunohistologic studies may reveal the presence of immune complexes; immune complex deposition around tubules occurs as a primary process or associated with immune glomerular injury. Tubulitis is seen when the inflammatory reaction extends into the tubular epithelium. Epithelial cell injury is often produced by such inflammatory processes. The urine sediment reveals white blood cells and white cell casts, which may include numerous polymorphonuclear leukocytes or eosinophils.

The most common cause of acute renal failure is injury to tubule epithelium. Primary tubule cell injury typically results from ischemia, toxic injury, or both. Cell injury results in disruption of the epithelium and its normal reabsorptive functions, and may lead to obstruction of tubule lumens. Cell exfoliation often occurs, and intact cells and cell fragments and debris can be seen in the urine sediment; these may be in the form of casts. Necrotic cells may be seen in situ along the tubule epithelium or in the tubule lumen, but often overt cell necrosis is not prominent. Apoptosis of tubule cells is seen after injury as well.

Glomerular Diseases

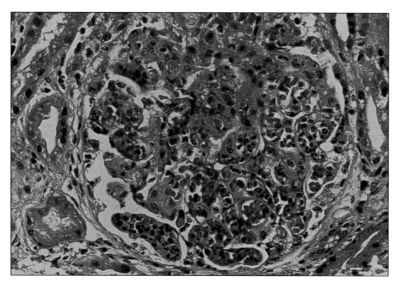

FIGURE 9-1 (*see* Color Plate)

Early postinfectious glomerulonephritis. Numerous polymorphonuclear leukocytes in glomerular capillary loops contribute to the hypercellular appearance of the glomerulus. There is also a segmental increase in mesangial cells (hematoxylin and eosin, original magnification × 400). This reactive inflammatory process occurs in response to glomerular deposition of immune complexes, including the large subepithelial "hump-like" deposits which are typical of post-infectious glomerulonephritis. The glomerulonephritis is usually self-limited and reversible, and especially with appropriate treatment of the underlying infection, long-term prognosis is excellent [1].

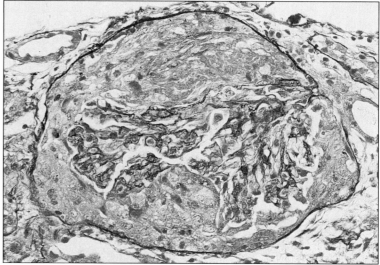

FIGURE 9-2 (*see* Color Plate)

A large epithelial crescent fills Bowman's space and compresses the capillary loops in the glomerular tuft. This silver stain highlights the glomerular mesangium and the basement membrane of the glomerular capillaries (silver stain, original magnification × 400). The patient presented with hematuria and acute renal failure. Immunostains were negative in this case, a finding consistent with a pauci-immune process. The differential diagnosis includes small vessel vasculitis, and anti-neutrophil cytoplasmic antibody may be positive. Crescentic glomerulonephritis may also occur with anti-glomerular basement membrane antibody disease, or as a complication of immune complex glomerulonephritis [2].

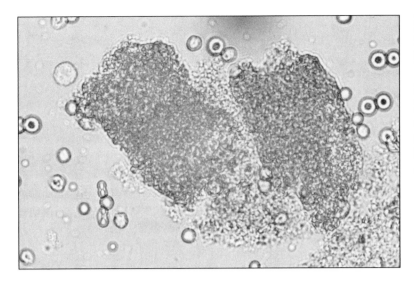

FIGURE 9-3 (*see* Color Plate)

Urine sediment of a patient with acute renal failure revealing red blood cells and some red blood cell casts (original magnification × 600). Biopsy in this case revealed crescentic glomerulonephritis. However, hematuria may be seen in any proliferative glomerulonephritis or with parenchymal infarcts. The "casts" assume the cylindrical shape of the renal tubules, and confirm an intrarenal source of the blood in the urine. Fragmented or dysmorphic red blood cells may be seen when the red cells have traversed through damaged glomerular capillaries.

Vascular Diseases

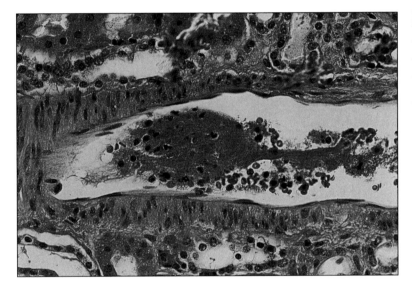

FIGURE 9-4 (*see* Color Plate)

An early thrombus is seen in a small renal artery in a patient with patchy cortical infarction (original magnification × 250). The patient presented with acute renal failure. The thrombosis may be due to a hypercoagulable state (*eg*, disseminated intravascular coaggulation) or endothelial injury (*eg*, hemolytic uremic syndrome). If the cortical necrosis is patchy, recovery of adequate renal function may occur [3].

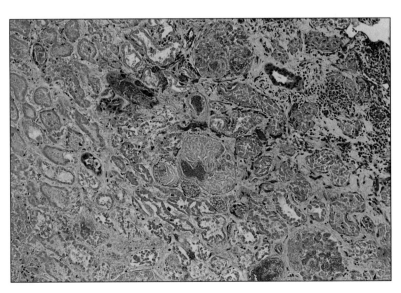

FIGURE 9-5 (*see* Color Plate)

A parenchymal infarct in a patient with renal vein thrombosis (hematoxylin and eosin, original magnification × 200). A few surviving tubules and a rim of inflammatory cells are seen at the periphery of the infarct. Infarcts may also be seen with arterial thromboses, and with severe injury to the microvasculature, as occurs in thrombotic microangiopathies [3]. If the process is extensive, acute cortical necrosis may occur, often leading to irreversible renal failure.

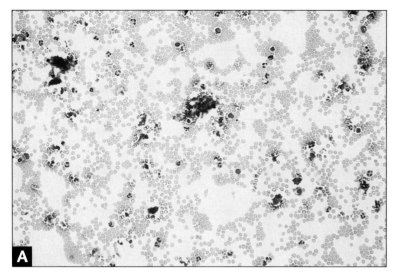

FIGURE 9-6 (*see* Color Plate)

A fine-needle aspirate in renal infarction. **A,** Low magnification shows many degenerating cells with a "dirty background" containing cellular debris and scattered neutrophils. Compare to acute tubular necrosis, which has only scattered degenerated or necrotic cells without the extensive necrosis and cell debris. Neutrophils may be numerous if the edge of an infarct is aspirated (May-Grunwald Giemsa, original magnification × 40). **B,** Diffusely degenerated and necrotic cells with condensed and disrupted cytoplasm and pyknotic nuclei, and an adjacent neutrophil. No significant numbers of viable tubule epithelial cells remain (May-Grunwald Giemsa, original magnification × 160).

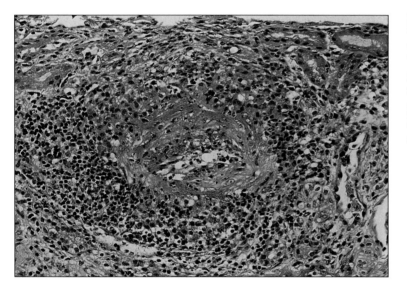

FIGURE 9-7 (*see* Color Plate)

A small artery with severe inflammation in a patient with a small vessel vasculitis. The wall of the vessel is infiltrated by lymphocytes, plasma cells, and eosinophils (hematoxylin and eosin, original magnification × 250). The patient was p-ANCA positive. ANCA may play a pathogenic role in the vasculitis process [4]. Vasculitis in the kidney is often part of a systemic syndrome, but may occur as an apparently renal-limited process.

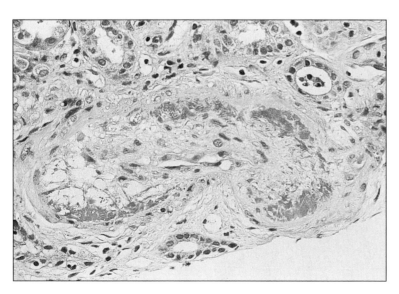

FIGURE 9-8 (*see* Color Plate)

Microangiopathic changes in a small artery, with endothelial activation, evidenced by the large endothelial cells with hyperchromatic nuclei and vacuolization. There is intimal edema with some cell proliferation, and a prominent band of fibrinoid necrosis is seen; the latter appears dark red-pink on this hematoxylin-eosin stain, and represents insudation of fibrin and plasma proteins into the wall of the injured vessel (original magnification × 250). The differential diagnosis includes hemolytic uremic syndrome, thrombotic thrombocytopenic purpura, malignant hypertension, scleroderma, and drug toxicity, the latter due most commonly to mitomycin C or cyclosporine/FK506 [5].

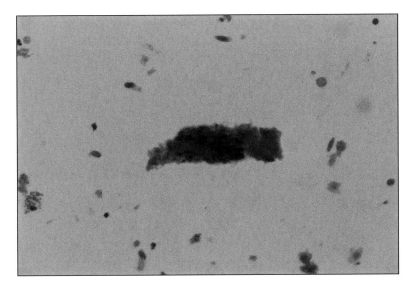

FIGURE 9-9 (*see* Color Plate)

A cast of necrotic tubular cells in urine sediment (Papanicolaou stain, original magnification × 400). The most likely causes of damage to the renal tubules with such findings in the urinary sediment are severe ischemia/infarction, or tubular necrosis due to exposure to toxins which injure the renal tubules. The latter include antibiotics, including aminoglycosides and cephalosporins, and chemotherapeutic agents.

Interstitial Disease

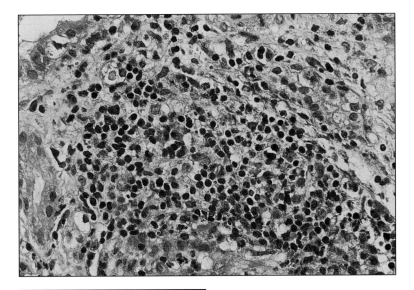

FIGURE 9-10 (*see* Color Plate)

Interstitial nephritis with edema and a mononuclear inflammatory infiltrate. Eosinophils in the infiltrate suggest a possible hypersensitivity reaction (hematoxylin and eosin, original magnification ×400). Drugs are the most common cause of such a reaction, which often presents with acute renal failure [6]. Inflammatory cells and cell casts may be seen in the urine sediment in these cases, as inflammatory cells infiltrate the tubular epithelium.

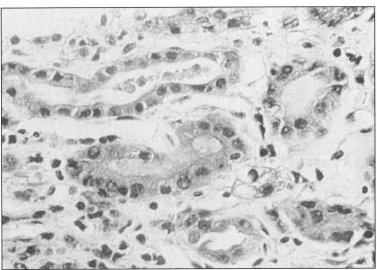

FIGURE 9-11 (*see* Color Plate)

Tubulitis, with infiltration of mononuclear cells into the tubular epithelium (hematoxylin and eosin, original magnification × 400). There is a mononuclear infiltrate and edema in the surrounding interstitium. Tubule cells may show evidence of lethal or sublethal injury as the inflammatory cells release damaging enzymes. Tubulitis is often seen in interstitial nephritis especially if the targets of the inflammatory reaction are tubular cell antigens or antigens deposited around the tubules. Immunofluorescence may reveal granular or linear deposits of immunoglobulin and complement around the tubules.

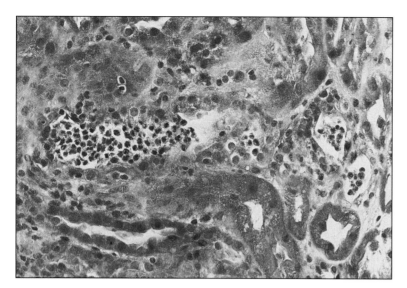

FIGURE 9-12 (*see* Color Plate)
Polymorphonuclear leukocytes forming a cast in a cortical tubule (hematoxylin and eosin, original magnification × 400). Note edema and inflammation in adjacent interstitium. These intratubular cells are highly suggestive of acute infection, and may be seen in distal as well as proximal nephron as part of an ascending infection. Intratubular PML may also be seen in vasculitis and other necrotizing glomerular processes, in which these cells escape across damaged areas of the inflamed glomerular tuft.

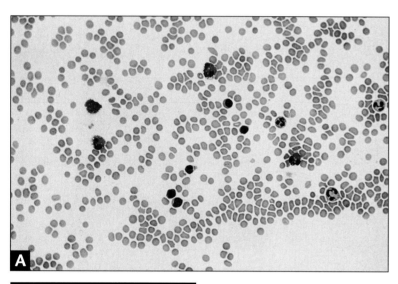

FIGURE 9-13 (*see* Color Plate)
Fine-needle aspirate of acute infectious interstitial nephritis (acute pyelonephritis). A 25-gauge needle attached to a 10-cc syringe was utilized to withdraw the aspirate into 4 cc of RPMI-based medium. The specimen was then cytocentrifuged and stained with May-Grunwald Giemsa. **A,** The renal aspirate contains large numbers of intrarenal neutrophils, which are focally undergoing degenerative changes with cytoplasmic vacuolization and nuclear breakdown. In bacterial infection there are many infiltrating neutrophils and there may be associated necrosis of tubule epithelial cells (original magnification × 80). **B,** A neutrophil contains phagocytosed bacteria within the cytoplasm; bacteria stain with Giemsa, so are readily detectable in this setting. Adjacent tubule epithelial cells have cytoplasmic granules but do not phagocytize bacteria (original magnification × 160).

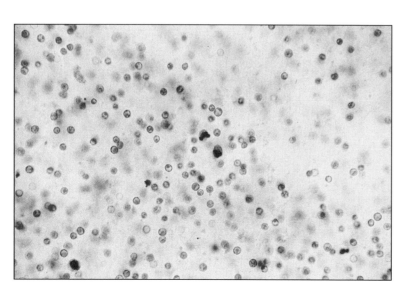

FIGURE 9-14 (*see* Color Plate)
Numerous polymorphonuclear leukocytes (PML) in the urine sediment of a patient with acute pyelonephritis (hematoxylin and eosin, original magnification × 400). Some red blood cells and tubular cells are seen in the background of this cytospin preparation. PML may be found in the urine with acute infection of the lower urinary tract as well, or as a contaminant from vaginal secretions in females. PML casts, on the other hand, are evidence that the cells are from the kidney.

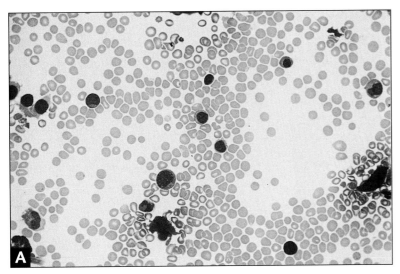

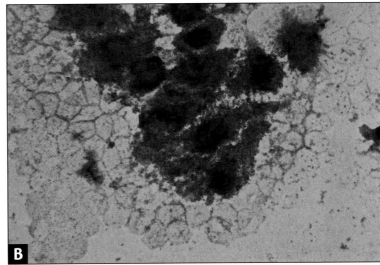

FIGURE 9-15 (*see* Color Plate)

Fine-needle aspirate from patient with intrarenal cytomegalovirus (CMV) infection. **A,** There are activated and transformed lymphocytes with immature nuclear chromatin and abundant blue cytoplasm that infiltrate the kidney in response to the infection; large granular lymphocytes (NK cells) may be seen as well, but few neutrophils. Similar activated lymphocytes, NK cells, and atypical monocytes can be observed within the peripheral blood. The tubule epithelial cells are virtually never seen to contain CMV inclusions in aspirate material, in contrast to core biopsy specimens. All intrarenal viral infections have a similar appearance, and immunostaining or in situ hybridization is required to identify specific viruses (May-Grunwald Giemsa, original magnification × 80). **B,** Tubular epithelial cells stained with antibody to CMV immediate and early nuclear proteins in active intrarenal CMV infection. With an immunoalkaline phosphatase method, cytoplasmic and prominent nuclear staining for these early proteins are observed in the tubular epithelium. In very early infection, neutrophils also may have cytoplasmic staining for these proteins (original magnification × 240).

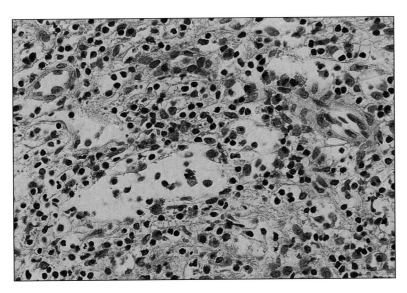

FIGURE 9-16 (*see* Color Plate)

Numerous eosinophils in an interstitial inflammatory infiltrate. Eosinophils may be diffuse within the infiltrate, but may also be clustered, forming "eosinophilic abscesses," as in this area (hematoxylin and eosin, original magnification × 400). Eosinophils may also be demonstrated in the urine sediment. Drugs most commonly producing acute interstitial nephritis as part of a hypersensitivity reaction include: penicillins, sulfonamides, and nonsteroidal anti-inflammatory drugs [6]. The patient had recently undergone a course of therapy with methicillin. The interstitial nephritis may be part of a systemic reaction which includes fever, rash, and eosinophilia.

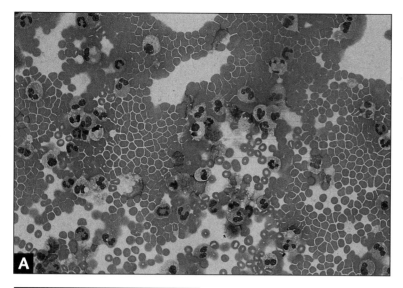

FIGURE 9-17 (*see* Color Plate)

Fine-needle aspirate of acute allergic interstitial nephritis. **A,** The aspirate contains numerous lymphocytes, occasional activated lymphocytes, and eosinophils without fully transformed lymphocytes, corresponding to the inflammatory component within the tubulointerstitium observed on routine renal biopsy. Monocytes often are present (May-Grunwald Giemsa, original magnification × 80). **B,** Higher magnification showing the typical infiltrating cells, including a monocyte, activated lymphocyte, and an eosinophil. A neutrophil is present, likely owing to blood contamination (May-Grunwald Giemsa, original magnification × 160).

Tubular Diseases

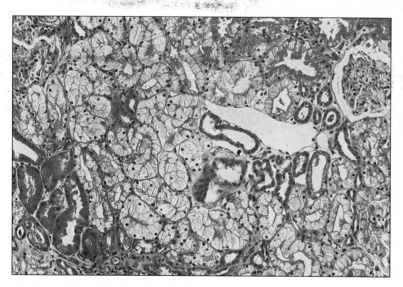

FIGURE 9-18 (*see* Color Plate)

Severe vacuolization of tubular cells in injured tubular epithelium (hematoxylin and eosin, original magnification × 400). The vacuoles reflect cell injury and derangement of homeostatic mechanisms that maintain the normal intracellular milieu. In this case, the vacuoles developed on exposure to intravenous immunoglobulin in a sucrose vehicle; the morphology is reminiscent of the severe changes produced by osmotic agents. While generally a nonspecific marker of cell injury, a distinctive pattern of "isometric" vacuolization, in which there are numerous intracellular vacuoles of uniform size (not shown here) is very typical of cyclosporine/FK506 effect [6].

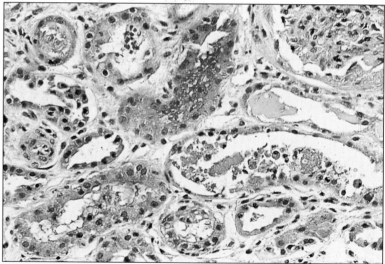

FIGURE 9-19 (*see* Color Plate)

Necrotic tubular cells and cell debris in tubular lumina. One tubule shows extensive cell loss, with tubular epithelium lined only by a very flattened layer of cytoplasm. The dilated lumen contains numerous necrotic tubular cells with pyknotic nuclei. Several tubules contain cell debris and one contains red blood cells (hematoxylin and eosin, original magnification × 250). Such changes are more often seen with toxic than with ischemic injury [6], unless the latter is very severe.

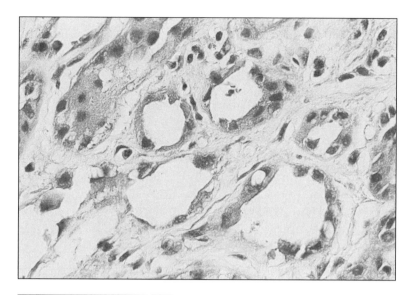

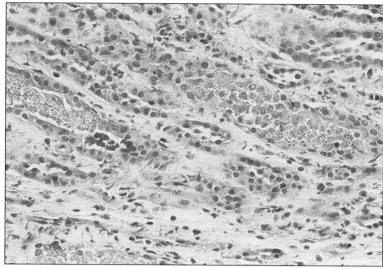

FIGURE 9-20 (*see* Color Plate)

This micrograph shows sites of cell exfoliation, attenuation of remaining cells, and reactive and regenerative changes (hematoxylin and eosin, original magnification × 400). Exfoliation occurs with disruption of cell-cell and cell-substrate adhesion, and may involve viable as well as non-viable cells [7]. Reactive and regenerative changes may include basophilia of cell cytoplasm, increased nuclear:cytoplasmic ratio, heterogeneity of nuclear size and appearance, hyperchromatic nuclei and mitotic figures.

FIGURE 9-21 (*see* Color Plate)

Outer medulla shows in situ cell necrosis and loss in medullary thick ascending limb (hematoxylin and eosin, original magnification × 250). Tubules contain cells and cell debris. Changes reflect ischemic injury. Impaction of cells and cast material may lead to tubular obstruction, especially in narrow regions of the nephron. Adhesion molecules on the surface of exfoliated cells may contribute to aggregation of cells within the tubule and adhesion of detached cells to in situ tubular cells [8].

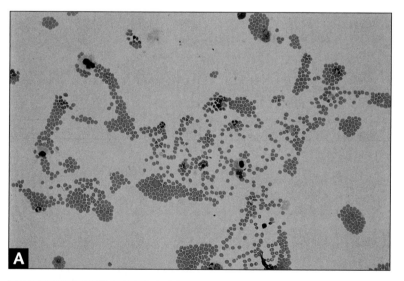

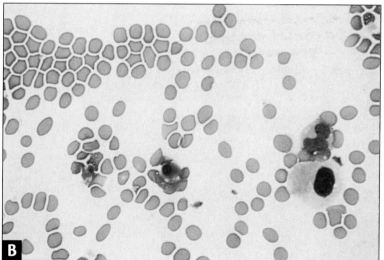

FIGURE 9-22 (*see* Color Plate)

Fine-needle aspirate showing acute tubular cell injury and necrosis. **A,** The aspirate shows scattered tubular epithelial cells with swelling and focal degenerative changes, and a minimal associated inflammatory infiltrate. There is no significant background cell debris (May-Grunwald Giemsa, original magnification × 40). **B,** One tubular cell is degenerated with reduction in cell size, condensed gray-blue cytoplasm, and a pyknotic nucleus. Another cell has more advanced necrosis with additional cytoplasmic disruption and a very small pyknotic nucleus. Compare the adjacent swollen damaged tubular cell which has not yet undergone necrosis (May-Grunwald Giemsa, original magnification × 160).

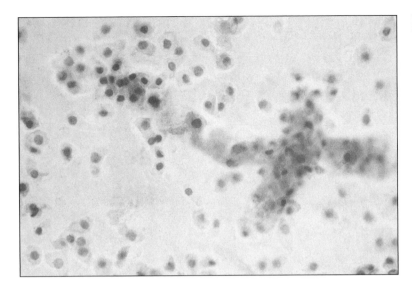

FIGURE 9-23 (*see* Color Plate)
Urine sediment from a patient with acute tubular injury showing tubular cells and cell casts (Papanicolaou stain, original magnification × 250). Many of these cells are morphologically intact, even by electron microscopy. Studies have shown that a significant percentage of the cells shed into the urine may exclude vital dyes, and may even grow when placed in culture, indicating that they remain viable. Such cells clearly detached from tubular basement membrane as a manifestation of sub-lethal injury [7].

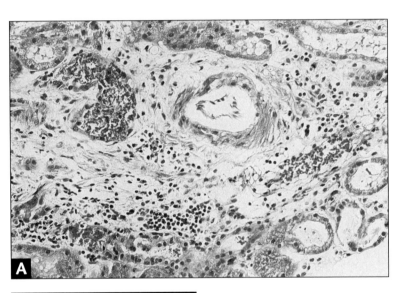

A

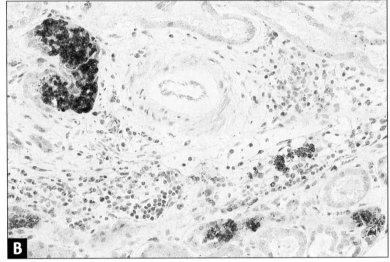

B

FIGURE 9-24 (*see* Color Plate)
Myoglobin casts in the tubules of a patient who abused cocaine. **A,** Hematoxylin and eosin stained casts have a dark red, coarsely granular appearance (original magnification × 250). **B,** Immunoperoxidase stain for myoglobin confirms positive staining in the casts (original magnification × 250). These casts may obstruct the nephron, especially with dehydration and low tubular fluid flow rates. Rhabdomyolysis with formation of intrarenal myoglobin casts may also occur with severe trauma, crush injury, or extreme exercise.

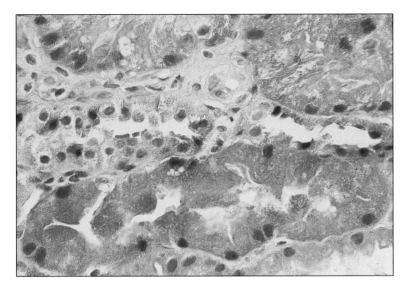

FIGURE 9-25 (*see* Color Plate)

Apoptosis of tubular cells following tubular cell injury. Note the shrunken cells with condensed nuclei and cytoplasm in the central tubule. The patient had presumed ischemic injury (hematoxylin and eosin, original magnification × 400). The role of apoptosis in injury to the renal tubule remains to be defined. The process may be difficult to quantitate, since apoptotic cells may rapidly disintegrate. In experimental models, the degree of apoptosis versus coaggulative necrosis occurring following injury is related to the severity and duration of injury, with milder injury showing more apoptosis [9].

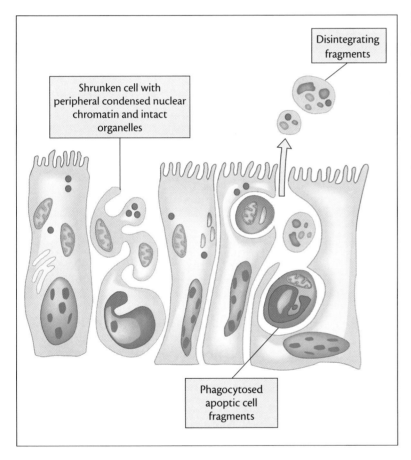

Disintegrating fragments

Shrunken cell with peripheral condensed nuclear chromatin and intact organelles

Phagocytosed apoptic cell fragments

FIGURE 9-26

Apoptosis-schematic of histologic changes in tubular epithelium. The process begins with condensation of the cytoplasm and of the nucleus, a process which involves endonucleases, which digest the DNA into ladder-like fragments characteristic of this process. The cell disintegrates into discrete membrane-bound fragments, so-called "apoptotic bodies." These fragments may be rapidly extruded into the tubular lumen or phagocytosed by neighboring epithelial cells or inflammatory cells. (*Modified from* Arends, *et al.* [10]; with permission.)

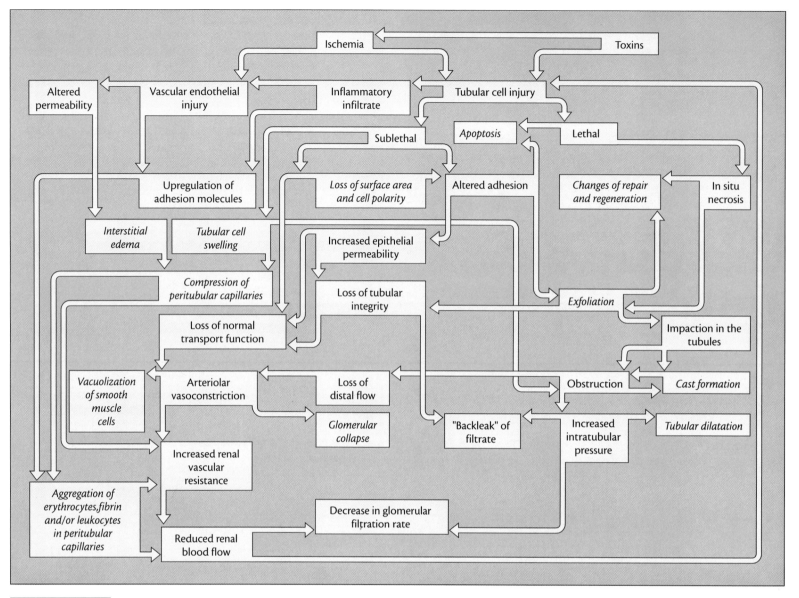

FIGURE 9-27

A schematic showing the relationship between morphologic and functional changes with injury to the renal tubule due to ischemia or nephrotoxins. Morphologic changes are shown in italics.

Histology reflects the altered hemodynamics, epithelial derangements, and obstruction which contribute to loss of renal function. (*Modified from* Racusen [11]; with permission.)

References

1. Popovic-Rolovic M, Kostic M, Antic-Peco A, *et al.*: Medium and long-term prognosis of patients with acute post-streptococcal glomerulonephritis. *Nephron* 1991, 58:393–399.

2. Jennette JC: Crescentic glomerulonephritis. In *Heptinstall's Pathology of the Kidney*, edn. 5. Edited by Jennette JC, JL Olson, M Schwarz, FG Silva. New York:Lippincott-Raven, 1998.

3. Racusen LC, Solez K: Renal cortical necrosis, infarction and atheroembolic disease. In *Renal Pathology*. Edited by Tisher C, B Brenner. Philadelphia:Lippincott-Raven, 1993:811.

4. Evert BH, Jennette JC, Falk RJ: The pathogenic role of antineutrophil cytoplasmic autoantibodies. *Am J Kidney Dis* 1991, 8:188–195.

5. Remuzzi G, Ruggenenti P: The hemolytic uremic syndrome. *Kidney Int* 1995, 47:2–19.

6. Nadasdy T, Racusen LC: Renal injury caused by therapeutic and diagnostic agents, and abuse of analgesics and narcotics. In *Heptinstalls Pathology of the Kidney*, edn. 5. Edited by Jennette JC, JL Olson, MM Schwartz, FG Silva. New York:Lippincott-Raven, 1998.

7. Racusen LC, Fivush BA, Li Y-L, *et al.*: Dissociation of tubular detachment and tubular cell death in clinical and experimental "acute tubular necrosis." *Lab Invest* 1991, 64:546–556.

8. Goligorsky MS, Lieberthal W, Racusen L, Simon EE: Integrin receptors in renal tubular epithelium: New insights into pathophysiology of acute renal failure. *Am J Physiol* 1993, 264:F1–F8.

9. Schumer KM, Olsson CA, Wise GJ, Buttyan R: Morphologic, biochemical and molecular evidence of apoptosis during the reperfusion phase after brief periods of renal ischemia. *Am J Pathol* 1992, 140:831–838.

10. Arends MJ, Wyllie AH: Apoptosis: Mechanisms and role in pathology. *Int Rev Exp Pathol* 1991, 32:225–254.

11. Racusen LC: Pathology of acute renal failure: Structure/function correlations. *Advances in Renal Replacement Therapy*, 1997 4(Suppl. 2): 3–16.

Acute Renal Failure in the Transplanted Kidney

Kim Solez
Lorraine C. Racusen

Acute renal failure (ARF) in the transplanted kidney represents a high-stakes area of nephrology and of transplantation practice. A correct diagnosis can lead to rapid return of renal function; an incorrect diagnosis can lead to loss of the graft and severe sequelae for the patient. The diagnostic possibilities are many (Fig. 10-1) and treatments quite different, although the clinical presentations of new-onset functional renal impairment and of persistent nonfunctioning after transplant may be identical.

In transplant-related ARF percutaneous kidney allograft biopsy is crucial in differentiating such diverse entities as acute rejection (Figs. 10-2 to 10-9), acute tubular necrosis (Figs. 10-10 to 10-14), cyclosporine toxicity (Figs. 10-15 and 10-16), posttransplant lymphoproliferative disorder (Fig. 10-17), and other, rarer, conditions.

In the case of acute rejection, standardization of transplant biopsy interpretation and reporting is necessary to guide therapy and to establish an objective endpoint for clinical trials of new immunosuppressive agents. The Banff Classification of Renal Allograft Pathology [1] is an internationally accepted standard for the assessment of renal allograft biopsies sponsored by the International Society of Nephrology Commission of Acute Renal Failure. The classification had its origins in a meeting held in Banff, Alberta, in the Canadian Rockies, in August, 1991, where subsequent meetings have been held every 2 years. Hot topics likely to influence the Banff Classification of Renal Allograft Pathology in 1999 and beyond are shown in Figs. 10-17 to 10-19.

Acute Rejection

DIAGNOSTIC POSSIBILITIES IN TRANSPLANT-RELATED ACUTE RENAL FAILURE

1. Acute (cell-mediated) rejection
2. Delayed-appearing antibody-mediated rejection
3. Acute tubular necrosis
4. Cyclosporine or FK506 toxicity
5. Urine leak
6. Obstruction
7. Viral infection
8. Post-transplant lymphoproliferative disorder
9. Vascular thrombosis
10. Prerenal azotemia

FIGURE 10-1

Diagnostic possibilities in transplant-related acute renal failure.

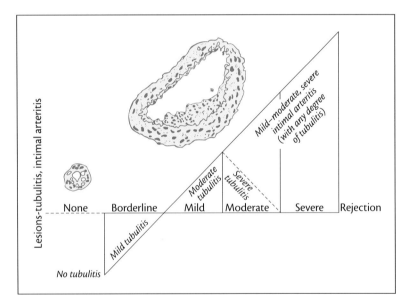

FIGURE 10-2

Diagnosis of rejection in the Banff classification makes use of two basic lesions, tubulitis and intimal arteritis. The 1993–1995 Banff classification depicted in this figure is the standard in use in virtually all current clinical trials and in many individual transplant units. In this construct, rejection is regarded as a continuum of mild, moderate, and severe forms. The 1997 Banff classification is similar, having the same threshold for rejection diagnosis, but it recognizes three different histologic types of acute rejection: tubulointersititial, vascular, and transmural. The quotation marks emphasize the possible overlap of features of the various types (*eg*, the finding of tubulitis should not dissuade the pathologist from conducting a thorough search for intimal arteritis).

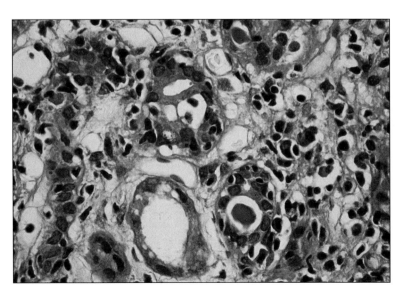

FIGURE 10-3

Tubulitis is not absolutely specific for acute rejection. It can be found in mild forms in acute tubular necrosis, normally functioning kidneys, and in cyclosporine toxicity and in conditions not related to rejection. Therefore, quantitation is necessary. The number of lymphocytes situated between and beneath tubular epithelial cells is compared with the number of tubular cells to determine the severity of tubulitis. Four lymphocytes per most inflamed tubule cross section or per ten tubular cells is required to reach the threshold for diagnosing rejection. In this figure, the two tubule cross sections in the center have eight mononuclear cells each. Rejection with intimal arteritis or transmural arteritis can occur without any tubulitis whatsoever, although usually in well-established rejection both tubulitis and intimal arteritis are observed.

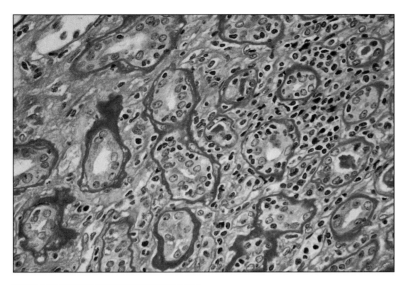

FIGURE 10-4 (*see* Color Plate)

In this figure the tubules with lymphocytic invasion are atrophic with thickened tubular basement membranes. There are 13 or 14 lymphocytes per tubular cross section. This is an example of how a properly performed periodic acid-Schiff (PAS) stain should look. The Banff classification is critically dependent on proper performance of PAS staining. The invading lymphocytes are readily apparent and countable in the tubules. In the Banff 1997 classification one avoids counting lymphocytes in atrophic tubules, as tubulitis there is more "nonspecific" than in nonatrophed tubules. (*From* Solez *et al.* [1]; with permission.)

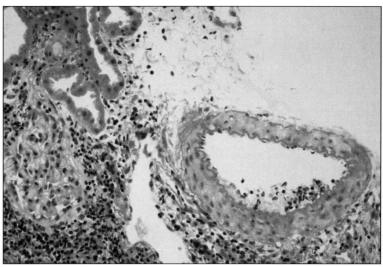

FIGURE 10-5

Intimal arteritis in a case of acute rejection. Note that more than 20 lymphocytes are present in the thickened intima. With this lesion, however, even a single lymphocyte in this site is sufficient to make the diagnosis. Thus, the pathologist must search for subtle intimal arteritis lesions, which are highly reliable and specific for rejection. (*From* Solez *et al.* [1]; with permission.)

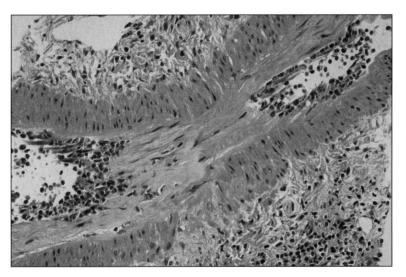

FIGURE 10-6

Artery in longitudinal section shows a more florid intimal arteritis than that in Figure 10-5. Aggregation of lymphocytes is also seen in the lumen, but this is a nonspecific change. The reporting for some clinical trials has involved counting lymphocytes in the most inflamed artery, but this has not been shown to correlate with clinical severity or outcome, whereas the presence or absence of the lesion has been shown to have such a correlation. (*From* Solez *et al.* [1]; with permission.)

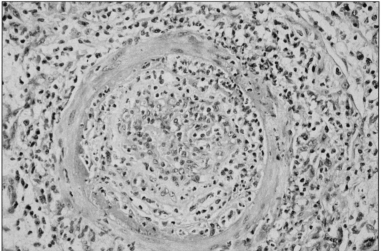

FIGURE 10-7

Transmural arteritis with fibrinoid change. In addition to the influx of inflammatory cells there has been proliferation of modified smooth muscle cells migrated from the media to the greatly thickened intima. Note the fibrinoid change at lower left and the penetration of the media by inflammatory cells at the upper right. Patients with these types of lesions have a less favorable prognosis, greater graft loss, and poorer long-term function as compared with patients with intimal arteritis alone. These sorts of lesions are also common in antibody-mediated rejection (*see* Fig. 10-9).

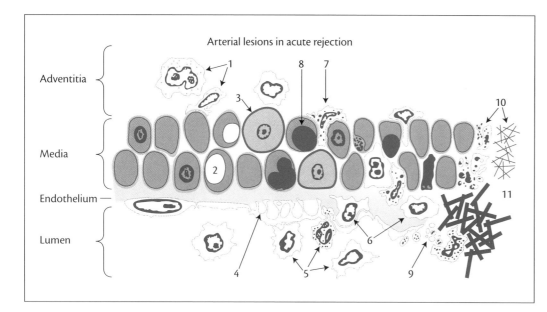

FIGURE 10-8

Diagram of arterial lesions of acute rejection. The initial changes (1–5) before intimal arteritis (6) occurs are completely nonspecific. These early changes are probably mechanistically related to the diagnostic lesions but can occur as a completely self-limiting phenomenon unrelated to clinical rejection. Lesions 7 to 10 are those characteristic of "transmural" rejection. Lesion 1 is perivascular inflammation; lesion 2, myocyte vacuolization; lesion 3, apoptosis; lesion 4, endothelial activation and prominence; lesion 5, leukocyte adherence to the endothelium; lesion 6 (specific), penetration of inflammatory cells under the endothelium (intimal arteritis); lesion 7, inflammatory cell penetration of the media; lesion 8, necrosis of medial smooth muscle cells; lesion 9, platelet aggregation; lesion 10, fibrinoid change; and lesion 11 is thrombosis.

The figure label: *Arterial lesions in acute rejection* — Adventitia, Media, Endothelium, Lumen.

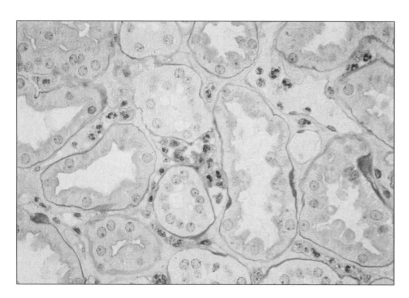

FIGURE 10-9 (*see* Color Plate)

Antibody-mediated rejection with aggregates of polymorphonuclear leukocytes (polymorphs) in peritubular capillaries. This lesion is a feature of both classic hyperacute rejection and of later appearing antibody-mediated rejection, which is by far the more common entity. Antibody- and cell-mediated rejection can coexist, so one may find both tubulitis and intimal arteritis along with this lesion; however many cases of antibody-mediated rejection have a paucity of tubulitis [2]. The polymorph aggregates can be subtle, another reason for looking with care at the biopsy that appears to show "nothing."

Acute Tubular Necrosis

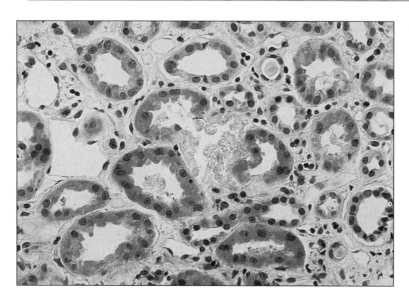

FIGURE 10-10 (*see* Color Plate)

Acute tubular necrosis in the allograft. Unlike "acute tubule necrosis" in native kidney, in this condition actual necrosis appears in the transplanted kidney but in a very small proportion of tubules, often less than one in 300 tubule cross sections. Where the necrosis does occur it tends to affect the entire tubule cross section, as in the center of this field [3].

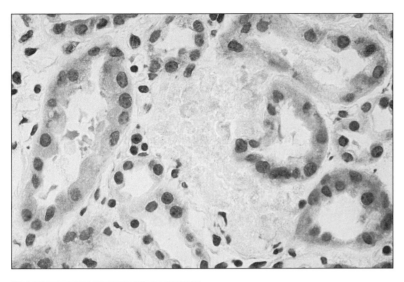

FIGURE 10-11 (*see* Color Plate)

A completely necrotic tubule in the center of the picture in a case of acute tubular necrosis (ATN) in an allograft. The tubule is difficult to identify because, in contrast to the appearance in native kidney ATN, no residual tubular cells survive; the epithelium is 100% necrotic.

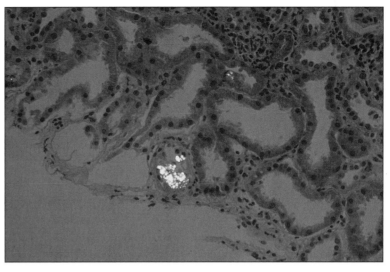

FIGURE 10-12 (*see* Color Plate)

Calcium oxalate crystals seen under polarized light. These are very characteristic of transplant acute tubular necrosis (ATN), probably because they relate to some degree to the duration of uremia, which is often much longer in transplant ATN (counting the period of uremia before transplantation) than in native ATN. With prolonged uremia elevation of plasma oxalate is greater and more persistent and consequently tissue deposition is greater [4].

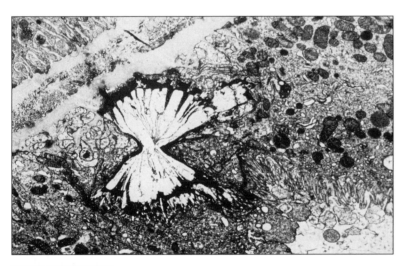

FIGURE 10-13

Calcium oxalate crystals seen by electron microscopy in transplant acute tubular necrosis.

FEATURES OF TRANSPLANT ACUTE TUBULAR NECROSIS (ATN) WHICH DIFFERENTIATE IT FROM NATIVE KIDNEY ATN

1. Apparently intact proximal tubular brush border
2. Occasional foci of necrosis of entire tubular cross sections
3. More extensive calcium oxalate deposition
4. Significantly fewer tubular casts
5. Significantly more interstitial inflammation
6. Less cell-to-cell variation in size and shape ("tubular cell unrest")

FIGURE 10-14

Features of transplant acute tubular necrosis that differentiate it from the same condition in native kidney [3].

Cyclosporine Toxicity

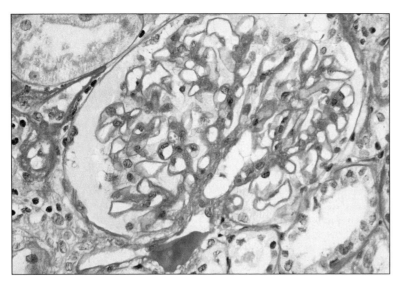

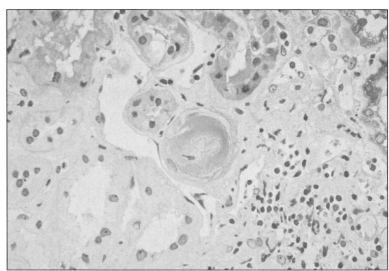

FIGURE 10-15

Cyclosporine nephrotoxicity with new-onset hyaline arteriolar thickening in the renin-producing portion of the afferent arteriole [5]. This lesion can be highly variable in extent and severity from section to section of the biopsy specimen, and it represents one of the strong arguments for examining multiple sections. The lesion is reversible if cyclosporine levels are reduced. Tacrolimus (FK506) produces an identical picture.

FIGURE 10-16 (*see* Color Plate)

Bland hyaline arteriolar thickening of donor origin in a renal allograft recipient never treated with cyclosporine. This phenomenon provides a strong argument for doing implantation biopsies; otherwise, donor changes can be mistaken for cyclosporine toxicity.

Posttransplant Lymphoproliferative Disorder

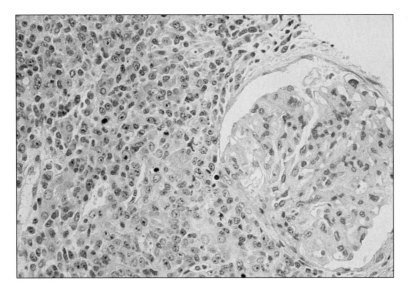

FIGURE 10-17

Posttransplant lymphoproliferative disorder (PTLD). The least satisfying facet of the 1997 Fourth Banff Conference on Allograft Pathology was the continued lack of good tools for the renal pathologist trying to distinguish the more subtle forms of PTLD from rejection. PTLD is rare, but, if misdiagnosed and treated with increased (rather than decreased) immunosuppression, it can quickly lead to death. The fact that both rejection and PTLD can occur simultaneously makes the challenge even greater [6]. It is hoped that newer techniques will make the diagnosis of this important condition more accurate in the future [7–9]. This figure shows an expansile plasmacytic infiltrate in a case of PTLD. However, most cases of PTLD are the result of Epstein-Barr virus–induced lymphoid proliferation.

Subclinical Rejection

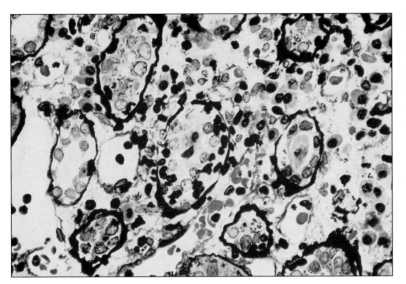

FIGURE 10-18 (*see* Color Plate)

Subclinical rejection. Subclinical rejection characterized by moderate to severe tubulitis may be found in as many as 35% of normally functioning grafts. Far from representing false-positive readings, such findings now appear to represent bona fide smoldering rejection that, if left untreated, is associated with increased incidence of chronic renal functional impairment and graft loss [10,11]. The important debate for the future is when to perform protocol biopsies to identify subclinical rejection and how best to treat it. This picture shows severe tubulitis in a normally functioning graft 15 months after transplantation. In the tubule in the center are 30 lymphocytes (versus 14 tubule cells). A year and a half later the patient developed renal functional impairment.

Thrombotic Microangiopathy

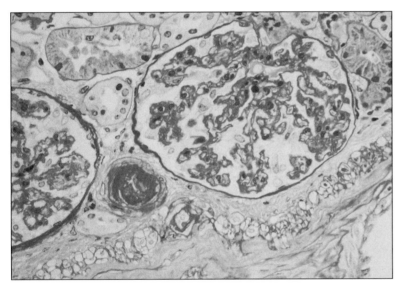

FIGURE 10-19

Thrombotic microangiopathy in renal allografts. A host of different conditions and influences can lead to arteriolar and capillary thrombosis in renal allografts and these are as various as the first dose reaction to OKT3, HIV infection, episodes of cyclosporine toxicity, and antibody-mediated rejection [2, 12, 13]. It is hoped that further study will allow for more accurate diagnosis in patients manifesting this lesion. The figure shows arteriolar thrombosis and ischemic capillary collapse in a case of transplant thrombotic microangiopathy.

Peritubular Capillary Basement Membrane Changes in Chronic Rejection

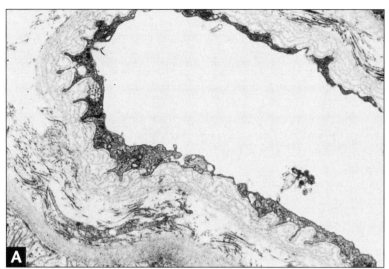 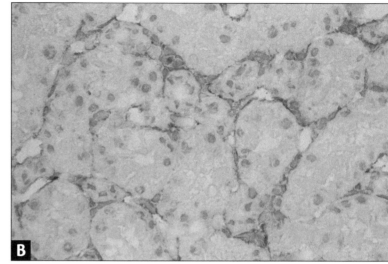

FIGURE 10-20 (*see* Color Plate)

Peritubular capillary basement membrane ultrastructural changes, **A**, and staining for VCAM-1 as specific markers for chronic rejection, **B** [14–16]. Splitting and multilayering of peritubular capillary basement membranes by electron microscopy holds promise as a relatively specific marker for chronic rejection [14,15]. VCAM-1 staining by immunohistology in these same structures may also be of diagnostic utility [16]. Ongoing studies of large numbers of patients using these parameters will test the value of these parameters which may eventually be added to the Banff classification. **A**, Multilayering of peritubular capillary basement membrane in a case of chronic rejection; **B**, shows staining of peritubular capillaries for VCAM-1 by immunoperoxidase in chronic rejection.

References

1. Solez K, Axelsen RA, Benediktsson H, *et al.*: International standardization of criteria for the histologic diagnosis of renal allograft rejection: The Banff working classification of kidney transplant pathology. *Kidney Int* 1993, 44:411–422.

2. Trpkov K, Campbell P, Pazderka F, *et al.*: Pathologic features of acute renal allograft rejection associated with donor-specific antibody, analysis using the Banff grading schema. *Transplantation* 1996, 61(11):1586–1592.

3. Solez K, Racusen LC, Marcussen N, *et al.*: Morphology of ischemic acute renal failure, normal function, and cyclosporine toxicity in cyclosporine-treated renal allograft recipients. *Kidney Int* 1993, 43(5):1058–1067.

4. Salyer WR, Keren D:Oxalosis as a complication of chronic renal failure. *Kidney Int* 1973, 4(1):61–66.

5. Strom EH, Epper R, Mihatsch MJ: Cyclosporin-associated arteriolopathy: The renin producing vascular smooth muscle cells are more sensitive to cyclosporin toxicity. *Clin Nephrol* 1995, 43(4):226–231.

6. Trpkov K, Marcussen N, Rayner D, *et al.*: Kidney allograft with a lymphocytic infiltrate: Acute rejection, post-transplantation lymphoproliferative disorder, neither, or both entities? *Am J Kidney Dis* 1997, 30(3):449–454.

7. Sasaki TM, Pirsch JD, D'Alessandro AM, *et al.*: Increased β 2-microglobulin (B2M) is useful in the detection of post-transplant lymphoproliferative disease (PTLD). *Clin Transplant* 1997, 11(1):29–33.

8. Chetty R, Biddolph S, Kaklamanis L, *et al.*: bcl-2 protein is strongly expressed in post-transplant lymphoproliferative disorders. *J Pathol* 1996, 180(3):254–258.

9. Wood A, Angus B, Kestevan P, *et al.*: Alpha interferon gene deletions in post-transplant lymphoma. *Br J Haematol* 1997, 98(4):1002–1003.

10. Nickerson P, Jeffrey J, McKenna R, *et al.*: Do renal allograft function and histology at 6 months posttransplant predict graft function at 2 years? *Transplant Proc* 1997, 29(6):2589–2590.

11. Rush D: Subclinical rejection. Presentation at Fourth Banff Conference on Allograft Pathology, March 7–12, 1997.

12. Wiener Y, Nakhleh RE, Lee MW, *et al.*: Prognostic factors and early resumption of cyclosporin A in renal allograft recipients with thrombotic microangiopathy and hemolytic uremic syndrome. *Clin Transplant* 1997, 11(3):157–162.

13. Frem GJ, Rennke HG, Sayegh MH: Late renal allograft failure secondary to thrombotic microangiopathy—human immunodeficiency virus nephropathy. *J Am Soc Nephrol* 1994, 4(9):1643–1648.

14. Monga G, Mazzucco G, Messina M, *et al.*: Intertubular capillary changes in kidney allografts: A morphologic investigation on 61 renal specimens. *Mod Pathol* 1992, 5(2):125–130.

15. Mazzucco G, Motta M, Segoloni G, Monga G: Intertubular capillary changes in the cortex and medulla of transplanted kidneys and their relationship with transplant glomerulopathy: An ultrastructural study of 12 transplantectomies. *Ultrastruct Pathol* 1994, 18(6):533–537.

16. Solez K, Racusen LC, Abdulkareem F, *et al.*: Adhesion molecules and rejection of renal allografts. *Kidney Int* 1997, 51(5):1476–1480.

Renal Injury Due To Environmental Toxins, Drugs, and Contrast Agents

Marc E. De Broe

The kidneys are susceptible to toxic or ischemic injury for several reasons. Thus, it is not surprising that an impressive list of exogenous drugs and chemicals can cause clinical acute renal failure (ARF) [1]. On the contrary, the contribution of environmental toxins to ARF is rather limited. In this chapter, some of the most common drugs and exogenous toxins encountered by the nephrologist in clinical practice are discussed in detail.

The clinical expression of the nephrotoxicity of drugs and chemicals is highly variable and is influenced by several factors. Among these is the direct toxic effect of drugs and chemicals on a particular type of nephron cell, the pharmacologic activity of some substances and their effects on renal function, the high metabolic activity (*ie*, vulnerability) of particular segments of the nephron, the multiple transport systems, which can result in intracellular accumulation of drugs and chemicals, and the high intratubule concentrations with possible precipitation and crystallization of particular drugs.

General Nephrotoxic Factors

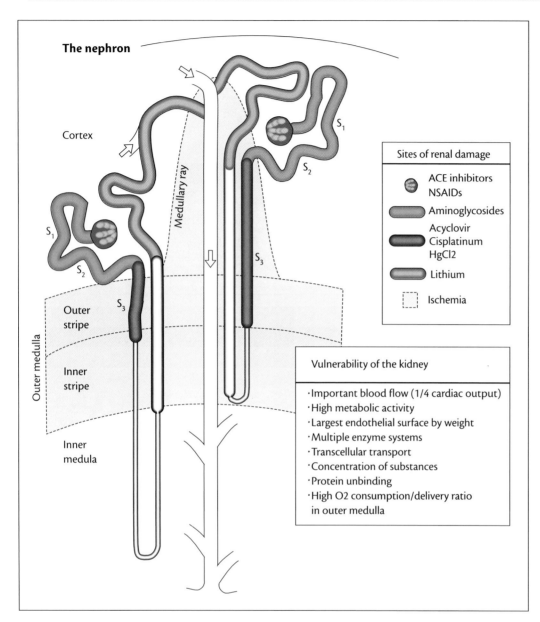

The nephron

Cortex

Medullary ray

S_1
S_2

S_1
S_2
S_3

Outer stripe
Inner stripe

Outer medulla

Inner medula

Sites of renal damage

- ACE inhibitors NSAIDs
- Aminoglycosides
- Acyclovir Cisplatinum HgCl2
- Lithium
- Ischemia

Vulnerability of the kidney

- Important blood flow (1/4 cardiac output)
- High metabolic activity
- Largest endothelial surface by weight
- Multiple enzyme systems
- Transcellular transport
- Concentration of substances
- Protein unbinding
- High O2 consumption/delivery ratio in outer medulla

FIGURE 11-1

Sites of renal damage, including factors that contribute to the kidney's susceptibility to damage. ACE—angiotensin-converting enzyme; NSAID—nonsteroidal anti-inflammatory drugs; $HgCl_2$—mercuric chloride.

DRUGS AND CHEMICALS ASSOCIATED WITH ACUTE RENAL FAILURE

Mechanisms

M1 Reduction in renal perfusion through alteration of intrarenal hemodynamics

M2 Direct tubular toxicity

M3 Heme pigment–induced toxicity (rhabdomyolysis)

M4 Intratubular obstruction by precipitation of the agents or its metabolites or byproducts

M5 Allergic interstitial nephritis

M6 Hemolytic-uremic syndrome

M1	M2	M3	M4	M5*	M6	Drugs
✓	✓				✓	Cyclosporine, tacrolimus
✓	✓					Amphotericin B, radiocontrast agents
✓				✓		Nonsteroidal anti-inflammatory drugs
✓						Angiotensin-converting enzyme inhibitors, interleukin-2†
✓	✓		✓			Methotrexate§
	✓					Aminoglycosides, cisplatin, foscarnet, heavy metals, intravenous immunoglobulin⁵, organic solvents, pentamidine
		✓			✓	Cocaine
		✓				Ethanol, lovastatin**
			✓	✓		Sulfonamides
			✓			Acyclovir, Indinavir, chemotherapeutic agents, ethylene glycol***
				✓		Allopurinol, cephalosporins, cimetidine, ciprofloxacin, furosemide, penicillins, phenytoin, rifampin, thiazide diuretics
					✓	Conjugated estrogens, mitomycin, quinine

* Many other drugs in addition to the ones listed can cause renal failure by this mechanism.

† Interleukin-2 produces a capillary leak syndrome with volume contractions.

§ Uric acid crystals form as a result of tumor lysis.

⁵ The mechanism of this agent is unclear but may be due to additives.

** Acute renal failure is most likely to occur when lovastatin is given in combination with cyclosporine.

*** Ethylene glycol–induced toxicity can cause calcium oxalate crystals.

FIGURE 11-2

Drugs and chemicals associated with acute renal failure. (*Apapted from* Thadhani, *et al.* [2].)

Aminoglycosides

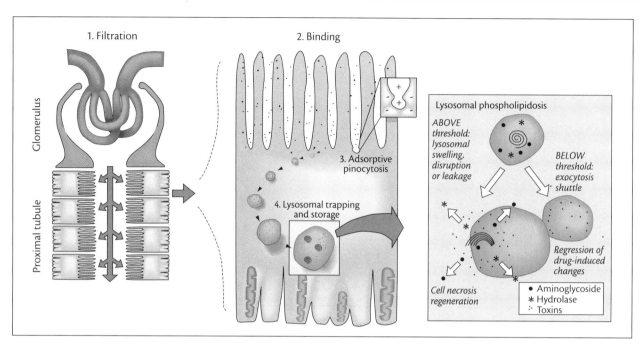

FIGURE 11-3

Renal handling of aminoglycosides: 1) glomerular filtration; 2) binding to the brush border membranes of the proximal tubule; 3) pinocytosis; and 4) storage in the lysosomes [3].

Nephrotoxicity and otovestibular toxicity remain frequent side effects that seriously limit the use of aminoglycosides, a still important class of antibiotics. Aminoglycosides are highly charged, polycationic, hydrophilic drugs that cross biologic membranes little, if at all [4,5]. They are not metabolized but are eliminated unchanged almost entirely by the kidneys. Aminoglycosides are filtered by the glomerulus at a rate almost equal to that of water. After entering the luminal fluid of proximal renal tubule, a small but toxicologically important portion of the filtered drug is reabsorbed and stored in the proximal tubule cells. The major transport of aminoglycosides into proximal tubule cells involves interaction with acidic, negatively charged phospholipid-binding sites at the level of the brush border membrane.

After charge-mediated binding, the drug is taken up into the cell in small invaginations of the cell membrane, a process in which megalin seems to play a role [6]. Within 1 hour of injection, the drug is located at the apical cytoplasmic vacuoles, called endocytotic vesicles. These vesicles fuse with lysosomes, sequestering the unchanged aminoglycosides inside those organelles.

Once trapped in the lysosomes of proximal tubule cells, aminoglycosides electrostatically attached to anionic membrane phospholipids interfere with the normal action of some enzymes (ie, phospholipases and sphingomyelinase). In parallel with enzyme inhibition, undigested phospholipids originating from the turnover of cell membranes accumulate in lysosomes, where they are normally digested. The overall result is lysosomal phospholipidosis due to nonspecific accumulation of polar phospholipids as "myeloid bodies," so called for their typical electron microscopic appearance. (*Adapted from* De Broe [3].)

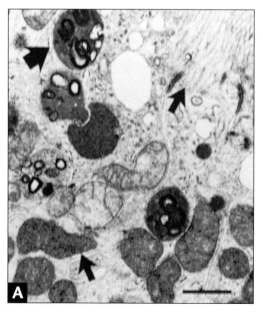
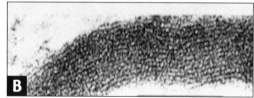

FIGURE 11-4

Ultrastructural appearance of proximal tubule cells in aminoglycoside-treated patients (4 days of therapeutic doses). Lysosomes (*large arrow*) contain dense lamellar and concentric structures. Brush border, mitochondria (*small arrows*) and peroxisomes are unaltered. At higher magnification the structures in lysosomes show a periodic pattern. The bar in **A** represents 1 μm, in part **B**, 0.1 μm [7].

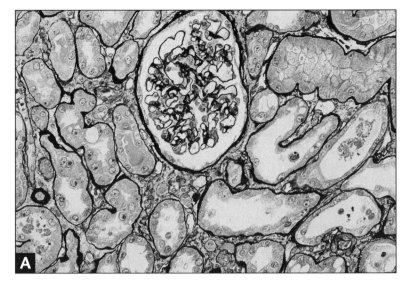

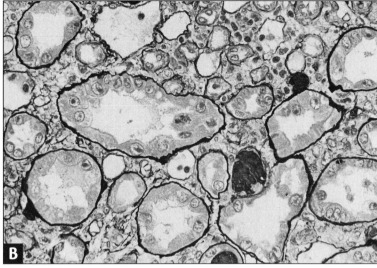

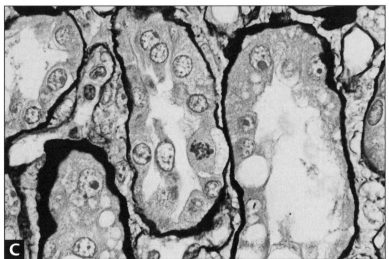

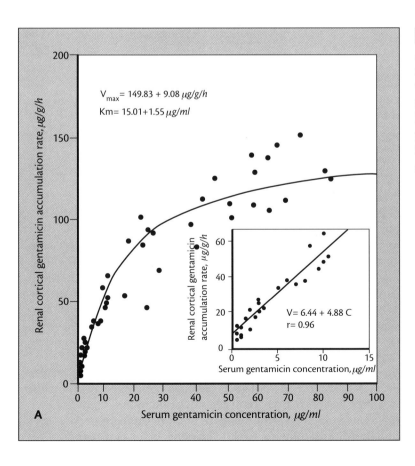

FIGURE 11-5 (*see* Color Plate)

Administration of aminoglycosides for days induces progression of lysosomal phospholipidosis. The overloaded lysosomes continue to swell, even if the drug is then withdrawn. In vivo this overload may result in loss of integrity of the membranes of lysosomes and release of large amounts of lysosomal enzymes, phospholipids, and aminoglycosides into the cytosol, but this has not been proven. Thus, these aminoglycosides can gain access to and injure other organelles, such as mitochondria, and disturb their functional integrity, which leads rapidly to cell death. As a consequence of cell necrosis, **A,** intratubular obstruction by cell debris increased intratubule pressure, a decrease in the glomerular filtration rate and cellular infiltration, **B,** may ensue. In parallel with these lethal processes in the kidney, a striking regeneration process is observed that is characterized by a dramatic increase in tubule cell turnover and proliferation, **C,** in the cortical interstitial compartment.

FIGURE 11-6

A, Relationship between constant serum levels and concomitant renal cortical accumulation of gentamicin after a 6 hour intravenous infusion in rats. The rate of accumulation is expressed in micrograms of aminoglycoside per gram of wet kidney cortex per hour, due to the linear accumulation in function of time. Each point represents one rat whose aminoglycosides were measured in both kidneys at the end of the infusion and the serum levels assayed twice during the infusion [8].

(Continued on next page)

V_{max} = 149.83 + 9.08 $\mu g/g/h$

Km = 15.01 + 1.55 $\mu g/ml$

V = 6.44 + 4.88 C

r = 0.96

Renal cortical gentamicin accumulation rate, $\mu g/g/h$ (y-axis, inset)

Serum gentamicin concentration, $\mu g/ml$ (x-axis, inset)

Renal cortical gentamicin accumulation rate, $\mu g/g/h$ (y-axis)

Serum gentamicin concentration, $\mu g/ml$ (x-axis)

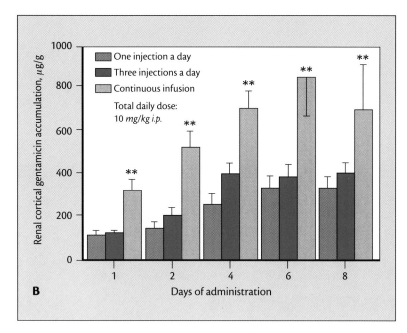

B

FIGURE 11-6 (*Continued*)

B, Kidney cortical concentrations of gentamicin in rats given equal daily amounts of aminoglycoside in single injections, three injections, or by continuous infusion over 8 days. Each block represents the mean of seven rats ±SD. Significance is shown only between cortical levels achieved after continuous infusion and single injections (asterisk—$P < 0.05$; double asterisk—$P < 0.01$) [9].

In rats, nephrotoxicity of gentamicin is more pronounced when the total daily dose is administered by continuous infusion rather than as a single injection. Thus, a given daily drug does not produce the same degree of toxicity when it is given by different routes. Indeed, renal cortical uptake is "less efficient" at high serum concentration than at low ones. A single injection results in high peak serum levels that overcome the saturation limits of the renal uptake mechanism. The high plasma concentrations are followed by fast elimination and, finally, absence of the drug for a while. This contrasts with the continuous low serum levels obtained with more frequent dosing when the uptake at the level of the renal cortex is not only more efficient but remains available throughout the treatment period. V_{max}—maximum velocity.

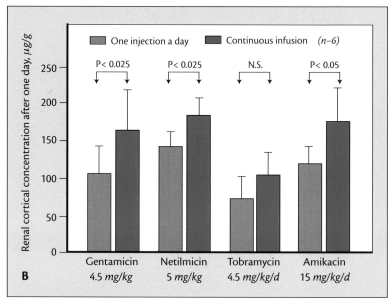

B

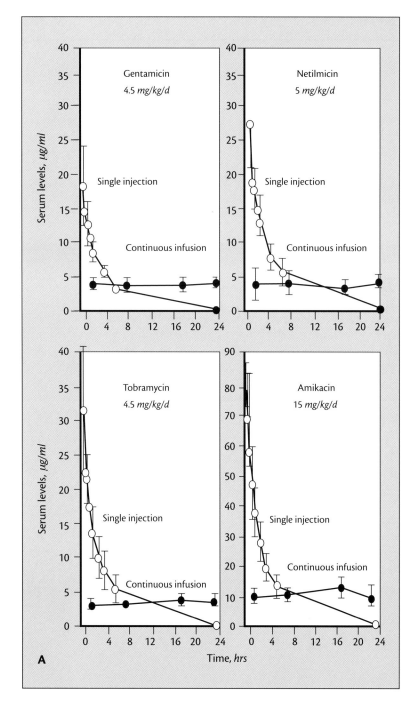

A

FIGURE 11-7

Course of serum concentrations, **A**, and of renal cortical concentrations, **B**, of gentamicin, netilmicin, tobramycin, and amikacin after dosing by a 30-minute intravenous injection or continuous infusion over 24 hours [10,11].

Two trials in humans found that the dosage schedule had a critical effect on renal uptake of gentamicin, netilmicin [10], amikacin, and tobramycin [11]. Subjects were patients with normal renal function (serum creatinine concentration between 0.9 and 1.2 mg/dL, proteinuria lower than 300 mg/24 h) who had renal cancer and submitted to nephrectomy. Before surgery, patients received gentamicin (4.5 mg/kg/d), netilmicin (5 mg/kg/d), amikacin (15 mg/kg/d), or tobramycin (4.5 mg/kg/d) as a single injection or as a continuous intravenous infusion over 24 hours. The single-injection schedule resulted in 30% to 50% lower cortical drug concentrations of netilmicin, gentamicin, and amikacin as compared with continuous infusion. For tobramycin, no difference in renal accumulation could be found, indicating the linear cortical uptake of this particular aminoglycoside [8]. These data, which supported decreased nephrotoxic potential of single-dose regimens, coincided with new insights in the antibacterial action of aminoglycosides (concentration-dependent killing of gram-negative bacteria and prolonged postantibiotic effect) [12]. N.S.—not significant.

RISK FACTORS FOR AMINOGLYCOSIDE NEPHROTOXICITY

Patient-Related Factors	Aminoglycoside-Related Factors	Other Drugs
Older age*	Recent aminoglycoside therapy	Amphotericin B
Preexisting renal disease		Cephalosporins
Female gender	Larger doses*	Cisplatin
Magnesium, potassium, or calcium deficiency*	Treatment for 3 days or more*	Clindamycin
Intravascular volume depletion*		Cyclosporine
Hypotension*	Dose regimen*	Foscarnet
Hepatorenal syndrome		Furosemide
Sepsis syndrome		Piperacillin
		Radiocontrast agents
		Thyroid hormone

* Similar to experimental data.

FIGURE 11-8

Risk factors for aminoglycoside nephrotoxicity. Several risk factors have been identified and classified as patient related, aminoglycoside related, or related to concurrent administration of certain drugs.

The usual recommended aminoglycoside dose may be excessive for older patients because of decreased renal function and decreased regenerative capacity of a damaged kidney. Preexisting renal disease clearly can expose patients to inadvertent overdosing if careful dose adjustment is not performed. Hypomagnesemia, hypokalemia, and calcium deficiency may be predisposing risk factors for consequences of aminoglycoside-induced damage [13]. Liver disease is an important clinical risk factor for aminoglycoside nephrotoxicity, particularly in patients with cholestasis [13]. Acute or chronic endotoxemia amplifies the nephrotoxic potential of the aminoglycosides [14].

PREVENTION OF AMINOGLYCOSIDE NEPHROTOXICITY

Identify risk factor
  Patient related
  Drug related
  Other drugs
Give single daily dose of gentamicin, netilmicin, or amikacin
Reduce the treatment course as much as possible
Avoid giving nephrotoxic drugs concurrently
Make interval between aminoglycoside courses as long as possible
Calculate glomerular filtration rate out of serum creatinine concentration

FIGURE 11-9

Prevention of aminoglycoside nephrotoxicity. Coadministration of other potentially nephrotoxic drugs enhances or accelerates the nephrotoxicity of aminoglycosides. Comprehension of the pharmacokinetics and renal cell biologic effects of aminoglycosides, allows identification of aminoglycoside-related nephrotoxicity risk factors and makes possible secondary prevention of this important clinical nephrotoxicity.

Amphotericin B

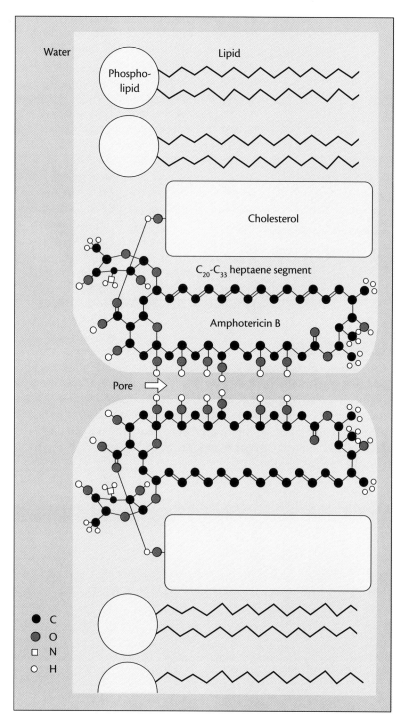

FIGURE 11-10

Proposed partial model for the amphotericin B (AmB)–induced pore in the cell membrane. AmB is an amphipathic molecule: its structure enhances the drug's binding to sterols in the cell membranes and induces formation of aqueous pores that result in weakening of barrier function and loss of protons and cations from the cell. The drug acts as a counterfeit phospholipid, with the C_{15} hydroxyl, C_{16} carboxyl, and C_{19} mycosamine groups situated at the membrane-water interface, and the C_1 to C_{14} and C_{20} to C_{33} chains aligned in parallel within the membrane. The heptaene chain seeks a hydrophobic environment, and the hydroxyl groups seek a hydrophilic environment. Thus, a cylindrical pore is formed, the inner wall of which consists of the hydroxyl-substituted carbon chains of the AmB molecules and the outer wall of which is formed by the heptaene chains of the molecules and by sterol nuclei [15].

RISK FACTORS IN THE DEVELOPMENT OF AMPHOTERICIN NEPHROTOXICITY

Age
Concurrent use of diuretics
Abnormal baseline renal function
Larger daily doses
Hypokalemia
Hypomagnesemia
Other nephrotoxic drugs (aminoglycosides, cyclosporine)

FIGURE 11-11

Risk factors for development of amphotericin B (AmB) nephrotoxicity. Nephrotoxicity of AmB is a major problem associated with clinical use of this important drug. Disturbances in both glomerular and tubule function are well described. The nephrotoxic effect of AmB is initially a distal tubule phenomenon, characterized by a loss of urine concentration, distal renal tubule acidosis, and wasting of potassium and magnesium, but it also causes renal vasoconstriction leading to renal ischemia. Initially, the drug binds to membrane sterols in the renal vasculature and epithelial cells, altering its membrane permeability. AmB-induced vasoconstriction and ischemia to very vulnerable sections of the nephron, such as medullary thick ascending limb, enhance the cell death produced by direct toxic action of AmB on those cells. This explains the salutary effect on AmB nephrotoxicity of salt loading, furosemide, theophylline, or calcium channel blockers, all of which improve renal blood flow or inhibit transport in the medullary thick ascending limb.

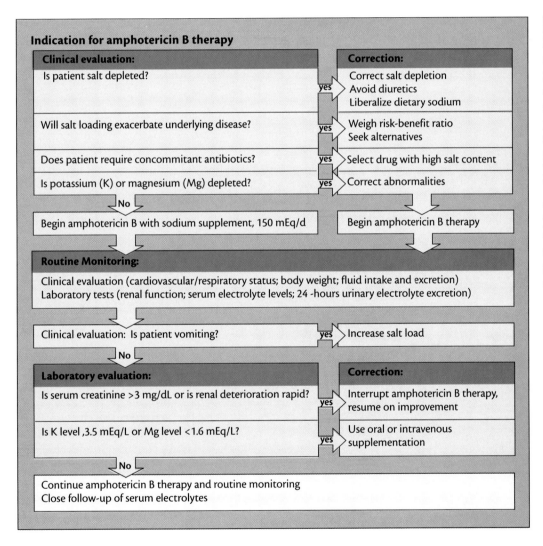

FIGURE 11-12

Proposed approach for management of amphotericin B (AmB) therapy. Several new formulations of amphotericin have been developed either by incorporating amphotericin into liposomes or by forming complexes to phospholipid. In early studies, nephrotoxicity was reduced, allowing an increase of the cumulative dose. Few studies have established a therapeutic index between antifungal and nephrotoxic effects of amphotericin. To date, the only clinically proven intervention that reduces the incidence and severity of nephrotoxicity is salt supplementation, which should probably be given prophylactically to all patients who can tolerate it. (*From* Bernardo JF, *et al*. [16]; with permission.)

Cyclosporine

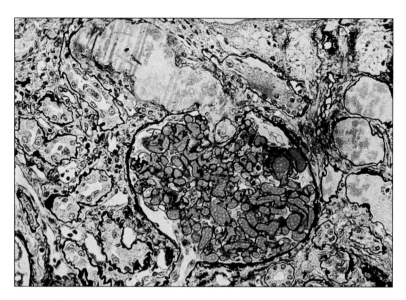

FIGURE 11-13 (*see* Color Plate)

Intravascular coagulation in a cyclosporine-treated renal transplant recipient. Cyclosporine produces a dose-related decrease in renal function in experimental animals and humans [17] that is attributed to the drug's hemodynamic action to produce vasoconstriction of the afferent arteriole entering the glomerulus. When severe enough, this can decrease glomerular filtration rate. Although the precise pathogenesis of the renal hemodynamic effects of cyclosporine are unclear, endothelin, inhibition of nitric oxide,

release of vasoconstrictor prostaglandins such as thromboxane A$_2$, and activation of the sympathetic nervous system, are among the candidates for cyclosporine-induced vasoconstriction [18].

The diagnosis of cyclosporine-induced acute renal dysfunction is not difficult when the patient has no other reason for reduced renal function (*eg*, psoriasis, rheumatoid arthritis). In renal transplant recipients, however, the situation is completely different. In this clinical setting, the clinician must differentiate between cyclosporine injury and acute rejection. The incidence of this acute cyclosporine renal injury can be enhanced by extended graft preservation, preexisting histologic lesions, donor hypotension, or preoperative complications. The gold standard for this important distinction remains renal biopsy.

In addition, cyclosporine has been associated with hemolytic-uremic syndrome with thrombocytopenia, red blood cell fragmentation, and intravascular (intraglomerular) coagulation. Again, this drug-related intravascular coagulation has to be differentiated from that of acute rejection. The absence of clinical signs and of rejection-related interstitial edema and cellular infiltrates can be helpful.

Vanrenterghem and coworkers [19] found a high incidence of venous thromboembolism shortly after (several of them within days) cadaveric kidney transplantation in patients treated with cyclosporine, in contrast to those treated with azathioprine. Recent studies [20] have shown that impaired fibrinolysis, due mainly to excess plasminogen activator inhibitor (PAI-1), may also contribute to this imbalance in coagulation and anticoagulation during cyclosporine treatment.

Lithium-Induced Acute Renal Failure

SIGNS AND SYMPTOMS OF TOXIC EFFECTS OF LITHIUM

Toxic Effect	Plasma Lithium Level	Signs and Symptoms
Mild	1–1.5 mmol/L	Impaired concentration, lethargy, irritability, muscle weakness, tremor, slurred speech, nausea
Moderate	1.6–2.5 mmol/L	Disorientation, confusion, drowsiness, restlessness, unsteady gait, coarse tremor, dysarthria, muscle fasciculation, vomiting
Severe	>2.5 mmol/L	Impaired consciousness (with progression to coma), delirium, ataxia, generalized fasciculations, extrapyramidal symptoms, convulsions, impaired renal function

FIGURE 11-14

Symptoms and signs of toxic effects of lithium. Lithium can cause acute functional and histologic (usually reversible) renal injury. Within 24 hours of administration of lithium to humans or animals, sodium diuresis occurs and impairment in the renal concentrating capacity becomes apparent. The defective concentrating capacity is caused by vasopressin-resistant (exogenous and endogenous) diabetes insipidus. This is in part related to lithium's inhibition of adenylate cyclase and impairment of vasopressin-induced generation of cyclic adenosine monophosphatase.

Lithium-induced impairment of distal urinary acidification has also been defined.

Acute lithium intoxication in humans and animals can cause acute renal failure. The clinical picture features nonspecific signs of degenerative changes and necrosis of tubule cells [21]. The most distinctive and specific acute lesions lie at the level of the distal tubule [22]. They consist of swelling and vacuolization of the cytoplasm of the distal nephron cells plus periodic acid-Schiff–positive granular material in the cytoplasm (shown to be glycogen) [23]. Most patients receiving lithium have side effects, reflecting the drug's narrow therapeutic index.

DRUG INTERACTIONS WITH LITHIUM

Salt depletion strongly impairs renal elimination of lithium.
Salt loading increases absolute and fractional lithium clearance.

Diuretics	
Acetazolamide	Increased lithium clearance
Thiazides	Increased plasma lithium level due to decreased lithium clearance
Loop diuretics	Acute increased lithium clearance
Amiloride	Usually no change in plasma lithium level; may be used to treat lithium-induced polyuria
Nonsteroidal anti-inflammatory drugs	Increased plasma lithium level due to decreased renal lithium clearance (exceptions are aspirin and sulindac)
Bronchodilators (amino-phylline, theophylline)	Decreased plasma lithium level due to increased renal lithium clearance
Angiotensin-converting enzyme inhibitors	May increase plasma lithium level
Cyclosporine	Decreased lithium clearance

FIGURE 11-15

Drug interactions with lithium [24]. Acute renal failure, with or without oliguria, can be associated with lithium treatment, and with severe dehydration. In this case, acute renal failure can be considered a prerenal type; consequently, it resolves rapidly with appropriate fluid therapy. Indeed, the histologic appearance in such cases is remarkable for its lack of significant abnormalities. Conditions that stimulate sodium retention and consequently lithium reabsorption, such as low salt intake and loss of body fluid by way of vomiting, diarrhea, or diuretics, decreasing lithium clearance should be avoided. With any acute illness, particularly one associated with gastrointestinal symptoms such as diarrhea, lithium blood levels should be closely monitored and the dose adjusted when necessary. Indeed, most episodes of acute lithium intoxication are largely predictable, and thus avoidable, provided that precautions are taken [25].

Removing lithium from the body as soon as possible the is the mainstay of treating lithium intoxication. With preserved renal function, excretion can be increased by use of furosemide, up to 40 mg/h, obviously under close monitoring for excessive losses of sodium and water induced by this loop diuretic. When renal function is impaired in association with severe toxicity, extracorporeal extraction is the most efficient way to decrease serum lithium levels. One should, however, remember that lithium leaves the cells slowly and that plasma levels rebound after hemodialysis is stopped, so that longer dialysis treatment or treatment at more frequent intervals is required.

Inhibitors of the Renin-Angiotensin System

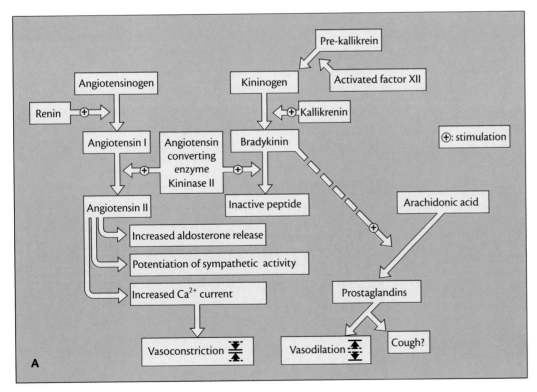

efferent arteriolar vascular tone and in general is reversible after withdrawing the angiotensin-converting enzyme (ACE) inhibitor [27].

Inhibition of the ACE kinase II results in at least two important effects: depletion of angiotensin II and accumulation of bradykinin [28]. The role of the latter effect on renal perfusion pressure is not clear, **A**.

To understand the angiotensin I converting enzyme inhibitor–induced drop in glomerular filtration rate, it is important to understand the physiologic role of the renin-angiotensin system in the regulation of renal hemodynamics, **B**. When renal perfusion drops, renin is released into the plasma and lymph by the juxtaglomerular cells of the kidneys. Renin cleaves angiotensinogen to form angiotensin I, which is cleaved further by converting enzyme to form angiotensin II, the principal effector molecule in this system. Angiotensin II participates in glomerular filtration rate regulation in a least two ways. First, angiotensin II increases arterial pressure—directly and acutely by causing vasoconstriction and more "chronically" by increasing body fluid volumes through stimulation of renal sodium retention; directly through an effect on the tubules, as well as by stimulating thirst

FIGURE 11-16

Soon after the release of this useful class of antihypertensive drugs, the syndrome of functional acute renal insufficiency was described as a class effect. This phenomenon was first observed in patients with renal artery stenosis, particularly when the entire renal mass was affected, as in bilateral renal artery stenosis or in renal transplants with stenosis to a solitary kidney [26]. Acute renal dysfunction appears to be related to loss of postglomerular

(Continued on next page)

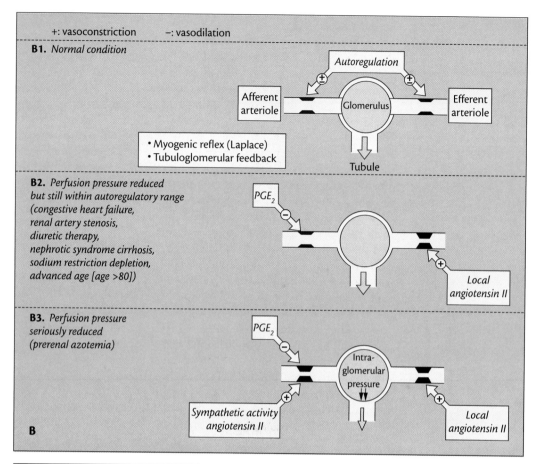

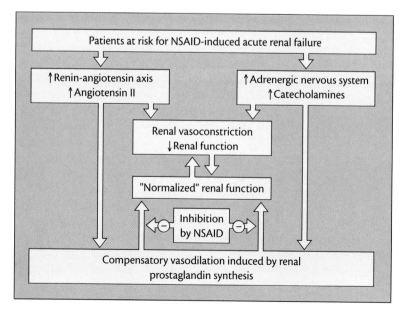

+: vasoconstriction   −: vasodilation

B1. *Normal condition*

Autoregulation

Afferent arteriole

Glomerulus

Efferent arteriole

• Myogenic reflex (Laplace)
• Tubuloglomerular feedback

Tubule

B2. *Perfusion pressure reduced but still within autoregulatory range (congestive heart failure, renal artery stenosis, diuretic therapy, nephrotic syndrome cirrhosis, sodium restriction depletion, advanced age [age >80])*

PGE₂

Local angiotensin II

B3. *Perfusion pressure seriously reduced (prerenal azotemia)*

PGE₂

Intraglomerular pressure

Sympathetic activity angiotensin II

Local angiotensin II

B

FIGURE 11-16 *(Continued)*

and indirectly via aldosterone. Second, angiotensin II preferentially constricts the efferent arteriole, thus helping to preserve glomerular capillary hydrostatic pressure and, consequently, glomerular filtration rate.

When arterial pressure or body fluid volumes are sensed as subnormal, the renin-angiotensin system is activated and plasma renin activity and angiotensin II levels increase. This may occur in the context of clinical settings such as renal artery stenosis,

dietary sodium restriction or sodium depletion as during diuretic therapy, congestive heart failure, cirrhosis, and nephrotic syndrome. When activated, this reninangiotensin system plays an important role in the maintenance of glomerular pressure and filtration through preferential angiotensin II–mediated constriction of the efferent arteriole. Thus, under such conditions the kidney becomes sensitive to the effects of blockade of the renin-angiotensin system by angiotensin I–converting enzyme inhibitor or angiotensin II receptor antagonist.

The highest incidence of renal failure in patients treated with ACE inhibitors was associated with bilateral renovascular disease [27]. In patients with already compromised renal function and congestive heart failure, the incidence of serious changes in serum creatinine during ACE inhibition depends on the severity of the pretreatment heart failure and renal failure.

Volume management, dose reduction, use of relatively short-acting ACE inhibitors, diuretic holiday for some days before initiating treatment, and avoidance of concurrent use of nonsteroidal anti-inflammatory drug (hyperkalemia) are among the appropriate measures for patients at risk.

Acute interstitial nephritis associated with angiotensin I–converting enzyme inhibition has been described [29]. (*Adapted from* Opie [30]; with permission.)

Nonsteroidal Anti-inflammatory Drugs

Patients at risk for NSAID-induced acute renal failure

↑Renin-angiotensin axis ↑Angiotensin II

↑Adrenergic nervous system ↑Catecholamines

Renal vasoconstriction ↓Renal function

"Normalized" renal function

Inhibition by NSAID

Compensatory vasodilation induced by renal prostaglandin synthesis

FIGURE 11-17

Mechanism by which nonsteroidal anti-inflammatory drugs (NSAIDs) disrupt the compensatory vasodilatation response of renal prostaglandins to vasoconstrictor hormones in patients with prerenal conditions. Most of the renal abnormalities encountered clinically as a result of NSAIDs can be attributed to the action of these compounds on prostaglandin production in the kidney [31].

Sodium chloride and water retention are the most common side effects of NSAIDs. This should not be considered drug toxicity because it represents a modification of a physiologic control mechanism without the production of a true functional disorder in the kidney.

PREDISPOSING FACTORS FOR NSAID-INDUCED ACUTE RENAL FAILURE

Severe heart disease (congestive heart failure)
Severe liver disease (cirrhosis)
Nephrotic syndrome (low oncotic pressure)
Chronic renal disease
Age 80 years or older
Protracted dehydration (several days)

FIGURE 11-18

Conditions associated with risk for nonsteroidal anti-inflammatory drugs (NSAID)-induced acute renal failure. NSAIDs can induce acute renal decompensation in patients with various renal and extrarenal clinical conditions that cause a decrease in blood perfusion to the kidney [32]. Renal prostaglandins play an important role in the maintenance of homeostasis in these patients, so disruption of counter-regulatory mechanisms can produce clinically important, and even severe, deterioration in renal function.

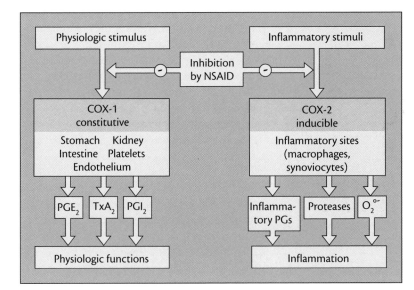

FIGURE11-19

Inhibition by nonsteroidal anti-inflammatory drugs (NSAIDs) on pathways of cyclo-oxygenase (COX) and prostaglandin synthesis [33]. The recent demonstration of the existence of functionally distinct isoforms of the cox enzyme has major clinical significance, as it now appears that one form of cox is operative in the gastric mucosa and kidney for prostaglandin generation (COX-1) whereas an inducible and functionally distinct form of cox is operative in the production of prostaglandins in the sites of inflammation and pain (COX-2) [33]. The clinical therapeutic consequence is that an NSAID with inhibitory effects dominantly or exclusively upon the cox isoenzyme induced at a site of inflammation may produce the desired therapeutic effects without the hazards of deleterious effects on the kidneys or gastrointestinal tract. PG—prostaglandin; TxA_2—thromboxane A_2.

EFFECTS OF NSAIDS ON RENAL FUNCTION

Renal Syndrome	Mechanism	Risk Factors	Prevention/Treatment [34]
Sodium retention and edema	↓ Prostaglandin	NSAID therapy (most common side effect)	Stop NSAID
Hyperkalemia	↓ Prostaglandin	Renal disease	Stop NSAID
	↓ Potassium to distal tubule	Heart failure	Avoid use in high-risk patients
		Diabetes	
	↓ Aldosterone/renin-angiotensin	Multiple myeloma	
		Potassium therapy	
		Potassium-sparing diuretic	
Acute deterioration of renal function	↓ Prostaglandin and disruption of hemodynamic balance	Liver disease	Stop NSAID
		Renal disease	Avoid use in high-risk patients
		Heart failure	
		Dehydration	
		Old age	Stop NSAID
			Dialysis and steroids (?)
Nephrotic syndrome with: Interstitial nephritis	↑ Lymphocyte recruitment and activation	Fenoprofen	Stop NSAID
			Avoid long-term analgesic use
Papillary necrosis	Direct toxicity	Combination aspirin and acetaminophen abuse	

FIGURE 11-20

Summary of effects of nonsteroidal anti-inflammatory drugs (NSAIDs) on renal function [31].

All NSAIDs can cause another type of renal dysfunction that is associated with various levels of functional impairment and characterized by the nephrotic syndrome together with interstitial nephritis.

Characteristically, the histology of this form of NSAID–induced nephrotic syndrome consists of minimal-change glomerulonephritis with tubulointerstitial nephritis. This is an unusual combination of findings and in the setting of protracted NSAID use is virtually pathognomic of NSAID-related nephrotic syndrome.

A focal diffuse inflammatory infiltrate can be found around the proximal and distal tubules. The infiltrate consists primarily of cytotoxic T lymphocytes but also contains other T cells, some B cells, and plasma cells. Changes in the glomeruli are minimal and resemble those of classic minimal-change glomerulonephritis with marked epithelial foot process fusion.

Hyperkalemia, an unusual complication of NSAIDs, is more likely to occur in patients with pre-existing renal impairment, cardiac failure, diabetes, or multiple myeloma or in those taking potassium supplements, potassium-sparing diuretic therapy, or intercurrent use of an angiotensin-converting enzyme inhibitor. The mechanism of NSAID hyperkalemia—suppression of prostaglandin-mediated renin release—leads to a state of hyporeninemic hypoaldosteronism. In addition, NSAIDs, particularly indomethacin, may have a direct effect on cellular uptake of potassium.

The renal saluretic response to loop diuretics is partially a consequence of intrarenal prostaglandin production. This component of the response to loop diuretics is mediated by an increase in renal medullary blood flow and an attendant reduction in renal concentrating capacity. Thus, concurrent use of an NSAID may blunt the diuresis induced by loop diuretics.

Contrast Medium–Associated Nephrotoxicity

RISK FACTORS THAT PREDISPOSE TO CONTRAST ASSOCIATED NEPHROPATHY

Confirmed	Suspected	Disproved
Chronic renal failure	Hypertension	Myeloma
Diabetic nephropathy	Generalized atherosclerosis	Diabetes without nephropathy
Severe congestive heart failure	Abnormal liver function tests	
Amount and frequency of contrast media	Hyperuricemia	
Volume depletion or hypotension	Proteinuria	

FIGURE 11-21

Risk factors that predispose to contrast-associated nephropathy. In random populations undergoing radiocontrast imaging the incidence of contrasts associated nephropathy defined by a change in serum creatinine of more than 0.5 mg/dL or a greater than 50% increase over baseline, is between 2% and 7%. For confirmed high-risk patients (baseline serum creatinine values greater than 1.5 mg/dL) it rises to 10% to 35%. In addition, there are suspected risk factors that should be taken into consideration when considering the value of contrast-enhanced imaging.

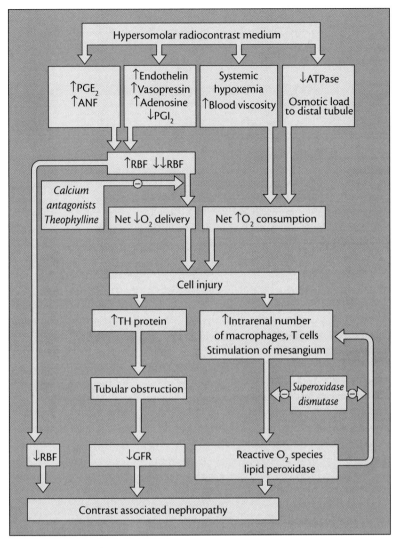

FIGURE 11-22

A proposed model of the mechanisms involved in radiocontrast medium–induced renal dysfunction. Based on experimental mod-

els, a consensus is developing to the effect that contrast-associated nephropathy involves combined toxic and hypoxic insults to the kidney [35]. The initial glomerular vasoconstriction that follows the injection of radiocontrast medium induces the liberation of both vasoconstrictor (endothelin, vasopressin) and vasodilator (prostaglandin E_2 [PGE_2], adenosine, atrionatiuretic factor {ANP}) substances. The net effect is reduced oxygen delivery to tubule cells, especially those in the thick ascending limb of Henle. Because of the systemic hypoxemia, raised blood viscosity, inhibition of sodium-potassium–activated ATPase and the increased osmotic load to the distal tubule at a time of reduced oxygen delivery, the demand for oxygen increases, resulting in cellular hypoxia and, eventually cell death. Additional factors that contribute to the acute renal dysfunction of contrast-associated nephropathy are the tubule obstruction that results from increased secretion of Tamm-Horsfall proteins and the liberation of reactive oxygen species and lipid peroxidation that accompany cell death. As noted in the figure, calcium antagonists and theophylline (adenosine receptor antagonist) are thought to act to diminish the degree of vasoconstriction induced by contrast medium.

The clinical presentation of contrast-associated nephropathy involves an asymptomatic increase in serum creatinine within 24 hours of a radiographic imaging study using contrast medium, with or without oliguria [36].

We have recently reviewed the clinical outcome of 281 patients with contrast-associated nephropathy according to the presence or absence of oliguric acute renal failure at the time of diagnosis. Of oliguric acute renal failure patients, 32% have persistent elevations of serum creatinine at recovery and half require permanent dialysis. In the absence of oliguric acute renal failure the serum creatinine value does not return to baseline in 24% of patients, approximately a third of whom require permanent dialysis. Thus, this is not a benign condition but rather one whose defined risks are not only permanent dialysis but also death. GFR—glomerular filtration rate; RBF—renal blood flow; TH—Tamm Horsfall protein.

PREVENTION OF CONTRAST ASSOCIATED NEPHROPATHY

Hydrate patient before the study (1.5 mL/kg/h) 12 h before and after.

Hemodynamically stabilize hemodynamics.

Minimize amount of contrast medium administered.

Use nonionic, iso-osmolar contrast media for patients at high risk (*see* Figure 11-21).

FIGURE 11-23

Prevention of contrast-associated nephropathy. The goal of management is the prevention of contrast-associated nephropathy.

Thus it is important to select the least invasive diagnostic procedure that provides the most information, so that the patient can make an informed choice from the available clinical alternatives.

Since radiographic contrast imaging is frequently performed for diabetic nephropathy, congestive heart failure, or chronic renal failure, concurrent administration of renoprotective agents has become an important aspect of imaging. A list of maneuvers that minimize the risk of contrast-associated nephropathy is contained in this table. The correction of prestudy volume depletion and the use of active hydration before and during the procedure are crucial to minimizing the risk of contrast-associated nephropathy. Limiting the total volume of contrast medium and using nonionic, isoosmolar media have proven to be protective for high-risk patients. Pretreatment with calcium antagonists is an intriguing but unsubstantiated approach.

References

1. Bennett WM, Porter GA: Overview of clinical nephrotoxicity. In *Toxicology of the Kidney*, edn 2. Edited by Hook JB, Goldstein RS. Raven Press, 1993:61–97.

2. Thadhani R, Pascual M, Bonventre JV: Acute renal failure. *N Engl J Med* 1996, 334:1448–1460.

3. De Broe ME: Prevention of aminoglycoside nephrotoxicity. In *Proc EDTA-ERA*. Edited by Davison AM, Guillou PJ. London:BailliÈre Tindal, 1985:959–973.

4. Lietman PS: Aminoglycosides and spectinoycin: aminocylitols. In *Principles and Practice of Infectious Diseases*, edn 2, Part I. Edited by Mandel GL, Doublas RG Jr, Bennett JE. New York: John Wiley & Sons, 1985:192–206.

5. Kaloyanides GJ, Pastoriza-Munoz E: Aminoglycoside nephrotoxicity. *Kidney Int* 1980, 18:571–582.

6. Molitoris BA. Cell biology of aminoglycoside nephrotoxicity: newer aspects. *Curr Opin Nephrol Hypertens* 1997, 6:384–388.

7. De Broe ME, Paulus GJ, Verpooten GA, *et al.*: Early effects of gentamicin, tobramycin, and amikacin on the human kidney. *Kidney Int* 1984, 25:643–652.

8. Giuliano RA, Verpooten GA, Verbist L, *et al.*: In vivo uptake kinetics of aminoglycosides in the kidney cortex of rats. *J Pharmacol Exp Ther* 1986, 236:470–475.

9. Giuliano RA, Verpooten GA, De Broe ME: The effect of dosing strategy on kidney cortical accumulation of aminoglycosides in rats. *Am J Kidney Dis* 1986, 8:297–303.

10. Verpooten GA, Giuliano RA, Verbist L, *et al.*: A once-daily dosage schedule decreases the accumulation of gentamicin and netilmicin in the renal cortex of humans. *Clin Pharmacol Ther* 1989, 44:1–5.

11. De Broe ME, Verbist L, Verpooten GA: Influence of dosage schedule on renal cortical accumulation of amikacin and tobramycin in man. *J Antimicrob Chemother* 1991, 27 (suppl C):41–47.

12. Bennett WM, Plamp CE, Gilbert DN, *et al.*: The influence of dosage regimen on experimental gentamicin nephrotoxicity: dissociation of peak serum levels from renal failure. *J Infect Dis* 1979, 140:576–580.

13. Moore RD, Smith CR, Lipsky JJ, *et al.*: Risk factors for nephrotoxicity in patients treated with aminoglycosides. *Ann Intern Med* 1984, 100:352–357.

14. Zager RA: A focus of tissue necrosis increases renal susceptibility to gentamicin administration. *Kidney Int* 1988; 33:84–90.

15. Andreoli TE: On the anatomy of amphotericin B-cholesterol pores in lipid bilayer membranes. *Kidney Int* 1973, 4:337–45.

16. Bernardo J, Sabra R, Branch RA: Amphotericin B. In *Clinical Nephrotoxins—Renal Injury From Drugs and Chemicals*. Edited by De Broe ME, Porter GA, Bennett WM, Verpooten GA. Dordrecht: Kluwer Academic, 1998:135–151.

17. Bennett WM: Mechanisms of acute and chronic nephrotoxicity from immunosuppressive drugs. *Renal Failure* 1996, 18:453–460.

18. de Mattos AM, Olyaei AJ, Bennett WM: Pharmacology of immunosuppressive medications used in renal diseases and transplantation. *Am J Kidney Dis* 1996, 28:631–667.

19. Vanrenterghem Y, Lerut T, Roels L, *et al.*: Thromboembolic complications and haemostatic changes in cyclosporin-treated cadaveric kidney allograft recipients. *Lancet* 1985, 1:999–1002.

20. Verpooten GA, Cools FJ, Van der Planken MG, *et al.*: Elevated plasminogen activator inhibitor levels in cyclosporin-treated renal allograft recipients. *Nephrol Dial Transplant* 1996, 11:347–351.

21. Vestergaard P, Amdisen A, Hansen AE, Schou M: Lithium treatment and kidney function. *Acta Psychiatry Scand* 1979; 60:504–520.

22. Johnson GF, Hunt G, Duggin GG, *et al.*: Renal function and lithium treatment: initial and follow-up tests in manic-depressive patients. *J Affective Disord* 1984; 6:249–263.

23. Coppen A, Bishop ME, Bailey JE, *et al.*: Renal function in lithium and non–lithium-treated patients with affective disorders. *Acta Psychiatry Scand* 1980; 62:343–355.

24. Battle DC, Dorhout-Mees EJ: Lithium and the kidney. In *Clinical nephrotoxins—renal injury from drugs and chemicals*. Edited by De Broe ME, Porter GA, Bennett WM, Verpooten GA. Dordrecht: Kluwer Academic, 1998:383–395.

25. Jorgensen F, Larsen S, Spanager E, *et al.*: Kidney function and quantitative histological changes in patients on long-term lithium therapy. *Acta Psychiatry Scand* 1984, 70:455–462.

26. Hricik DE, Browning PJ, Kopelman R, *et al.*: Captopril-induced functional renal insufficiency in patients with bilateral renal artery stenosis or renal artery stenosis in a solitary kidney. *N Engl J Med* 1983, 308:373–376.

27. Textor SC: ACE inhibitors in renovascular hypertension. *Cardiovasc Drugs Ther* 1990; 4:229–235.

28. de Jong PE, Woods LL: Renal injury from angiotensin I converting enzyme inhibitors. In *Clinical nephrotoxins—renal injury from drugs and chemicals*. Edited by De Broe ME, Porter GA, Bennett WM, Verpooten GA. Dordrecht: Kluwer Academic, 1998:239–250.

29. Smith WR, Neil J, Cusham WC, Butkus DE: Captopril associated acute interstitial nephritis. *Am J Nephrol* 1989, 9:230–235.

30. Opie LH: *Angiotensin-converting enzyme inhibitors*. New York: Willy-Liss, 1992; 3.

31. Whelton A, Watson J: Nonsteroidal anti-inflammatory drugs: effects on kidney function. In *Clinical Nephrotoxins—Renal Injury From drugs and Chemicals*. Edited by De Broe ME, Porter GA, Bennett WM, Verpooten GA. Dordrecht: Kluwer Academic, 1998:203–216.

32. De Broe ME, Elseviers MM: Analgesic nephropathy. *N Engl J Med* 1998, 338:446–452.

33. Mitchell JA, Akarasereenont P, Thiemermann C, *et al.*: Selectivity of nonsteroidal antiinflammatory drugs as inhibitors of constitutive and inducible cyclooxygenase. *Proc Natl Acad Sci USA* 1993, 90(24):11693–11697.

34. Bennett WM, Henrich WL, Stoff JS: The renal effects of nonsteroidal anti-inflammatory drugs: summary and recommendations. *Am J Kidney Dis* 1996, 28(1 Suppl 1):S56–S62.

35. Heyman SN, Rosen S, Brezis M: Radiocontrast nephropathy: a paradigm for the synergism between toxic and hypoxic insults in the kidney. *Exp Nephrol* 1994, 2:153.

36. Porter GA, Kremer D: Contrast associated nephropathy: presentation, pathophysiology and management. In *Clinical nephrotoxins—Renal Injury From Drugs and Chemicals*. Edited by De Broe ME, Porter GA, Bennett WM, Verpooten GA. Dordrecht: Kluwer Academic, 1998:317–331.

Diagnostic Evaluation of the Patient with Acute Renal Failure

Brian G. Dwinnell
Robert J. Anderson

Acute renal failure (ARF) is abrupt deterioration of renal function sufficient to result in failure of urinary elimination of nitrogenous waste products (urea nitrogen and creatinine). This deterioration of renal function results in elevations of blood urea nitrogen and serum creatinine concentrations. While there is no disagreement about the general definition of ARF, there are substantial differences in diagnostic criteria various clinicians use to define ARF (*eg*, magnitude of rise of serum creatinine concentration). From a clinical perspective, for persons with normal renal function and serum creatinine concentration, glomerular filtration rate must be dramatically reduced to result in even modest increments (*eg*, 0.1 to 0.3 mg/dL) in serum creatinine concentration. Moreover, several studies demonstrate a direct relationship between the magnitude of serum creatinine increase and mortality from ARF. Thus, the clinician must carefully evaluate all cases of rising serum creatinine.

The process of urine formation begins with delivery of blood to the glomerulus, filtration of the blood at the glomerulus, further processing of the filtrate by the renal tubules, and elimination of the formed urine by the renal collecting system. A derangement of any of these processes can result in the clinical picture of rapidly deteriorating renal function and ARF. As the causes of ARF are multiple and since subsequent treatment of ARF depends on a clear delineation of the cause, prompt diagnostic evaluation of each case of ARF is necessary.

CHAPTER

12

RATIONALE FOR ORGANIZED APPROACH TO ACUTE RENAL FAILURE

Common
 Present in 1%–2% of hospital admissions
 Develops after admission in 1%–5% of noncritically ill patients
 Develops in 5%–20% after admission to an intensive care unit
Multiple causes
 Prerenal
 Postrenal
 Renal
Therapy dependent upon diagnosing cause
 Prerenal: improve renal perfusion
 Postrenal: relieve obstruction
 Renal: identify and treat specific cause
Poor outcomes
 Twofold increased length of stay
 Two- to eightfold increased mortality
 Substantial morbidity

FIGURE 12-1

Rationale for an organized approach to acute renal failure (ARF). An organized approach to the patient with ARF is necessary, as this disorder is common and is caused by several insults that operate via numerous mechanisms. Successful amelioration of the renal failure state depends on early identification and treatment of the cause of the disorder [1–7]. If not diagnosed and treated and reversed quickly, it can lead to substantial morbidity and mortality.

PRESENTING FEATURES OF ACUTE RENAL FAILURE

Common
 Rising BUN or creatinine
 Oligoanuria
Less common
 Symptoms of uremia
 Characteristic laboratory abnormalities

FIGURE 12-2

Presenting features of acute renal failure (ARF). ARF usually comes to clinical attention by the finding of either elevated (or rising) blood urea nitrogen (BUN) or serum creatinine concentration. Less commonly, decreased urine output (less than 20 mL per hour) heralds the presence of ARF. It is important to acknowledge, however, that at least half of all cases of ARF are nonoliguric [2–6]. Thus, healthy urine output does not ensure normal renal function. Rarely, ARF comes to the attention of the clinician because of symptoms of uremia (*eg*, anorexia, nausea, vomiting, confusion, pruritus) or laboratory findings compatible with renal failure (metabolic acidosis, hyperkalemia, hyperphosphatemia, hypocalcemia, hyperuricemia, hypermagnesemia, anemia).

Blood Urea Nitrogen, Creatinine, and Renal Failure

OVERVIEW OF BLOOD UREA NITROGEN AND SERUM CREATININE

	Blood Urea Nitrogen	Serum Creatinine
Source	Protein that can be of exogenous or endogenous origin	Nonenzymatic hydrolysis of creatine released from skeletal muscle
Constancy of production	Variable	More stable
Renal handling	Completely filtered; significant tubular reabsorption	Completely filtered; some tubular secretion
Value as marker for glomerular filtration rate	Modest	Good in steady state
Correlation with uremic symptoms	Good	Poor

FIGURE 12-3

Overview of blood urea nitrogen (BUN) and serum creatinine. Given the central role of BUN and serum creatinine in determining the presence of renal failure, an understanding of the metabolism of these substances is needed. Urea nitrogen derives from the breakdown of proteins that are delivered to the liver. Thus, the urea nitrogen production rate can vary with exogenous protein intake and endogenous protein catabolism. Urea nitrogen is a small, uncharged molecule that is not protein bound, and as such, it is readily filtered at the renal glomerulus. Urea nitrogen undergoes renal tubular reabsorption by specific transporters. This tubular reabsorption limits the value of BUN as a marker for glomerular filtration. However, the BUN usually correlates with the symptoms of uremia. By contrast, the production of creatinine is usually more constant unless there has been a marked reduction of skeletal muscle mass (*eg*, loss of a limb, prolonged starvation) or diffuse muscle injury. Although creatinine undergoes secretion into renal tubular fluid, this is very modest in degree. Thus, a steady-stable serum creatinine concentration is usually a relatively good marker of glomerular filtration rate as noted in Figure 12-5.

BLOOD UREA NITROGEN (BUN)-CREATININE RATIO

> 10	< 10
Increased protein intake	Starvation
Catabolic state	Advanced liver disease
Fever	Postdialysis state
Sepsis	Drugs that impair tubular secretion
Trauma	Cimetidine
Corticosteroids	Trimethoprim
Tissue necrosis	Rhabdomyolysis
Tetracyclines	
Diminished urine flow	
Prerenal state	
Postrenal state	

FIGURE 12-4

The blood urea nitrogen (BUN)-creatinine ratio. Based on the information in Figure 12-3, the BUN-creatinine ratio often deviates from the usual value of about 10:1. These deviations may have modest diagnostic implications. As an example, for reasons as yet unclear, tubular reabsorption of urea nitrogen is enhanced in low-urine flow states. Thus, a high BUN-creatinine ratio often occurs in prerenal and postrenal (*see* Fig. 12-6) forms of renal failure. Similarly, enhanced delivery of amino acids to the liver (as with catabolism, corticosteroids, etc.) can enhance urea nitrogen formation and increase the BUN-creatinine ratio. A BUN-creatinine ratio lower than 10:1 can occur because of decreased urea nitrogen formation (*eg*, in protein malnutrition, advanced liver disease), enhanced creatinine formation (*eg*, with rhabdomyolysis), impaired tubular secretion of creatinine (*eg*, secondary to trimethoprim, cimetidine), or relatively enhanced removal of the small substance urea nitrogen by dialysis.

CORRELATION OF STEADY-STATE SERUM CREATININE CONCENTRATION AND GLOMERULAR FILTRATION RATE (GFR)

Creatinine (mg/dL)	GFR (mL/min)
1	100
2	50
4	25
8	12.5
16	6.25

FIGURE 12-5

Correlation of steady-state serum creatinine concentration and glomerular filtration rate (GFR).

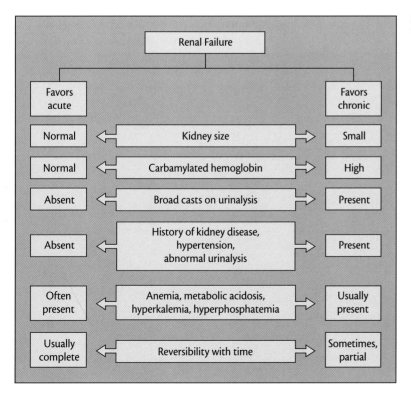

FIGURE 12-6

Categories of renal failure. Once the presence of renal failure is ascertained by elevated blood urea nitrogen (BUN) or serum creatinine value, the clinician must decide whether it is acute or chronic. When previous values are available for review, this judgment is made relatively easily. In the absence of such values, the factors depicted here may be helpful. Hemoglobin potentially undergoes nonenzymatic carbamylation of its terminal valine [8]. Thus, similar to the hemoglobin A1C value as an index of blood sugar control, the level of carbamylated hemoglobin is an indicator of the degree and duration of elevated BUN, but, this test is not yet widely available. The presence of small kidneys strongly suggests that renal failure is at least in part chronic. From a practical standpoint, because even chronic renal failure often is partially reversible, the clinician should assume and evaluate for the presence of acute reversible factors in all cases of acute renal failure.

Categorization of Causes of Acute Renal Failure

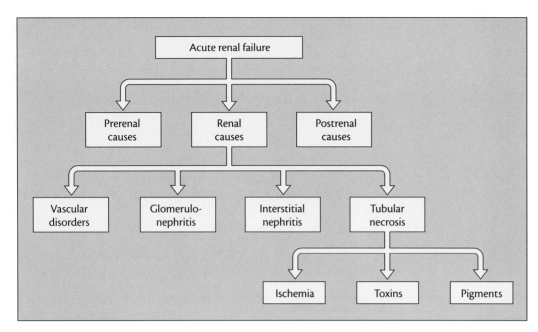

FIGURE 12-7

Acute renal failure (ARF). This figure depicts the most commonly used schema to classify and diagnostically approach the patient with ARF [1, 6, 9]. The most common general cause of ARF (60% to 70% of cases) is prerenal factors. Prerenal causes include those secondary to renal hypoperfusion, which occurs in the setting of extracellular fluid loss (eg, with vomiting, nasogastric suctioning, gastrointestinal hemorrhage, diarrhea, burns, heat stroke, diuretics, glucosuria), sequestration of extracellular fluid (eg, with pancreatitis, abdominal surgery, muscle crush injury, early sepsis), or impaired cardiac output. In most prerenal forms of ARF, one or more of the vasomotor mechanisms noted in Figure 12-8 is operative. The diagnostic criteria for prerenal ARF are delineated in Figure 12-9. Once prerenal forms of ARF have been ruled out, postrenal forms (ie, obstruction to urine flow) should be considered. Obstruction to urine flow is a less common (5% to 15% of cases) cause of ARF but is nearly always amenable to therapy. The site of obstruction can be intrarenal (eg, crystals or proteins obstructing the terminal collecting tubules) or extrarenal (eg, blockade of the renal pelvis, ureters, bladder, or urethra). The diagnosis of postrenal forms of ARF is supported by data outlined in Figure 12-10. After pre- and postrenal forms of ARF have been considered, attention should focus on the kidney. When considering renal forms of ARF, it is helpful to think in terms of renal anatomic compartments (vasculature, glomeruli, interstitium, and tubules). Acute disorders involving any of these compartments can lead to ARF.

VASOMOTOR MECHANISMS CONTRIBUTING TO ACUTE RENAL FAILURE

Decreased Renal Perfusion Pressure	Afferent Arteriolar Constriction	Efferent Arteriolar Dilation
Extracellular fluid volume loss or sequestration	Sepsis	Converting enzyme inhibitors
Impaired cardiac output	Medications (NSAIDs, cyclosporine, contrast medium, amphotericin, alpha-adrenergic agonists)	Angiotensin II receptor antagonists
Antihypertensive medications	Hypercalcemia	
Sepsis	Postoperative state	
	Hepatorenal syndrome	

FIGURE 12-8

Vasomotor mechanisms contributing to acute renal failure (ARF). Most prerenal forms of ARF have operational one or more of the vasomotor mechanisms depicted here [6]. Collectively, these factors lead to diminished glomerular filtration and ARF. NSAIDs—nonsteroidal anti-inflammatory drugs.

FIGURE 12-9

DIAGNOSIS OF POSSIBLE PRERENAL CAUSES OF ACUTE RENAL FAILURE

History	Examination	Laboratory/Other
Extracellular fluid loss or sequestration from skin, gastrointestinal and/or renal source (see Fig. 12-15)	Orthostatic hypotension and tachycardia	Normal urinalysis
Orthostatic lightheadedness	Dry mucous membranes	Urinary indices compatible with normal tubular function (see Fig. 12-14)
Thirst	No axillary moisture	Elevated BUN-creatinine ratio
Oliguria	Decreased skin turgor	Improved renal function with correction of the underlying cause
Symptoms of heart failure	Evidence of congestive heart failure	Rarely, chest radiography, cardiac ultrasound, gated blood pool scan, central venous and/or Swan-Ganz wedge pressure recordings
Edema	Presence of edema	

Diagnosis of possible prerenal causes of acute renal failure (ARF). Prerenal events are the most common factors that lead to contemporary ARF. The historical, physical examination, and laboratory and other investigations involved in identifying a prerenal form of ARF are outlined here [1]. BUN—blood urea nitrogen.

FIGURE 12-10

DIAGNOSIS OF POSSIBLE POSTRENAL CAUSES OF ACUTE RENAL FAILURE

History	Examination	Laboratory/Other
Very young or very old age	Distended bladder	Abnormal urinalysis
Nocturia	Enlarged prostate	Elevated BUN-creatinine ratio
Decreased size or force of urine stream	Abnormal pelvic examination	Elevated postvoiding residual volume
Anticholinergic or alpha-adrenergic agonist medications		Abnormal renal ultrasound, CT or MRI findings
Bladder, prostate, pelvic, or intra-abdominal cancer		Improvement after drainage
Fluctuating urine volume		
Oligoanuria		
Suprapubic pain		
Urolithiasis		
Medication known to produce crystalluria (sulfonamides, acyclovir, methotrexate, protease inhibitors)		

Diagnosis of possible postrenal causes of acute renal failure (ARF). Postrenal causes of ARF are less common (5% to 15% of ARF population) but are nearly always amenable to therapy. This figure depicts the historical, physical examination and tests that can lead to an intrarenal (crystal deposition) or extrarenal (blockade of the collecting system) form of obstructive uropathy [1, 6, 9, 10]. BUN—blood urea nitrogen; CT—computed tomography; MRI—magnetic resonance imaging.

FIGURE 12-11

POSTOPERATIVE ACUTE RENAL FAILURE

Frequency	Predisposing Factors	Preventive Strategies
Elective surgery 1%–5%	Comorbidity results in decreased renal reserve	Avoid nephrotoxins
Emergent or vascular surgery 5%–10%	The surgical experience decreases renal function (volume shifts, vasoconstriction)	Minimize hospital-acquired infections (invasive equipment)
	A second insult usually occurs (sepsis, reoperation, nephrotoxin, volume/cardiac issue)	Selective use of volume expansion, vasodilators, inotropes
		Preoperative hemodynamic optimization in selected cases
		Increase tissue oxygenation delivery to supranormal levels in selected cases

Postoperative acute renal failure (ARF). The postoperative setting of ARF is very common. This figure depicts data on the frequency, predisposing factors, and potential strategies for preventing postoperative ARF [11, 12].

Diagnostic Steps in Evaluating Acute Renal Failure

STEPWISE APPROACH TO DIAGNOSIS OF ACUTE RENAL FAILURE

Step 1	Step 2	Step 3	Step 4
History	Consider urinary diagnostic indices (*see* Fig. 12-16)	Consider selected therapeutic trials	Consider renal biopsy
Record review			Consider empiric therapy for suspected diagnosis
Physical examination	Consider need for further evaluation to exclude urinary tract obstruction		
Urinary bladder catherization (if oligoanuric)	Consider need for more data to assess intravascular volume or cardiac output status		
Urinalysis (*see* Fig. 12-15)	Consider need for additional blood tests		
	Consider need for evaluation of renal vascular status		

FIGURE 12-12

Stepwise approach to diagnosis of acute renal failure (ARF). The multiple causes, predisposing factors, and clinical settings demand a logical, sequential approach to each case of ARF. This figure presents a four-step approach to assessing ARF patients in an effort to delineate the cause in a timely and cost-effective manner. Step 1 involves a focused history, record review, and examination. The salient features of these analyses are noted in more detail in Figure 12-13. In many cases, a single bladder catheterization is needed to assess the degree of residual volume, which should be less than 30 to 50 mL. Urinalysis is a critical part of the initial evaluation of all patients with ARF. Generally, a relatively normal urinalysis suggests either a prerenal or postrenal cause, whereas a urinalysis containing cells and casts is most compatible with a renal cause. A detailed schema of urinalysis interpretation in the setting of ARF is depicted in Figure 12-15. Usually, after Step 1 the clinician has a reasonably good idea of the likely cause of the ARF. Sometimes, the information noted under Step 2 is needed to ascertain definitively the cause of the ARF. More details of Step 2 are depicted in Figure 12-14. Oftentimes, urinary diagnostic indices (*see* Fig. 12-16),

are helpful in differentiating between prerenal (intact tubular function) and acute tubular necrosis (impaired tubular function) as the cause of renal failure. Sometimes, further evaluation (usually ultrasonography, less commonly computed tomography or magnetic resonance imaging) is needed to exclude the possibility of bilateral ureteric obstruction (or single ureteric obstruction in patients with a single kidney). Occasionally, additional studies such as central venous pressure or left ventricular filling pressure determinations are needed to better assess whether prerenal factors are contributing to the ARF. When the cause of the ARF continues to be difficult to ascertain and renal vascular disorders (*see* Fig. 12-17 and 12-18), glomerulonephritis (*see* Fig. 12-19) or acute interstitial nephritis (*see* Fig. 12-20) remain possibilities, additional blood analyses and other tests described in Figures 12-18 through 12-20 may be indicated. Sometimes, selected therapeutic trials (eg, volume expansion, maneuvers to increase cardiac index, ureteric stent or nephrostomy tube relief of obstruction) are necessary to document the cause of ARF definitively. Empiric therapy (eg, corticosteroids for suspected acute allergic interstitial nephritis) is given as both a diagnostic and a therapeutic maneuver in selected cases. Rarely, despite all efforts, the cause of the ARF remains unknown and renal biopsy is necessary to establish a definitive diagnosis.

FIRST STEP IN EVALUATION OF ACUTE RENAL FAILURE

History

Disorders that suggest or predispose to renal failure: hypertension, diabetes mellitus, human immunodeficiency virus, vascular disease, abnormal urinalyses, family history of renal disease, medication use, toxin or environmental exposure, infection, heart failure, vasculitis, cancer

Disorders that suggest or predispose to volume depletion: vomiting, diarrhea, pancreatitis, gastrointestinal bleeding, burns, heat stroke, fever, uncontrolled diabetes mellitus, diuretic use, orthostatic hypotension, nothing-by-mouth status, nasogastric suctioning

Disorders that suggest or predispose to obstruction: stream abnormalities, nocturia, anticholingeric medications, stones, urinary tract infections, bladder or prostate disease, intra-abnominal malignancy, suprapubic or flank pain, anuria, fluctuating urine volumes

Symptoms of renal failure: anorexia, vomiting, reversed sleep pattern, puritus

Record review

Recent events (procedures, surgery)

Medications (*see* Fig. 12-22)

Vital signs

Intake and output

Body weights

Blood chemistries and hemogram

Physical examination

Skin: rash suggestive of allergy, palpable purpura of vasculitis, livedo reticularis and digital infarctions suggesting atheroemboli

Eyes: hypertension, diabetes mellitus, Hollenhorst plaques, vasculitis, candidemia

Lungs: rales, rubs

Heart: evidence of heart failure, pericardial disease, jugular venous pressure

Vascular system: bruits, pulses, abdominal aortic aneurysm

Abdomen: flank or suprapubic masses, ascites, costovertebral angle pain

Extremities: edema, pulses, compartment syndromes

Nervous system: focal findings, asterixis, mini-mental status examination

Consider bladder catheterization

Urinalysis (*see* Fig. 12-13)

FIGURE 12-13

First step in evaluation of acute renal failure.

SECOND STEP IN EVALUATION OF ACUTE RENAL FAILURE

FIGURE 12-14

Second step in evaluation of acute renal failure.

Urine diagnostic indices (*see* Fig. 12-16)

Consider need for further evaluation for obstruction

Ultrasonography, computed tomography, or magnetic resonance imaging

Consider need for additional blood tests

Vasculitis/glomerulopathy: human immunodeficiency virus infections, antineutrophilic cytoplasmic antibodies, antinuclear antibodies, serologic tests for hepatitis, systemic bacterial endocarditis and streptococcal infections, rheumatoid factor, complement, cryoglobins

Plasma cell disorders: urine for light chains, serum analysis for abnormal proteins

Drug screen/level, additional chemical tests

Consider need for evaluation of renal vascular supply

Isotope scans, Doppler sonography, angiography

Consider need for more data to assess volume and cardiac status

Swan-Ganz catheterization

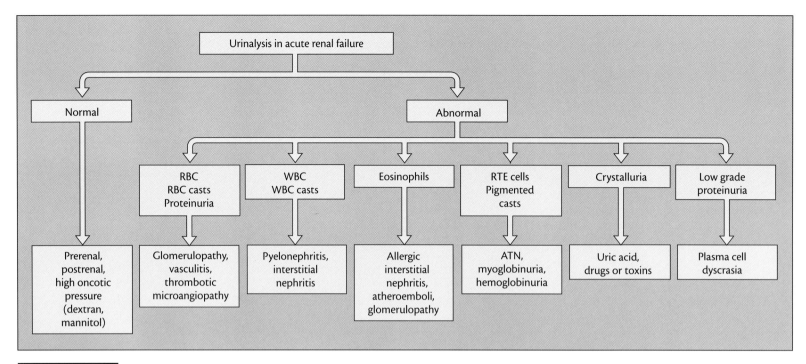

FIGURE 12-15

Urinalysis in acute renal failure (ARF). A normal urinalysis suggests a prerenal or postrenal form of ARF; however, many patients with ARF of postrenal causes have some cellular elements on urinalysis. Relatively uncommon causes of ARF that usually present with oligoanuria and a normal urinalysis are mannitol toxicity and large doses of dextran infusion. In these disorders, a "hyperoncotic state" occurs in which glomerular capillary oncotic pressure, combined with the intratubular hydrostatic pressure, exceeds the glomerular capillary hydrostatic pressure and stop glomerular filtration. Red blood cells (RBCs) can be seen with all renal forms of ARF. When RBC casts are present, glomerulonephritis or vasculitis is most likely.

White blood cells (WBCs) can also be present in small numbers in the urine of patients with ARF. Large numbers of WBCs and WBC casts strongly suggest the presence of either pyelonephritis or acute interstitial nephritis. Eosinolphiluria (Hansel's stain) is often present in either allergic interstitial nephritis or atheroembolic disease [13, 14]. Renal tubular epithelial (RTE) cells and casts and pigmented granular casts typically are present in pigmenturia-associated ARF (see Fig. 12-21) and in established acute tubular necrosis (ATN). The presence of large numbers of crystals on urinalysis, in conjunction with the clinical history, may suggest uric acid, sulfonamides, or protease inhibitors as a cause of the renal failure.

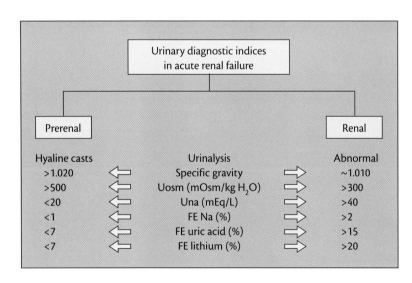

FIGURE 12-16

Urinary diagnostic indices in acute renal failure (ARF). These indices have traditionally been used in the setting of oliguria, to help differentiate between prerenal (intact tubular function) and acute tubular necrosis (ATN, impaired tubular function). Several caveats to interpretation of these indices are in order [1]. First, none of these is completely sensitive or specific in differentiating the prerenal from the ATN form of ARF. Second, often a continuum exists between early prerenal conditions and late prerenal conditions that lead to ischemic ATN. Most of the data depicted here are derived from patients relatively late in the progress of ARF when the serum creatinine concentrations were 3 to 5 mg/dL. Third, there is often a relatively large "gray area," in which the various indices do not give definitive results. Finally, some of the indices (eg, fractional excretion of endogenous lithium [FE lithium]) are not readily available in the clinical setting. The fractional excretion (FE) of a substance is determined by the formula: U/P substance ÷ U/P creatinine × 100. U/P—urine-plasma ratio.

Vascular Mechanisms Involved in Acute Renal Failure

VASCULAR CAUSES OF ACUTE RENAL FAILURE

Arterial	Venous
Large vessels	Occlusion
Renal artery stenosis	Clot
Thrombosis	Tumor
Cross-clamping	
Emboli	
Atheroemboli	
Endocarditis	
Atrial fibrillation	
Mural thrombus	
Tumor	
Small vessels	
Cortical necrosis malignant hypertension	
Scleroderma	
Vasculitis	
Antiphospholipid syndrome	
Thrombotic microangiopathies	
Hemolytic-uremic syndrome	
Thrombotic thrombocytopenic purpura	
Postpartum	
Medications (mitomycin C, cyclosporine, tacrolimus)	

FIGURE 12-17

Vascular causes of acute renal failure (ARF). Once prerenal and postrenal causes of ARF have been excluded, attention should be focused on the kidney. One useful means of classifying renal causes of ARF is to consider the anatomic compartments of the kidney. Thus, disorders of the renal vasculature (see Fig. 12-18), glomerulus (see Fig. 12-19), interstitium (see Fig. 12-20) and tubules can all result in identical clinical pictures of ARF [1]. This figure depicts the disorders of the renal arterial and venous systems that can result in ARF [15].

DIAGNOSIS OF POSSIBLE VASCULAR CAUSE OF ACUTE RENAL FAILURE

History	Examination	Laboratory/Other
Factors that predispose to vascular disease (smoking, hypertension, diabetes mellitus, hyperlipidemia)	Marked hypertension	Thrombocytopenia
	Atrial fibrillation	Microangiopathic hemolysis
	Scleroderma	Coagulopathy
Claudication, stroke, myocardial infarction	Palpable purpura	Urinalysis with hematuria and low-grade proteinuria
Surgical procedure on aorta	Abdominal aortic aneurysm	Abnormal renal isotope scan and/or Doppler ultrasonography
Catheterization procedure involving aorta	Diminished pulses	
Selected clinical states (scleroderma, pregnancy)	Infarcted toes	Renal angiography
Selected medications, toxins (cyclosporine, mitomycin C, cocaine, tacrolimus)	Hollendhorst plaques	Renal or extrarenal tissue analysis
Constitutional symptoms	Vascular bruits	
	Stigmata of bacterial endocarditis	
	Illeus	

FIGURE 12-18

Diagnosis of a possible vascular cause of acute renal failure (ARF). This figure depicts the historical, physical examination, and testing procedures that often lead to diagnosis of a "vascular cause" of ARF [1, 15, 16].

Acute Glomerulonephritis

DIAGNOSIS OF A POSSIBLE ACUTE GLOMERULAR PROCESS AS THE CAUSE OF ACUTE RENAL FAILURE

History	Examination	Laboratory/Other
Recent infection	Hypertension	Urinalysis with hematuria, red cell casts, and proteinuria
Sudden onset of edema, dyspnea	Edema	Serologic or culture evidence of recent infection
Systemic disorder (eg, lupus erythematosus, Wegener's granulomatosis, Goodpasture's syndrome)	Rash	
	Arthropathy	
	Prominent pulmonary findings	Laboratory evidence of immune-mediated process (low complement, cryoglobulinemia, antinuclear antibody, anti-DNA, rheumatoid factor, anti–glomerular basement membrane antibody, antineutrophilic cytoplasmic antibody)
No evidence of other causes of renal failure	Stigmata of bacterial endocarditis or visceral abscess	
		Renal tissue examination

FIGURE 12-19

Diagnosis of a possible acute glomerular process as the cause of acute renal failure (ARF). Acute glomerulonephritis is a relatively rare cause of ARF in adults. In the pediatric age group, acute glomerulonephritis and a disorder of small renal arteries (hemolytic-uremic syndrome) are relatively common causes. This figure depicts the historical, examination, and laboratory findings that collectively may support a diagnosis of acute glomerulonephritis as the cause of ARF [16, 17].

Interstitial Nephritis

DIAGNOSIS OF POSSIBLE ACUTE INTERSTITIAL NEPHRITIS AS THE CAUSE OF ACUTE RENAL FAILURE

History	Examination	Laboratory/Other
Medication exposure	Fever	Abnormal urinalysis (white blood cells or cell casts, eosinophils, eosinophilic casts, low-grade proteinuria, sometimes hematuria)
Severe pyelonephritis	Rash	Eosinophilia
Systemic infection	Back or flank pain	Urinary diagnositc indices compatible with a renal cause of renal failure (see Fig. 12-16)
		Uptake on gallium or indium scan
		Renal biopsy

FIGURE 12-20

Diagnosis of possible acute interstitial nephritis as the cause of acute renal failure (ARF). This figure outlines the historical, physical examination and other investigative methods that can lead to identification of acute interstitial nephritis as the cause of ARF [18].

Acute Tubular Necrosis

DIAGNOSIS OF POSSIBLE PIGMENT-ASSOCIATED FORMS OF ACUTE RENAL FAILURE

Myoglobinuria			Hemoglobinuria		
History	Examination	Laboratory	History	Examination	Laboratory
Trauma to muscles	Can be normal	Serum creatinine disproportionately elevated related to BUN	Condition associated with intravascular hemolysis (red cell trauma, antibody-mediated hemolysis, direct red cell toxicity, sickle cell disease)	Can be normal	Normocytic anemia
Condition known to predispose to nontraumatic rhabdomyolysis	Muscle edema, weakness, pain	Elevated (10-fold) enzymes (CK, SGOT, LDH, adolase)		Pallor	High red cell LDH fraction
	Neurovascular entrapment or compartment syndromes in severe cases	Elevations of plasma potassium, uric acid, phosphorus, and hypocalcemia		Flank pain	Reticulocytosis
Muscle pain or stiffness					Low haptoglobin
Dark urine	Flank pain	Urinalysis with pigmented granular casts, (+) stick reaction for blood in the absence of hematuria, and myoglobin test if available			Urinalysis with pigmented granular casts, (+) stick reaction for blood in absence of hemataria and reddish brown or pink plasma
		Clear plasma			

FIGURE 12-21

Diagnosis of possible pigment-associated forms of acute renal failure (ARF). Once prerenal and postrenal forms of ARF have been ruled out and renal vascular, glomerular, and interstitial processes seem unlikely, a diagnosis of acute tubular necrosis (ATN) is probable. A diagnosis of ATN is thus one of exclusion (of other causes of ARF). In the majority of cases when ATN is present, one or more of the three predisposing conditions have been identified to be operational. These conditions include renal ischemia due to a prolonged prerenal state, nephrotoxin exposure, and sometimes pigmenturia. A diagnosis of ATN is supported by the absence of other causes of ARF, the presence of one or more predisposing factors, and the presence of urinary diagnostic indices and urinalysis suggested of ATN (*see* Figs. 12-15 and 12-16). A pigmenturic disorder (myloglobinuria or hemoglobinuria) can predispose to ARF. This figure depicts the historical, physical examination, and supporting diagnostic tests that often lead to a diagnosis of pigment-associated ARF [19]. BUN—blood urea nitrogen; CK—creatinine kinase; SGOT—serum glutamic-oxaloacetic transaminase; LDH—lactic dehydrogenase.

Nephrotoxin Acute Renal Failure

NEPHROTOXIC ACUTE RENAL FAILURE

Prerenal
Diuretics
Interleukin 2
CEIs
Antihypertensive agents

Tubular toxicity
Aminoglyosides
Cisplatin
Vancomycin
Foscarnet
Pentamidine
Radiocontrast
Amphotercin
Heavy metals

Vasoconstriction
NSAIDs
Radiocontrast agents
Cyclosporine
Tacrolimus
Amphotericin

Endothelial injury
Cyclosporine
Mitomycin C
Tacrolimus
Cocaine
Conjugated estrogens
Quinine

Crystalluria
Sulfonamides
Methotrexate
Acyclovir
Triamterene
Ethylene glycol
Protease inhibitors

Glomerulopathy
Gold
Penicillamine
NSAIDs

Interstitial nephritis
Multiple

FIGURE 12-22

Nephrotoxin acute renal failure (ARF). A variety of nephrotoxins have been implicated in causing 20% to 30% of all cases of ARF. These potential nephrotoxins can act through a variety of mechanisms to induce renal dysfunction [6, 20, 21]. CEI—converting enzyme inhibitor; NSAID—nonsteroidal anti-inflammatory drugs.

References

1. Anderson RJ, Schrier RW: Acute renal failure. In *Diseases of the Kidney*. Edited by Schrier RW, Gottschalk CW. Boston: Little, Brown; 1997:1069–1113.

2. Hou SH, Bushinsky D, Wish JB, Harrington JT: Hospital-acquired renal insufficiency: A prospective study. *Am J Med* 1983, 74:243–248.

3. Shusterman N, Strom BL, Murray TG, *et al.*: Risk factors and outcome of hospital-acquired acute renal failure. *Am J Med* 1987, 83:65–71.

4. Levy EM, Viscoli CM, Horwitz RI: The effect of acute renal failure on mortality. *JAMA* 1996, 275:1489–1494.

5. Liaño F, Pascual J: Epidemiology of acute renal failure: A prospective, multicenter, community-based study. *Kid Int* 1996, 50:811–818.

6. Thadhani R, Pascual M, Bonventre JV: Acute renal failure. *New Engl J Med* 1996, 334:1448–1460.

7. Feest TG, Round A, Hamad S: Incidence of severe acute renal failure in adults: Results of a community-based study. *Br Med J* 1993, 306:481–483.

8. Davenport A: Differentiation of acute from chronic renal impairment by detection of carbamylated hemoglobin. *Lancet* 1993, 341:1614–1616.

9. Mendell JA, Chertow GM: A practical approach to acute renal failure. *Med Clin North Am* 1997, 81:731–748.

10. Kopp JB, Miller KD, Mican JM, *et al.*: Crystalluria and urinary tract abnormalities associated with indinovir. *Ann Intern Med* 1997, 127:119–125.

11. Charlson ME, MacKenzie CR, Gold JP, Shires T: Postoperative changes in serum creatinine. *Ann Surg* 1989, 209:328–335.

12. Kellerman PS: Perioperative care of the renal patient. *Arch Intern Med* 1994, 154:1674–1681.

13. Nolan CR, Anger MS, Kelleher SP: Eosinophiluria —a new method of detection and definition of the clinical spectrum. *N Engl J Med* 1986, 315:1516–1519.

14. Wilson DM, Salager TL, Farkouh ME: Eosinophiluria in atheroembolic renal disease. *Am J Med* 1991, 91:186–191.

15. Abuelo JG: Diagnosing vascular causes of acute renal failure. *Ann Intern Med* 1995, 123:601–614.

16. Falk RJ, Jennette JC: ANCA small-vessel vasculitis. *J Am Soc Nephrol* 1997, 8:314–322.

17. Kobrin S, Madacio MP: Acute poststreptococcal glomerulonephritis and other bacterial infection-related glomerulonephritis. In *Diseases of the Kidney*. Edited by Schrier RW, Gottschalk CW. Boston: Little, Brown; 1997:1579–1594.

18. Eknoyan G: Acute tubulointerstitial nephritis. In *Diseases of the Kidney*. Edited by Schrier RW, Gottschalk CW. Boston: Little, Brown; 1997:1249–1272.

19. Don BR, Rodriguez RA, Humphreys MH: Acute renal failure associated with pigmenturia as crystal deposits. In *Diseases of the Kidney*. Edited by Schrier RW, Gottschalk CW. Boston: Little, Brown; 1997:1273–1302.

20. Chaudbury O, Ahmed Z: Drug-induced nephrotoxicity. *Med Clin North Am* 1997, 81:705–717.

21. Palmer B, Henrich WL: Nephrotoxicity of nonsteroidal anti-inflammatory agents, analgesics, and angiotensin converting enzyme inhibitors. In *Diseases of the Kidney*. Edited by Schrier RW, Gottschalk CW. Boston: Little, Brown; 1997:1167–1188.

Pathophysiology of Ischemic Acute Renal Failure: Cytoskeletal Aspects

Bruce A. Molitoris
Robert Bacallao

Ischemia remains the major cause of acute renal failure (ARF) in the adult population [1]. Clinically a reduction in glomerular filtration rate (GFR) secondary to reduced renal blood flow can reflect prerenal azotemia or acute tubular necrosis (ATN). More appropriate terms for ATN are *acute tubular dysfunction* or *acute tubular injury*, as necrosis only rarely is seen in renal biopsies, and renal tubular cell injury is the hallmark of this process. Furthermore, the reduction in GFR during acute tubular dysfunction can now, in large part, be related to tubular cell injury. Ischemic ARF resulting in acute tubular dysfunction secondary to cell injury is divided into initiation, maintenance, and recovery phases. Recent studies now allow a direct connection to be drawn between these clinical phases and the cellular phases of ischemic ARF (Fig. 13-1). Thus, renal function can be directly related to the cycle of cell injury and recovery.

Renal proximal tubule cells are the cells most injured during renal ischemia (Fig. 13-2) [2,3]. Proximal tubule cells normally reabsorb 70% to 80% of filtered sodium ions and water and also serve to selectively reabsorb other ions and macromolecules. This vectorial transport across the cell from lumen to blood is accomplished by having a surface membrane polarized into apical (brush border membrane) and basolateral membrane domains separated by junctional complexes (Fig. 13-3) [4]. Apical and basolateral membrane domains are biochemically and functionally different with respect to many parameters, including enzymes, ion channels, hormone receptors, electrical resistance, membrane transporters, membrane lipids, membrane fluidity, and cytoskeletal associations. This epithelial cell polarity is essential for normal cell function, as demonstrated by the vectorial transport of sodium from the lumen to the blood (*see* Fig. 13-3). The establishment

CHAPTER

13

and maintenance of this specialized organization is a dynamic and ATP dependent multistage process involving the formation and maintenance of cell-cell and cell-substratum attachments and the targeted delivery of plasma membrane components to the appropriate domains [5]. These processes are very dependent on the cytoskeleton, in general, and the cytoskeletal membrane interactions mediated through F-actin (see Fig. 13-2, 13-3), in particular.

Ischemia in vivo and cellular ATP depletion in cell culture models ("chemical ischemia") are known to produce characteristic surface membrane structural, biochemical, and functional abnormalities in proximal tubule cells. These alterations occur in a duration-dependent fashion and are illustrated in Figures 13-2 and 13-3 and listed in Figure 13-4. Ischemia-induced alterations in the actin cytoskeleton have been postulated to mediate many of the aforementioned surface membrane changes [2,6,7]. This possible link between ischemia-induced actin cytoskeletal alterations and surface membrane structural and functional abnormalities is suggested by several lines. First, the actin cytoskeleton is known to play fundamental roles in surface membrane formation and stability, junctional complex formation and regulation, Golgi structure and function, and cell–extracellular membrane attachment [2,4,5,8]. Second, proximal tubule cell actin cytoskeleton is extremely sensitive to ischemia and ATP depletion [9,10]. Third, there is a strong correlation between the time course of actin and surface membrane alterations during ischemia or ATP depletion [2,9,10]. Finally, many of the characteristic surface membrane changes

induced by ischemia can be mimicked by F-actin disassembly mediated by cytochalasin D [11]. Although these correlations are highly suggestive of a central role for actin alterations in the pathophysiology of ischemia-induced surface membrane damage they fall short in providing mechanistic data that directly relate actin cytoskeletal changes to cell injury.

Proximal tubule cell injury during ischemia is also known to be principally responsible for the reduction in GFR. Figure 13-5 illustrates the three known pathophysiologic mechanisms that relate proximal tubule cell injury to a reduction in GFR. Particularly important is the role of the cytoskeleton in mediating these three mechanisms of reduced GFR. First, loss of apical membrane into the lumen and detachment of PTC result in substrate for cast formation. Both events have been related to actin cytoskeletal and integrin polarity alterations [12–15]. Cell detachment and the loss of integrin polarity are felt to play a central role in tubular obstruction (Fig. 13-6). Actin cytoskeletal-mediated tight junction opening during ischemia occurs and results in back-leak of glomerular filtrate into the blood. This results in ineffective glomerular filtration (Fig. 13-7). Finally, abnormal proximal sodium ion reabsorption results in large distal tubule sodium delivery and a reduction in GFR via tubuloglomerular feedback mechanisms [2,16,17].

In summary, ischemia-induced alterations in proximal tubule cell surface membrane structure and function are in large part responsible for cell and organ dysfunction. Actin cytoskeletal dysregulation during ischemia has been shown to be responsible for much of the surface membrane structural damage.

RELATIONSHIP BETWEEN THE CLINICAL AND CELLULAR PHASES OF ISCHEMIC ACUTE RENAL FAILURE

Clinical Phases	Cellular Phases
Prerenal azotemia	Vascular and cellular adaptation
↓	↓
Initiation	ATP depletion, cell injury
↓	↓
Maintenance	Repair, migration, apoptosis, proliferation
↓	↓
Recovery	Cellular differentiation

FIGURE 13-1

Relationship between the clinical and cellular phases of ischemic acute renal failure. Prerenal azotemia results from reduced renal blood flow and is associated with reduced organ function (decreased glomerular filtration rate), but cellular integrity is maintained through vascular and cellular adaptive responses. The initiation phase occurs when renal blood flow decreases to a level that results in severe cellular ATP depletion that, in turn, leads to acute cell injury. Severe cellular ATP depletion causes a constellation of cellular alterations culminating in proximal tubule cell injury, cell death, and organ dysfunction [2]. During the clinical phase known as maintenance, cells undergo repair, migration, apoptosis, and proliferation in an attempt to re-establish and maintain cell and tubule integrity [3]. This cellular repair and reorganization phase results in slowly improving cell and organ function. During the recovery phase, cell differentiation continues, cells mature, and normal cell and organ function return [18].

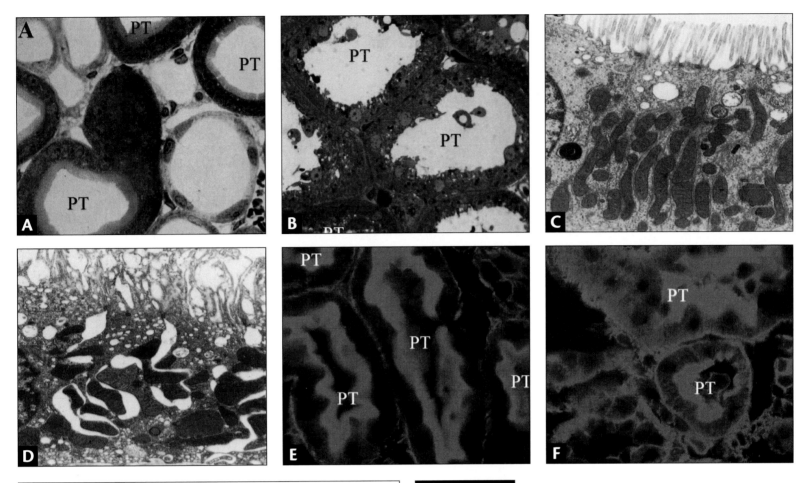

FIGURE 13-2

Ischemic acute renal failure in the rat kidney. Light A, B, transmission electron, C, D, and immunofluorescence E, F, microscopy of control renal cortical sections, A, C, E, and after moderate ischemia induced by 25 minutes of renal artery occlusion, B, D, F. Note the extensive loss of apical membrane structure, B, D, in proximal (PT) but not distal tubule cells. This has been shown to correlate with extensive alterations in F-actin as shown by FITC-phalloidin labeling, E, F. G, Drawing of a proximal tubule cell under physiologic conditions. Note the orderly arrangement of the actin cytoskeleton and its extensive interaction with the surface membrane at the zonula occludens (ZO, tight junction) zonula adherens (ZA, occludens junction), interactions with ankyrin to mediate Na+, K+-ATPase [2] stabilization and cell adhesion molecule attachment [5,8]. The actin cytoskeleton also mediates attachment to the extracellular matrix (ECM) via integrins [12,15]. Microtubules (MT) are involved in the polarized delivery of endocytic and exocytic vesicles to the surface membrane. Finally, F-actin filaments bundle together via actin-bundling proteins [19] to mediate amplification of the apical surface membrane via microvilli (MV). The actin bundle attaches to the surface membrane by the actin-binding proteins myosin I and ezrin [19,20].

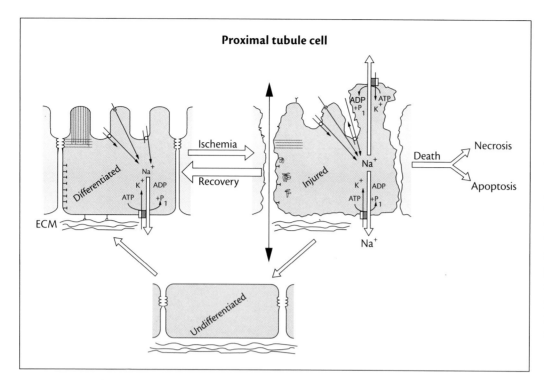

Proximal tubule cell

FIGURE 13-3

Fate of an injured proximal tubule cell. The fate of a proximal tubule cell after an ischemic episode depends on the extent and duration of the ischemia. Cell death can occur immediately via necrosis or in a more programmed fashion (apoptosis) hours to days after the injury. Fortunately, most cells recover either in a direct fashion or via an intermediate undifferentiated cellular pathway. Again, the severity of the injury determines the route taken by a particular cell. Adjacent cells are often injured to varying degrees, especially during mild to moderate ischemia. It is believed that the rate of organ functional recovery relates directly to the severity of cell injury during the initiation phase. ECM—extracellular membrane; Na+—sodium ion; K+—potassium ion; P₁—phosphate.

FIGURE 13-4

Ischemia induced proximal tubule cell alterations.

ISCHEMIA INDUCED PROXIMAL TUBULE CELL ALTERATIONS

Alterations	References
Surface Membrane Alterations	
1. Microvilli fusion, internalization, fragmentation and luminal shedding resulting in loss of surface membrane area and tubular obstruction	[21]
2. Loss of surface membrane polarity for lipids and proteins	[2,22,23]
3. Junctional complex dissociation with unregulated paracellular permeability (backleak)	[6,24–27]
4. Reduced PTC vectorial transport	[28]
Actin Cytoskeletal Alterations	
1. Polymerization of actin throughout the cell cytosol	[6,16,29]
2. Disruption and delocalization of F-actin structures including stress fibers, cortical actin and the junctional ring	[2,7,16]
3. Accumulation of intracellular F-actin aggregates containing surface membrane proteins—myosin I, the tight junction proteins ZO-1, ZO-2, cingulin	[20,30]
4. Disruption and dissociation of the spectrin cytoskeleton	[31,32]
5. Disruption of microtubules during early reflow in vivo	[33]
6. The cytoskeleton of proximal tubule cells, as compared to distal tubule cells, is more sensitive to ischemia in vivo and ATP depletion in vitro	[6,16,34]

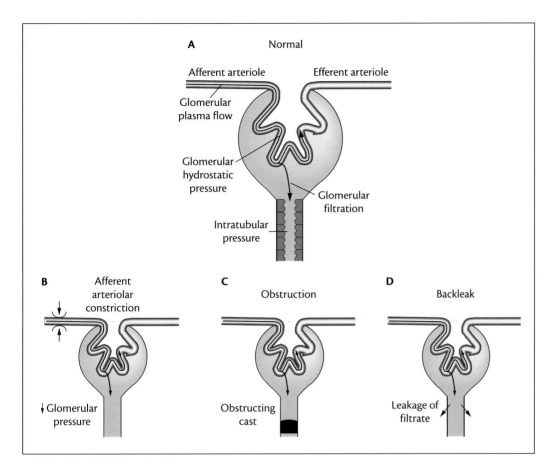

FIGURE 13-5

Mechanisms of proximal tubule cell—mediated reductions in glomerular filtration rate (GFR) following ischemic injury. **A,** GFR depends on four factors: 1) adequate blood flow to the glomerulus; 2) an adequate glomerular capillary pressure as determined by afferent and efferent arteriolar resistance; 3) glomerular permeability; and 4) low intratubular pressure. **B,** Afferent arteriolar constriction diminishes GFR by reducing blood flow—and, therefore, glomerular capillary pressure. This occurs in response to a high distal sodium delivery and is mediated by tubular glomerular feedback. **C,** Obstruction of the tubular lumen by cast formation increases tubular pressure and, when it exceeds glomerular capillary pressure, a marked decrease or no filtration occurs. **D,** Back-leak occurs when the paracellular space between cells is open for the flux of glomerular filtrate to leak back into the extracellular space and into the blood stream. This is believed to occur through open tight junctions.

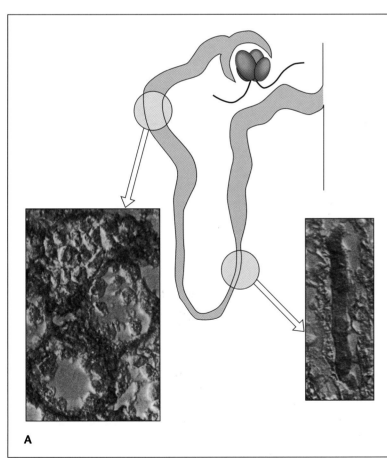

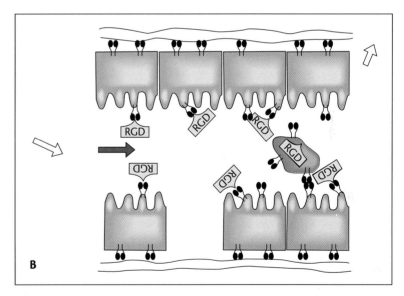

FIGURE 13-6

Overview of potential therapeutic effects of cyclic integrin-binding peptides. **A,** During ischemic injury, tubular obstruction occurs as a result of loss of apical membrane, cell contents, and detached cells released into the lumen. **B,** Also, basolateral integrins diffuse to the apical region of the cell. Biotinylated cyclic peptides containing the sequence cRGDDFV bind to desquamated cells in the ascending limb of the loop of Henle and in proximal tubule cells in ischemic rat kidneys. The desquamated cells can adhere to injured cells or aggregate, causing tubule obstruction.

(Continued on next page)

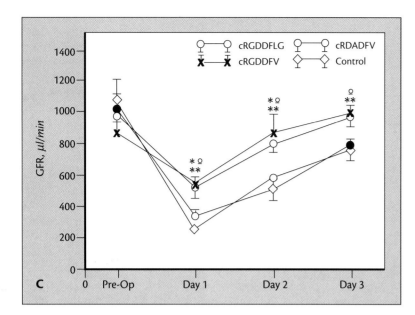

FIGURE 13-6 (*Continued*)

C, When cyclic peptides that contain the RGD canonical binding site of integrins are perfused intra-arterially, the peptides ameliorate the extent of acute renal failure, as demonstrated by a higher glomerular filtration rate (GFR) in rats receiving peptide containing the RGD sequence. **B**, Proposed mechanism of renal protection by cyclic RGD peptides. By adhering to the RGD binding sites of the integrins located on the apical plasma membrane or distributed randomly on desquamated cells, the cyclic peptide blocks cellular aggregation and tubular obstruction [12–15]. (*Courtesy of* MS Goligorski, MD.)

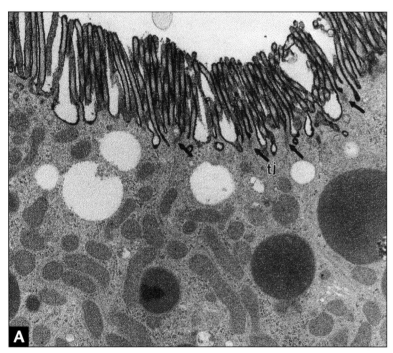

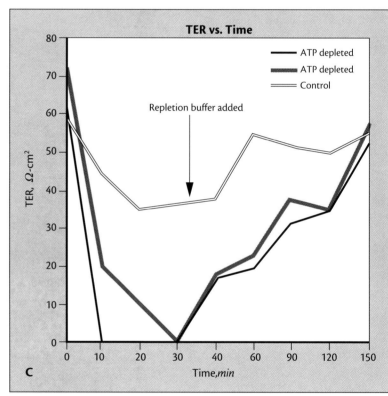

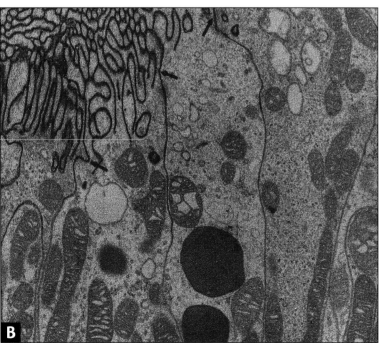

FIGURE 13-7

Functional and morphologic changes in tight junction integrity associated with ischemic injury or intracellular ATP depletion. **A** and **B**, Ruthenium red paracellular permeability in rat proximal tubules. **A**, In control kidneys, note the electron-dense staining of the brush border, which cuts off at the tight junctions (tj, *arrows*). **B**, Sections from a perfusion-fixed kidney after 20 minutes of renal artery cross-clamp [35]. The electron-dense staining can be seen at cell contact sites beyond the tight junction (*arrows*). The paracellular pathway is no longer sealed by the tight junction, permitting backleak of the electron-dense ruthenium red. **C**, Changes in the transepithelial resistance (TER) versus time during ATP depletion and ATP repletion [36]. Paracellular resistance to electron movement

(Continued on next page)

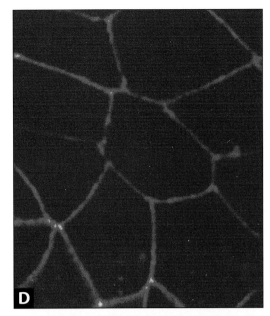

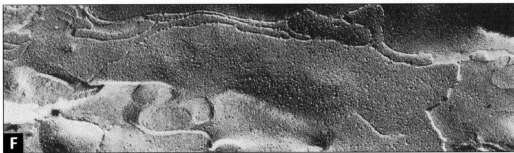

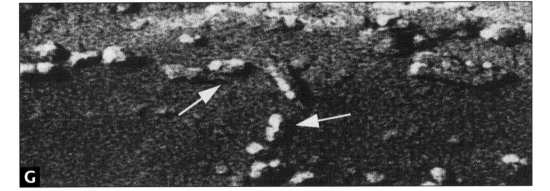

FIGURE 13-7 (*Continued*)

(the TER falls to zero with ATP depletion). The cellular junctional complex that controls the TER is the tight junction. When the TER falls to zero, this suggests that tight junction structural integrity has been compromised. **D** and **E**, Staining of renal epithelial cells with antibodies that bind to a component of the tight junction, ZO-1 [37]. **D**, ZO-1 staining in untreated Mardin-Darby carnine kidney (MDCK) cells. ZO-1 is located at the periphery of cells at cell contact sites, forming a continuous linear contour. **E**, In ATP–depleted cells the staining pattern is discontinuous. **F** and **G**, Ultrastructural analysis of the tight junction in MDCK cells. In untreated MDCK cells, electron micrographs of the tight junction shows a continuous ridge like structure in freeze fracture preparations [38]. In ATP depleted cells the strands are disrupted, forming aggregates (*arrows*). Note that the continuous strands are no longer present and large gaps are observable.

Acknowledgment

These studies were in part supported by the National Institute of Diabetes and Digestive and Kidney Diseases Grants DK 41126 (BAM) and DK4683 (RB) and by an American Heart Association Established Investigator Award (BAM), a VA Merrit Review Grant (BAM), and a NKF Clinical Scientist Award (RB).

References

1. Liaño F, Pascual J, Madrid Acute Renal Failure Study Group: Epidemiology of acute renal failure: A prospective, multicenter, community-based study. *Kidney Int* 1996, 50:811–818.

2. Molitoris BA, Wagner MC: Surface membrane polarity of proximal tubular cells: Alterations as a basis for malfunction. *Kidney Int* 1996, 49:1592–1597.

3. Thadhani R, Pascual M, Bonventre JV: Acute renal failure. *N Engl J Med* 1996, 334:1448–1457.

4. Drubin DG, Nelson WJ: Origins of cell polarity. *Cell* 1996, 84:335–344.

5. Mays RW, Nelson WJ, Marrs JA: Generation of epithelial cell polarity: Roles for protein trafficking, membrane-cytoskeleton, and E-cadherin–mediated cell adhesion. *Cold Spring Harbor Symposia on Quantitative Biol* 1995, 60:763–773.

6. Bacallao R, Garfinkel A, Monke S, *et al.*: ATP depletion: A novel method to study junctional properties in epithelial tissues. I. Rearrangement of the actin cytoskeleton. *J Cell Sci* 1994, 107:3301–3313.

7. Kroshian VM, Sheridan AM, Lieberthal W: Functional and cytoskeletal changes induced by sublethal injury in proximal tubular epithelial cells. *Am J Physiol* 1994, F21–F30.

8. Fish EM, Molitoris BA: Alterations in epithelial polarity and the pathogenesis of disease states. *N Engl J Med* 1994, 330:1580–1588.

9. Glaumann B, Glauman H, Berezesky IK, *et al.*: Studies on the cellular recovery from injury II. Ultrastructural studies on the recovery of the pars convoluta of the proximal tubule of the rat kidney from temporary ischemia. *Virchows Arch B* 1977, 24:1–18.

10. Kellerman PS, Norenberg SL, Jones GM: Early recovery of the actin cytoskeleton during renal ischemic injury *in vivo*. *Am J Kidney Dis* 1996, 16:33–42.

11. Kellerman PS, Clark RAF, Hoilien CA, *et al.*: Role of microfilaments in the maintenance of proximal tubule structural and functional integrity. *Am J Physiol* 1990, 259:F279–F285.

12. Noiri E, Gailit J, Gurrath M, *et al.*: Cyclic RGD peptides ameliorate ischemic acute renal failure in rats. *Kidney Int* 1994, 46:1050–1058.

13. Noiri E, Goligorsky MS, Som P: Radiolabeled RGD peptides as diagnostic tools in acute renal failure and tubular obstruction. *J Am Soc Nephrol* 1996, 7:2682–2688.

14. Romanov V, Noiri E, Czerwinski G, *et al.*: Two novel probes reveal tubular and vascular RGD binding sites in the ischemic rat kidney. *Kidney Int* 1997, 52:92–102.

15. Goligorsky MS, Noiri E, Romanov V, *et al.*: Therapeutic potential of RGD peptides in acute renal failure. *Kidney Int* 1997, 51:1487–1493.

16. Molitoris BA, Dahl R, Geerdes AE: Cytoskeleton disruption and apical redistribution of proximal tubule Na+,K+-ATPase during ischemia. *Am J Physiol* 1992, 263:F488–F495.

17. Alejandro V, Scandling JD, Sibley RK, *et al.*: Mechanisms of filtration failure during postischemic injury of the human kidney: A study of the reperfused renal allograft. *J Clin Invest* 1995, 95:820–831.

18. Bacallao R, Fine LG: Molecular events in the organization of renal tubular epithelium: From nephrogenesis to regeneration. *Am J Physiol* 1989, 257:F913–F924.

19. Molitoris BA: Putting the actin cytoskeleton into perspective: pathophysiology of ischemic alterations. *Am J Physiol* 1997, 272:F430–F433.

20. Wagner MC, Molitoris BA: ATP depletion alters myosin Ib cellular location in LLC-PK1 cells. *Am J Physiol* 1997, 272:C1680–C1690.

21. Venkatachalam MA, Jones DB, Rennke HG, *et al.*: Mechanism of proximal tubule brush border loss and regeneration following mild ischemia. *Lab Invest* 1981, 45:355–365.

22. Ritter D, Dean AD, Guan ZH, *et al.*: Polarized distribution of renal natriuretic peptide receptors in normal physiology and ischemia. *Am J Physiol* 1995, 269:F918–F925.

23. Alejandro VSJ, Nelson WJ, Huie P, *et al.*: Postischemic injury, delayed function and Na+/K+-ATPase distribution in the transplanted kidney. *Kidney Int* 1995, 48:1308–1315.

24. Donohoe JF, Venkatachalam MA, Benard DB, *et al.*: Tubular leakage and obstruction after renal ischemia: Structural-functional correlations. *Kidney Int* 1978, 13:208–222.

25. Molitoris BA, Falk SA, Dahl RH: Ischemic-induced loss of epithelial polarity. Role of the tight junction. *J Clin Invest* 1989, 84:1334–1339.

26. Mandel LJ, Bacallao R, Zampighi G: Uncoupling of the molecular fence and paracellular gate functions in epithelial tight junctions. *Nature* 1993, 361:552–555.

27. Kwon O, Nelson J, Sibley RK, *et al.*: Backleak, tight junctions and cell-cell adhesion in postischemic injury to the renal allograft (Abstract). *J Am Soc Nephrol* 1996, 7:A2907.

28. Molitoris BA. Na+-K+-ATPase that redistributes to apical membrane during ATP depletion remains functional. *Am J Physiol* 1993, 265:F693–F597.

29. Kellerman PS: Exogenous adenosine triphosphate (ATP) proximal tubule microfilament structure and function *in vivo* in a maleic acid model of ATP depletion. *J Clin Invest* 1993, 92:1940–1949.

30. Tsukamoto T, Nigam SK: ATP depletion causes tight junction proteins to form large, insoluble complexes with cytoskeletal proteins in renal epithelial cells. *J Biol Chem* 1997, 273:F463–F472.

31. Molitoris BA, Dahl R, Hosford M: Cellular ATP depletion induces disruption of the spectrin cytoskeletal network. *Am J Physiol* 1996, 271:F790–F798.

32. Edelstein CL, Ling H, Schrier RW: The nature of renal cell injury. *Kidney Int* 1997, 51:1341–1351.

33. Abbate M, Bonventre JV, Brown D: The microtubule network of renal epithelial cells is disrupted by ischemia and reperfusion. *Am J Physiol* 1994, 267:F971–F978.

34. Sheridan AM, Schwartz JH, Kroshian VM, *et al.*: Renal mouse proximal tubular cells are more susceptible than MDCK cells to chemical anoxia. *Am J Physiol* 1993, 265:F342–F350.

35. Molitoris BA, Falk SA, Dahl RH: Ischemia-induced loss of epithelial polarity. Role of the tight junction. *J Clin Invest* 1989, 84:1334–1339.

36. Doctor RB, Bacallao R, Mandel LJ: Method for recovering ATP content and mitochondrial function after chemical anoxia in renal cell cultures. *Am J Physiol* 1994, 266:C1803–C1811.

37. Stevenson BR, Siliciano JD, Mooseker MS, *et al.*: Identification of ZO-1: A high molecular weight polypeptide associated with the tight junction (zonula occludens) in a variety of epithelia. *J Cell Biol* 1986, 103:755–766.

38. Mandel LJ, Bacallao R, Zampighi G: Uncoupling of the molecular 'fence' and paracellular 'gate' functions in epithelial tight junctions. *Nature* 1993, 361:552–555.

Pathophysiology of Ischemic Acute Renal Failure

Michael S. Goligorsky
Wilfred Lieberthal

Acute renal failure (ARF) is a syndrome characterized by an abrupt and reversible kidney dysfunction. The spectrum of inciting factors is broad: from ischemic and nephrotoxic agents to a variety of endotoxemic states and syndrome of multiple organ failure. The pathophysiology of ARF includes vascular, glomerular and tubular dysfunction which, depending on the actual offending stimulus, vary in the severity and time of appearance. Hemodynamic compromise prevails in cases when noxious stimuli are related to hypotension and septicemia, leading to renal hypoperfusion with secondary tubular changes (described in Chapter 13). Nephrotoxic offenders usually result in primary tubular epithelial cell injury, though endothelial cell dysfunction can also occur, leading to the eventual cessation of glomerular filtration. This latter effect is a consequence of the combined action of tubular obstruction and activation of tubuloglomerular feedback mechanism. In the following pages we shall review the existing concepts on the phenomenology of ARF including the mechanisms of decreased renal perfusion and failure of glomerular filtration, vasoconstriction of renal arterioles, how formed elements gain access to the renal parenchyma, and what the sequelae are of such an invasion by primed leukocytes.

CHAPTER

14

Vasoactive Hormones

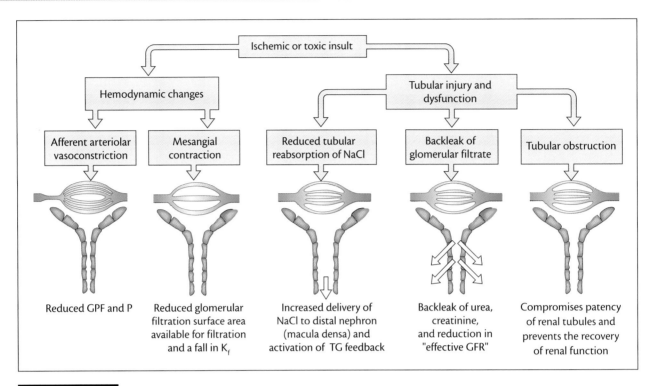

FIGURE 14-1

Pathophysiology of ischemic and toxic acute renal failure (ARF). The severe reduction in glomerular filtration rate (GFR) associated with established ischemic or toxic renal injury is due to the combined effects of alterations in intrarenal hemodynamics and tubular injury. The hemodynamic alterations associated with ARF include afferent arteriolar constriction and mesangial contraction, both of which directly reduce GFR. Tubular injury reduces GFR by causing tubular obstruction and by allowing backleak of glomerular filtrate. Abnormalities in tubular reabsorption of solute may contribute to intrarenal vasoconstriction by activating the tubuloglomerular (TG) feedback system. GPF—glomerular plasmaflow; P—glomerular pressure; K_f—glomerular ultrafiltration coefficient.

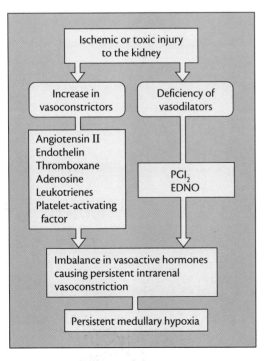

FIGURE 14-2

Vasoactive hormones that may be responsible for the hemodynamic abnormalities in acute tubule necrosis (ATN). A persistent reduction in renal blood flow has been demonstrated in both animal models of acute renal failure (ARF) and in humans with ATN. The mechanisms responsible for the hemodynamic alterations in ARF involve an increase in the intrarenal activity of vasoconstrictors and a deficiency of important vasodilators. A number of vasoconstrictors have been implicated in the reduction in renal blood flow in ARF. The importance of individual vasoconstrictor hormones in ARF probably varies to some extent with the cause of the renal injury. A deficiency of vasodilators such as endothelium-derived nitric oxide (EDNO) and/or prostaglandin I_2 (PGI_2) also contributes to the renal hypoperfusion associated with ARF. This imbalance in intrarenal vasoactive hormones favoring vasoconstriction causes persistent intrarenal hypoxia, thereby exacerbating tubular injury and protracting the course of ARF.

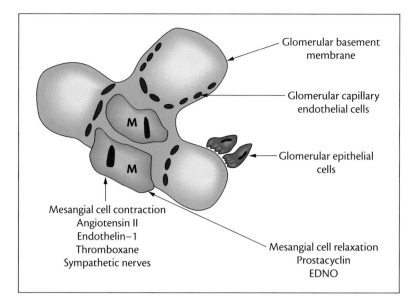

FIGURE 14-3

The mesangium regulates single-nephron glomerular filtration rate (SNGFR) by altering the glomerular ultrafiltration coefficient (K_f). This schematic diagram demonstrates the anatomic relationship between glomerular capillary loops and the mesangium. The mesangium is surrounded by capillary loops. Mesangial cells (M) are specialized pericytes with contractile elements that can respond to vasoactive hormones. Contraction of mesangium can close and prevent perfusion of anatomically associated glomerular capillary loops. This decreases the surface area available for glomerular filtration and reduces the glomerular ultrafiltration coefficient.

Glomerular basement membrane

Glomerular capillary endothelial cells

Glomerular epithelial cells

Mesangial cell contraction
Angiotensin II
Endothelin–1
Thromboxane
Sympathetic nerves

Mesangial cell relaxation
Prostacyclin
EDNO

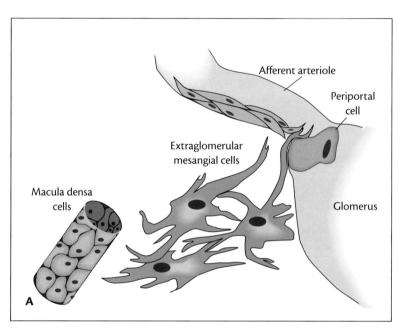

FIGURE 14-4

A, The topography of juxtaglomerular apparatus (JGA), including macula densa cells (MD), extraglomerular mesangial cells (EMC), and afferent arteriolar smooth muscle cells (SMC). Insets schematically illustrate, **B,** the structure of JGA; **C,** the flow of information within the JGA; and **D,** the putative messengers of tubuloglomerular feedback responses. AA—afferent arteriole; PPC—peripolar cell; EA—efferent arteriole; GMC—glomerular mesangial cells. (*Modified from* Goligorsky *et al.* [1]; with permission.)

Afferent arteriole

Periportal cell

Extraglomerular mesangial cells

Macula densa cells

Glomerus

A

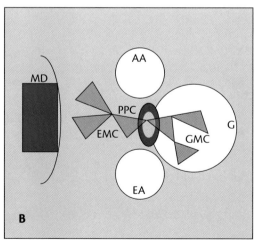

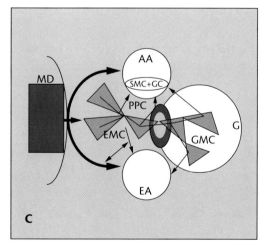

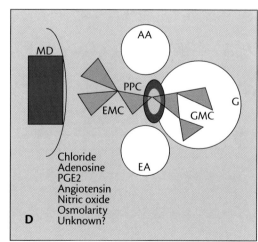

Chloride
Adenosine
PGE2
Angiotensin
Nitric oxide
Osmolarity
Unknown?

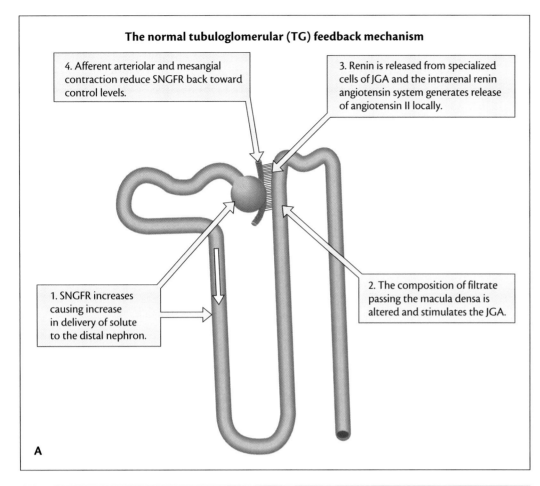

The normal tubuloglomerular (TG) feedback mechanism

4. Afferent arteriolar and mesangial contraction reduce SNGFR back toward control levels.

3. Renin is released from specialized cells of JGA and the intrarenal renin angiotensin system generates release of angiotensin II locally.

1. SNGFR increases causing increase in delivery of solute to the distal nephron.

2. The composition of filtrate passing the macula densa is altered and stimulates the JGA.

A

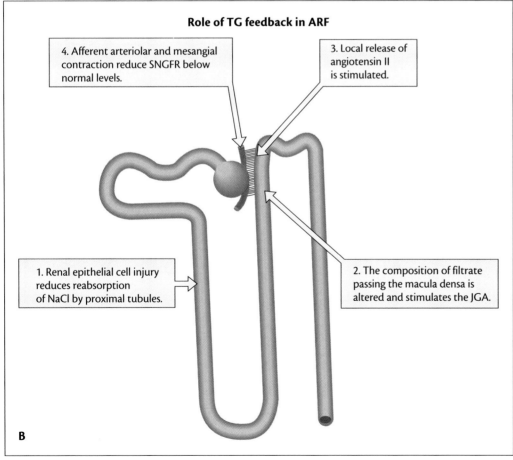

Role of TG feedback in ARF

4. Afferent arteriolar and mesangial contraction reduce SNGFR below normal levels.

3. Local release of angiotensin II is stimulated.

1. Renal epithelial cell injury reduces reabsorption of NaCl by proximal tubules.

2. The composition of filtrate passing the macula densa is altered and stimulates the JGA.

B

FIGURE 14-5

The tubuloglomerular (TG) feedback mechanism. **A,** Normal TG feedback. In the normal kidney, the TG feedback mechanism is a sensitive device for the regulation of the single nephron glomerular filtration rate (SNGFR). *Step 1*: An increase in SNGFR increases the amount of sodium chloride (NaCl) delivered to the juxtaglomerular apparatus (JGA) of the nephron. *Step 2*: The resultant change in the composition of the filtrate is sensed by the macula densa cells and initiates activation of the JGA. *Step 3*: The JGA releases renin, which results in the local and systemic generation of angiotensin II. *Step 4*: Angiotensin II induces vasocontriction of the glomerular arterioles and contraction of the mesangial cells. These events return SNGFR back toward basal levels. **B,** TG feedback in ARF. *Step 1*: Ischemic or toxic injury to renal tubules leads to impaired reabsorption of NaCl by injured tubular segments proximal to the JGA. *Step 2*: The composition of the filtrate passing the macula densa is altered and activates the JGA. *Step 3*: Angiotensin II is released locally. *Step 4*: SNGFR is reduced below normal levels. It is likely that vasoconstrictors other than angiotensin II, as well as vasodilator hormones (such as PGI_2 and nitric oxide) are also involved in modulating TG feedback. Abnormalities in these vasoactive hormones in ARF may contribute to alterations in TG feedback in ARF.

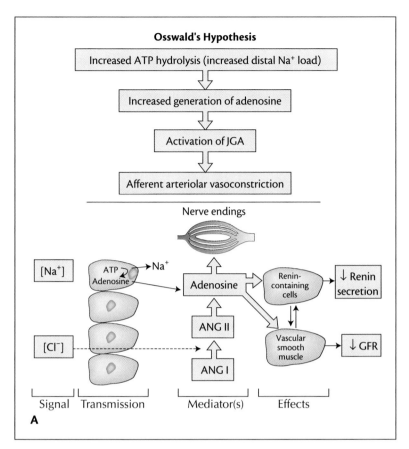

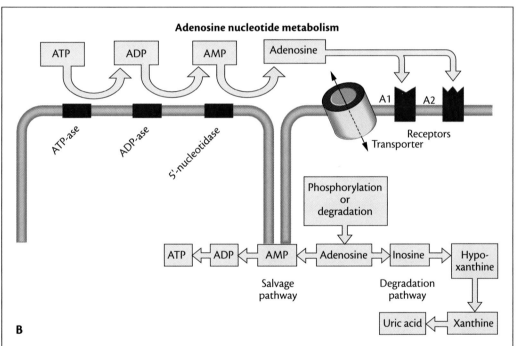

FIGURE 14-6

Metabolic basis for the adenosine hypothesis. **A,** Osswald's hypothesis on the role of adenosine in tubuloglomerular feedback. **B,** Adenosine metabolism: production and disposal via the salvage and degradation pathways. (**A,** *Modified from* Osswald *et al.* [2]; with permission.)

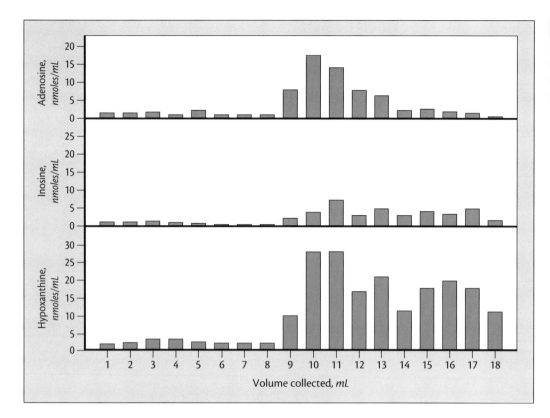

FIGURE 14-7

Elevated concentration of adenosine, inosine, and hypoxanthine in the dog kidney and urine after renal artery occlusion. (*Modified from* Miller *et al.* [3]; with permission.)

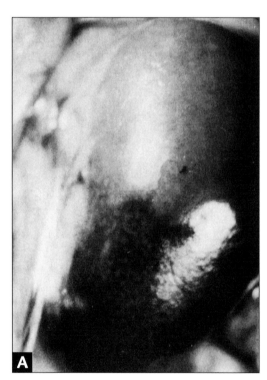

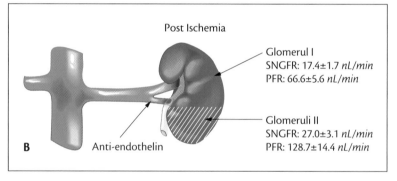

Post Ischemia

Glomerul I
SNGFR: 17.4±1.7 *nL/min*
PFR: 66.6±5.6 *nL/min*

Glomeruli II
SNGFR: 27.0±3.1 *nL/min*
PFR: 128.7±14.4 *nL/min*

Anti-endothelin

B

A

FIGURE 14-8

Endothelin (ET) is a potent renal vasoconstrictor. Endothelin (ET) is a 21 amino acid peptide of which three isoforms—ET-1, ET-2 and ET-3—have been described, all of which have been shown to be present in renal tissue. However, only the effects of ET-1 on the kidney have been clearly elucidated. ET-1 is the most potent vaso-constrictor known. Infusion of ET-1 into the kidney induces pro-found and long lasting vasoconstriction of the renal circulation. **A,** The appearance of the rat kidney during the infusion of ET-1 into the inferior branch of the main renal artery. The lower pole of the kidney perfused by this vessel is profoundly vasoconstricted and hypoperfused. **B,** Schematic illustration of function in separate populations of glomeruli within the same kidney. The entire kidney underwent 25 minutes of ischemia 48 hours before micropuncture. Glomeruli I are nephrons not exposed to endothelin antibody; Glomeruli II are nephrons that received infusion with antibody through the inferior branch of the main renal artery. SNGFR—sin-gle nephron glomerular filtration rate; PFR—glomerular renal plas-ma flow rate. (*From* Kon *et al.* [4]; with permission.)

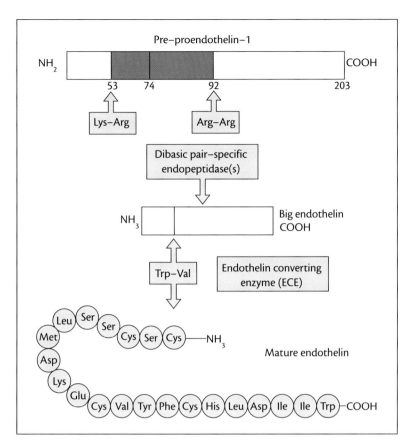

FIGURE 14-9

Biosynthesis of mature endothelin-1 (ET-1). The mature ET-1 peptide is produced by a series of biochemical steps. The precursor of active ET is pre-pro ET, which is cleaved by dibasic pair-specific endopeptidases and carboxypeptidases to yield a 39–amino acid intermediate termed big ET-1. Big ET-1, which has little vasoconstrictor activity, is then converted to the mature 21–amino acid ET by a specific endopeptidase, the endothelin-converting enzyme (ECE). ECE is localized to the plasma membrane of endothelial cells. The arrows indicate sites of cleavage of pre-pro ET and big ET.

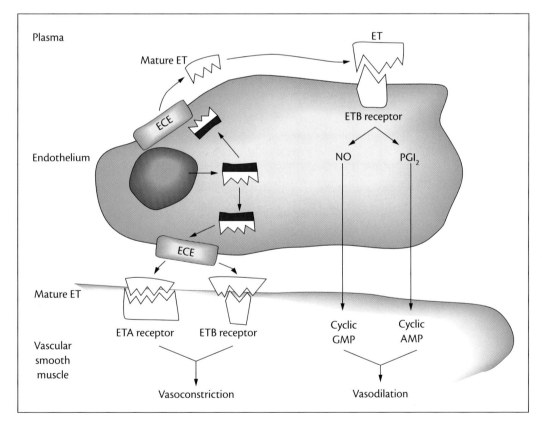

FIGURE 14-10

Regulation of endothelin (ET) action; the role of the ET receptors. Pre-pro ET is produced and converted to big ET. Big ET is converted to mature, active ET by endothelin-converting enzyme (ECE) present on the endothelial cell membrane. Mature ET secreted onto the basolateral aspect of the endothelial cell binds to two ET receptors (ET_A and ET_B); both are present on vascular smooth muscle (VSM) cells. Interaction of ET with predominantly expressed ET_A receptors on VSM cells induces vasoconstriction. ET_B receptors are predominantly located on the plasma membrane of endothelial cells. Interaction of ET-1 with these endothelial ET_B receptors stimulates production of nitric oxide (NO) and prostacyclin by endothelial cells. The production of these two vasodilators serves to counterbalance the intense vasoconstrictor activity of ET-1. PGI_2—prostaglandin I_2.

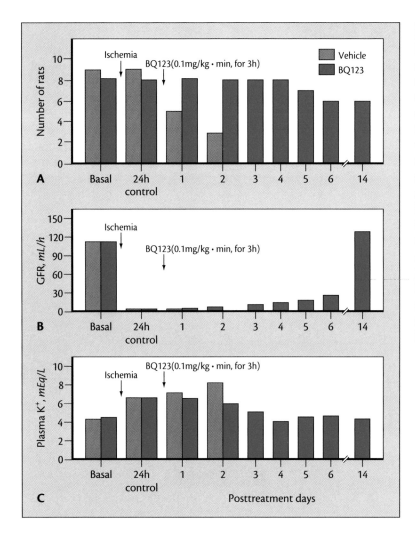

FIGURE 14-11

Endothelin-1 (ET-1) receptor blockade ameliorates severe ischemic acute renal failure (ARF) in rats. The effect of an ET_A receptor antagonist (BQ123) on the course of severe postischemic ARF was examined in rats. BQ123 (*light bars*) or its vehicle (*dark bars*) was administered 24 hours after the ischemic insult and the rats were followed for 14 days. **A**, Survival. All rats that received the vehicle were dead by the 3rd day after ischemic injury. In contrast, all rats that received BQ123 post-ischemia survived for 4 days and 75% recovered fully. **B**, Glomerular filtration rate (GFR). In both groups of rats GFR was extremely low (2% of basal levels) 24 hours after ischemia. In BQ123-treated rats there was a gradual increase in GFR that reached control levels by the 14th day after ischemia. **C**, Serum potassium. Serum potassium increased in both groups but reached significantly higher levels in vehicle-treated compared to the BQ123-treated rats by the second day. The severe hyperkalemia likely contributed to the subsequent death of the vehicle treated rats. In BQ123-treated animals the potassium fell progressively after the second day and reached normal levels by the fourth day after ischemia. (*Adapted from* Gellai *et al.* [5]; with permission.)

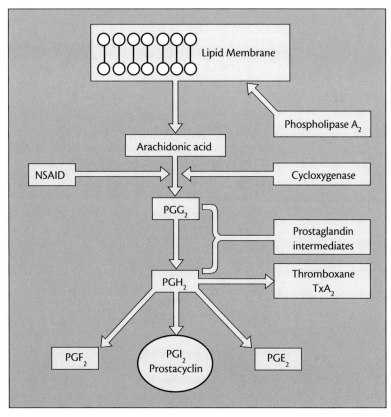

FIGURE 14-12

Production of prostaglandins. Arachidonic acid is released from the plasma membrane by phospholipase A_2. The enzyme cycloxygenase catalyses the conversion of arachidonate to two prostanoid intermediates (PGH_2 and PGG_2). These are converted by specific enzymes into a number of different prostanoids as well as thromboxane (TXA_2). The predominant prostaglandin produced varies with the cell type. In endothelial cells prostacyclin (PGI_2) (*in the circle*) is the major metabolite of cycloxygenase activity. Prostacyclin, a potent vasodilator, is involved in the regulation of vascular tone. TXA_2 is not produced in endothelial cells of normal kidneys but may be produced in increased amounts and contribute to the pathophysiology of some forms of acute renal failure (eg, cyclosporine A–induced nephrotoxicity). The production of all prostanoids and TXA_2 is blocked by nonsteroidal anti-inflammatory agents (NSAIDs), which inhibit cycloxygenase activity.

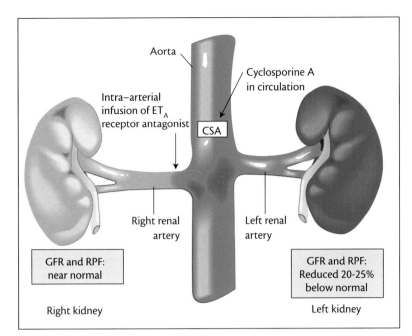

FIGURE 14-13

Endothelin (ET) receptor blockade ameliorates acute cyclosporine-induced nephrotoxicity. Cyclosporine A (CSA) was administered intravenously to rats. Then, an ET receptor anatgonist was infused directly into the right renal artery. Glomerular filtration rate (GFR) and renal plasma flow (RPF) were reduced by the CSA in the left kidney. The ET receptor antagonist protected GFR and RPF from the effects of CSA on the right side. Thus, ET contributes to the intrarenal vasoconstriction and reduction in GFR associated with acute CSA nephrotoxicity. (*From* Fogo *et al.* [6]; with permission.)

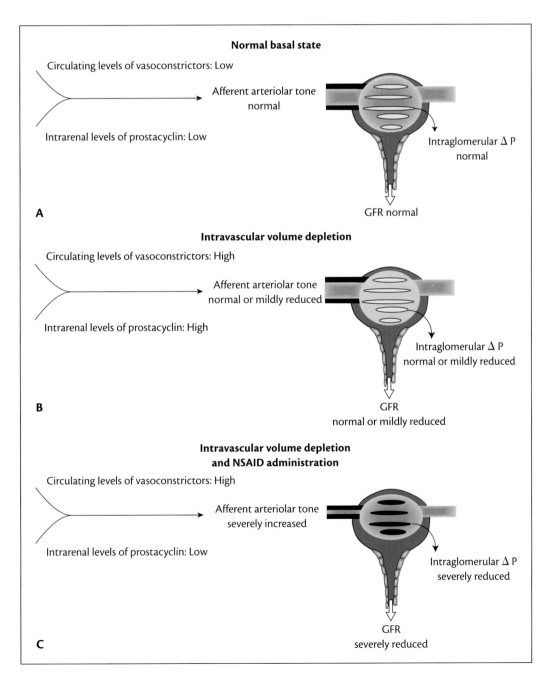

FIGURE 14-14

Prostacyclin is important in maintaining renal blood flow (RBF) and glomerular filtration rate (GFR) in "prerenal" states. A, When intravascular volume is normal, prostacyclin production in the endothelial cells of the kidney is low and prostacyclin plays little or no role in control of vascular tone. B, The reduction in absolute or "effective" arterial blood volume associated with all prerenal states leads to an increase in the circulating levels of a number of of vasoconstrictors, including angiotensin II, catecholamines, and vasopressin. The increase in vasoconstrictors stimulates phospholipase A_2 and prostacyclin production in renal endothelial cells. This increase in prostacyclin production partially counteracts the effects of the circulating vasoconstrictors and plays a critical role in maintaining normal or nearly normal RBF and GFR in prerenal states. C, The effect of cycloxygenase inhibition with nonsteroidal anti-inflammatory drugs (NSAIDs) in prerenal states. Inhibition of prostacyclin production in the presence of intravascular volume depletion results in unopposed action of prevailing vasoconstrictors and results in severe intrarenal vascasoconstriction. NSAIDs can precipitate severe acute renal failure in these situations.

A. VASODILATORS USED IN EXPERIMENTAL ACUTE RENAL FAILURE (ARF)

Vasodilator	ARF Disorder	Time Given in Relation to Induction	Observed Effect
Propranolol	Ischemic	Before, during, after	↓Scr, BUN if given before, during; no effect if given after
Phenoxybenzamine	Toxic	Before, during, after	Prevented fall in RBF
Clonidine	Ischemic	After	↓Scr, BUN
Bradykinin	Ischemic	Before, during	↑RBF, GFR
Acetylcholine	Ischemic	Before, after	↑RBF; no change in GFR
Prostaglandin E_1	Ischemic	After	↑RBF; no change in GFR
Prostaglandin E_2	Ischemic, toxic	Before, during	↑GFR
Prostaglandin I_2	Ischemic	Before, during, after	↑GFR
Saralasin	Toxic, ischemic	Before	↑RBF; no change in Scr, BUN
Captopril	Toxic, ischemic	Before	↑RBF; no change in Scr, BUN
Verapamil	Ischemic, toxic	Before, during, after	↑RBF, GFR in most studies
Nifedipine	Ischemic	Before	↑GFR
Nitrendipine	Toxic	Before, during	↑GFR
Diliazem	Toxic	Before, during, after	↑GFR; ↓recovery time
Chlorpromazine	Toxic	Before	↑GFR; ↓recovery time
Atrial natriuretic peptide	Ischemic, toxic	After	↑RBF, GFR

BUN—blood urea nitrogen; GFR—glomerular filtration rate; RBF—renal blood flow; Scr–serum creatinine.

B. VASODILATORS USED TO ALTER COURSE OF CLINICAL ACUTE RENAL FAILURE (ARF)

Vasodilator	ARF Disorder	Observed Effect	Remarks
Dopamine	Ischemic, toxic	Improved V, Scr if used early	Combined with furosemide
Phenoxybenzamine	Ischemic, toxic	No change in V, RBF	
Phentolamine	Ischemic, toxic	No change in V, RBF	
Prostaglandin A_1	Ischemic	No change in V, Scr	Used with dopamine
Prostaglandin E_1	Ischemic	↑RBF, no change v, C_{cr}	Used with NE
Dihydralazine	Ischemic, toxic	↑RBF, no change V, Scr	
Verapamil	Ischemic	↑C_{cr} or no effect	
Diltiazem	Transplant, toxic	↑C_{cr} or no effect	Prophylactic use
Nifedipine	Radiocontrast	No effect	
Atrial natriuretic peptide	Ischemic	↑C_{cr}	

C_{cr}—creatinine clearance; NE—norepinephrine; RBF—renal blood flow; Scr—serum creatinine; V—urine flow rate.

FIGURE 14-15

Vasodilators used in acute renal failure (ARF). **A,** Vasodilators used in experimental acute ARF. **B,** Vasodilators used to alter the course of clinical ARF. (*From* Conger [7]; with permission.)

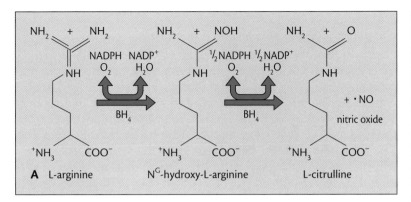

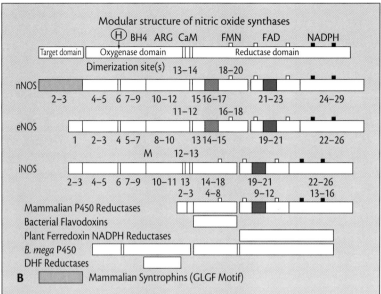

FIGURE 14-16

Chemical reactions leading to the generation of nitric oxide (NO), A, and enzymes that catalyze them, B. (*Modified from* Gross [8]; with permission.)

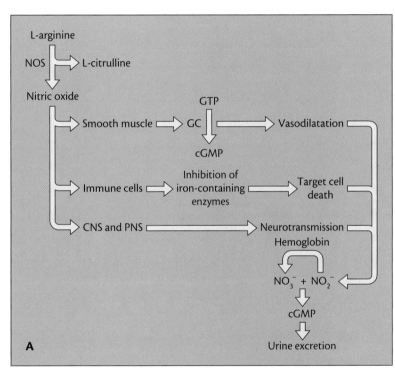

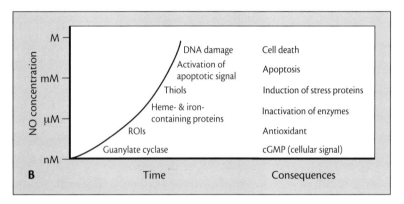

FIGURE 14-17

Major organ, A, and cellular, B, targets of nitric oxide (NO). A, Synthesis and function of NO. B, Intracellular targets for NO and pathophysiological consequences of its action. C, Endothelium-dependent vasodilators, such as acetylcholine and the calcium ionophore A23187, act by stimulating eNOS activity thereby increasing endothelium-derived nitric oxide (EDNO) production. In contrast, other vasodilators act independently of the endothelium. Some endothelium-independent vasodilators such as nitroprusside and nitroglycerin induce vasodilation by directly releasing nitric oxide in vascular smooth muscle cells. NO released by these agents, like EDNO, induces vasodilation by stimulating the production of cyclic guanosine monophosphate (cGMP) in vascular smooth muscle (VSM) cells. Atrial natriuretic peptide (ANP) is also an endothelium-independent vasodilator but acts differently from NO. ANP directly stimulates an isoform of guanylyl cyclase (GC) distinct from soluble GC (called particulate GC) in VSM. CNS—central nervous system; GTP—guanosine triphosphate; NOS—nitric oxide synthase; PGC—particulate guanylyl cyclase; PNS—peripheral nervous system; ROI—reduced oxygen intermediates; SGC—soluble guanylyl cyclase. (A, *From* Reyes *et al.* [9], with permission; B, *from* Kim *et al.* [10], with permission.)

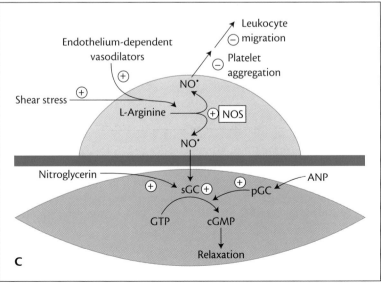

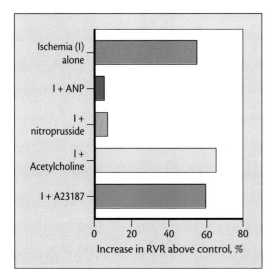

FIGURE 14-18

Impaired production of endothelium-dependent nitric oxide (EDNO) contributes to the vasoconstriction associated with established acute renal failure (ARF). Ischemia-reperfusion injury in the isolated erythrocyte-perfused kidney induced persistant intrarenal vasoconstriction. The endothelium-independent vasodilators (atrial natriuretic peptide [ANP] and nitroprusside) administered during the reflow period caused vasodilation and restored the elevated intrarenal vascular resistance (RVR) to normal. In marked contrast, two endothelium-dependent vasodilators (acetylcholine and A23187) had no effect on renal vascular resistance after ischemia-reflow. These data suggest that EDNO production is impaired following ischemic injury and that this loss of EDNO activity contributes to the vasoconstriction associated with ARF. (*Adapted from* Lieberthal [11]; with permission.)

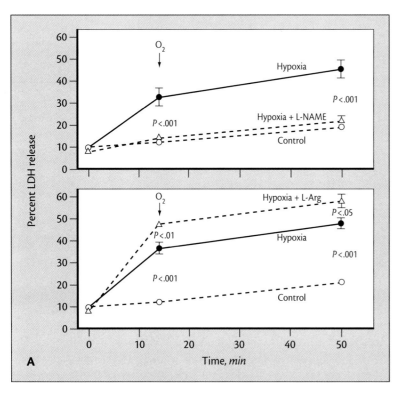

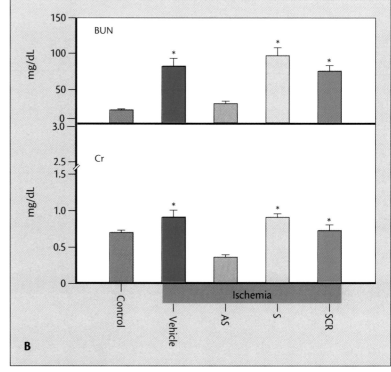

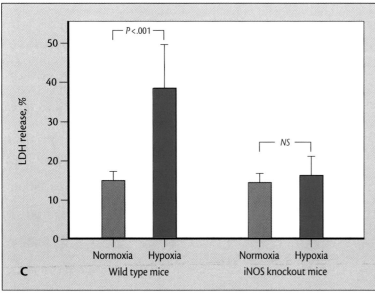

FIGURE 14-19

Deleterious effects of nitric oxide (NO) on the viability of renal tubular epithelia. **A**, Hypoxia and reoxygenation lead to injury of tubular cells (*filled circles*); inhibition of NO production improves the viability of tubular cells subjected to hypoxia and reoxygenation (*triangles* in *upper graph*), whereas addition of L-arginine enhances the injury (*triangles* in *lower graph*). **B**, Amelioration of ischemic injury in vivo with antisense oligonucleotides to the iNOS: blood urea nitrogen (BUN), and creatinine (CR) in rats subjected to 45 minutes of renal ischemia after pretreatment with antisense phosphorothioate oligonucleotides (AS) directed to iNOS or with sense (S) and scrambled (SCR) constructs. **C**, Resistance of proximal tubule cells isolated from iNOS knockout mice to hypoxia-induced injury. LDH—lactic dehydrogenase. (**A**, *From* Yu *et al.* [12], with permission; **B**, *from* Noiri *et al.* [13], with permission; **C**, *from* Ling *et al.* [14], with permission.)

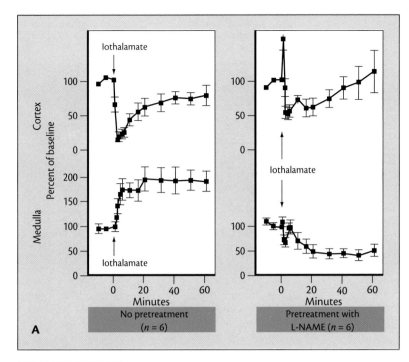

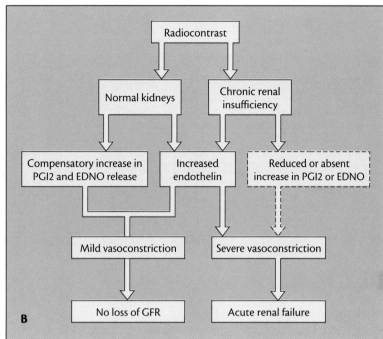

FIGURE 14-20

Proposed role of nitric oxide (NO) in radiocontrast-induced acute renal failure (ARF). **A,** Administration of iothalamate, a radiocontrast dye, to rats increases medullary blood flow. Inhibitors of either prostaglandin production (such as the NSAID, indomethacin) or inhibitors of NO synthesis (such as L-NAME) abolish the compensatory increase in medullary blood flow that occurs in response to radiocontrast administration. Thus, the stimulation of prostaglandin and NO production after radiocontrast administration is important in maintaining medullary perfusion and oxygenation after administration of contrast agents. **B,** Radiocontrast stimulates the production of vasodilators (such as prostaglandin [PGI$_2$] and endothelium-dependent nitric oxide [EDNO]) as well as endothelin and other vasoconstrictors within

the normal kidney. The vasodilators counteract the effects of the vasoconstrictors so that intrarenal vasoconstriction in response to radiocontrast is usually modest and is associated with little or no loss of renal function. However, in situations when there is pre-existing chronic renal insufficiency (CRF) the vasodilator response to radiocontrast is impaired, whereas production of endothelin and other vasoconstrictors is not affected or even increased. As a result, radiocontrast administration causes profound intrarenal vasoconstriction and can cause ARF in patients with CRF. This hypothesis would explain the predisposition of patients with chronic renal dysfunction, and especially diabetic nephropathy, to contrast-induced ARF. (**A,** *Adapted from* Agmon and Brezis [15], with permission; **B,** *from* Agmon *et al.* [16], with permission.)

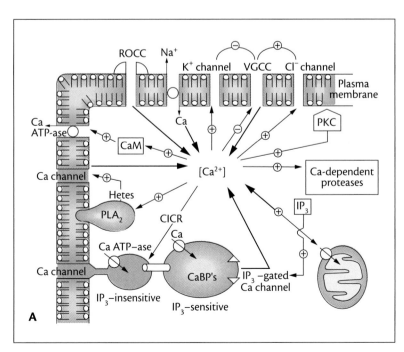

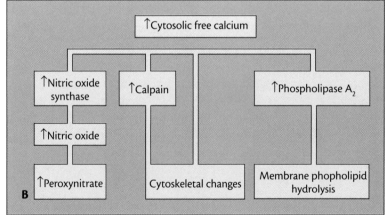

FIGURE 14-21

Cellular calcium metabolism and potential targets of the elevated cytosolic calcium. **A,** Pathways of calcium mobilization. **B,** Pathophysiologic mechanisms ignited by the elevation of cytosolic calcium concentration. (**A,** *Adapted from* Goligorsky [17], with permission; **B,** *from* Edelstein and Schrier [18], with permission.)

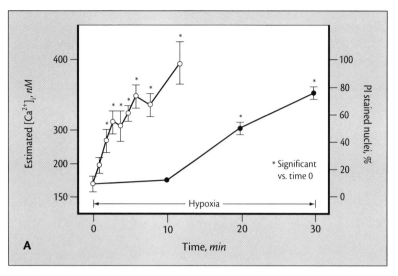

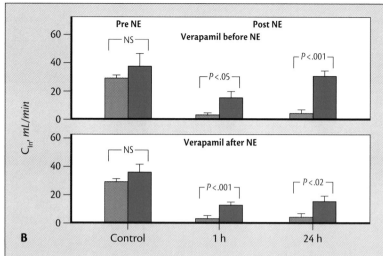

FIGURE 14-22

Pathophysiologic sequelae of the elevated cytosolic calcium (C^{2+}).
A, The increase in cytosolic calcium concentration in hypoxic rat
proximal tubules precedes the tubular damage as assessed by propidi-
um iodide (PI) staining. **B,** Administration of calcium channel inhibitor
verapamil before injection of norepinephrine (*cross-hatched bars*) significantly attenuated the drop in inulin clearance induced by norepinephrine alone (*open bars*). (**A,** *Adapted from* Kribben *et al.* [19], with
permission; **B,** *adapted from* Burke *et al.* [20], with permission.)

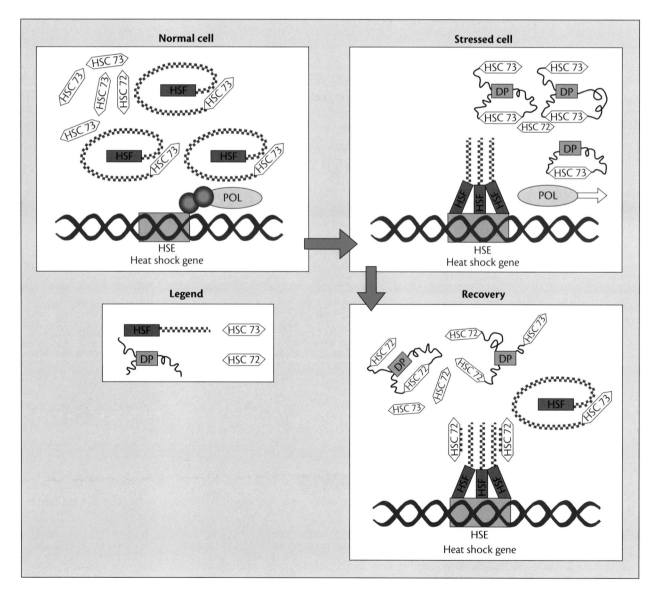

FIGURE 14-23

Dynamics of heat shock
proteins (HSP) in stressed
cells. Mechanisms of activation and feedback con-
trol of the inducible heat
shock gene. In the nor-
mal unstressed cell, heat
shock factor (HSF) is
rendered inactive by
association with the con-
stitutively expressed
HSP70. After hypoxia or
ATP depletion, partially
denatured proteins (DP)
become preferentially
associated with HSC73,
releasing HSF and allow-
ing trimerization and
binding to the heat shock
element (HSE) to initiate
the transcription of the
heat shock gene. After
translation, excess
inducible HSP (HSP72)
interacts with the trimer-
ized HSF to convert it
back to its monomeric
state and release it from
the HSE, thus turning off
the response. (*Adapted
from* Kashgarian [21];
with permission.)

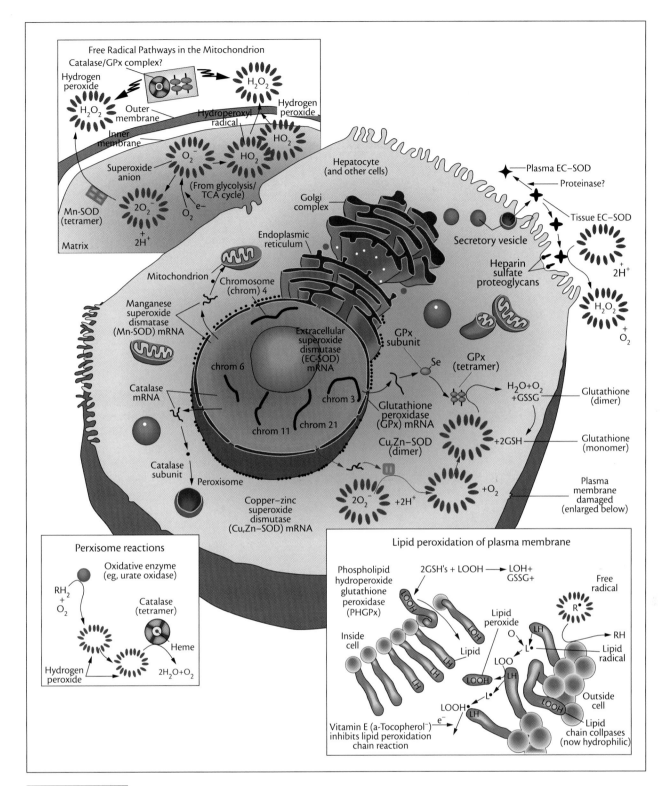

FIGURE 14-24

Cellular sources of reactive oxygen species (ROS) defense systems from free radicals. Superoxide and hydrogen peroxide are produced during normal cellular metabolism. ROS are constantly being produced by the normal cell during a number of physiologic reactions. Mitochondrial respiration is an important source of superoxide production under normal conditions and can be increased during ischemia-reflow or gentamycin-induced renal injury. A number of enzymes generate superoxide and hydrogen peroxide during their catalytic cycling. These include cycloxygenases and lipoxygenes that catalyze prostanoid and leukotriene synthesis. Some cells (such as leukocytes, endothelial cells, and vascular smooth muscle cells) have NADH/ or NADPH oxidase enzymes in the plasma membrane that are capable of generating superoxide. Xanthine oxidase, which converts hypoxathine to xanthine, has been implicated as an important source of ROS after ischemia-reperfusion injury. Cytochrome p450, which is bound to the membrane of the endoplasmic reticulum, can be increased by the presence of high concentrations of metabolites that are oxidized by this cytochrome or by injurious events that uncouple the activity of the p450. Finally, the oxidation of small molecules including free heme, thiols, hydroquinines, catecholamines, flavins, and tetrahydropterins, also contribute to intracellular superoxide production. (*Adapted from* [22]; with permission.)

EVIDENCE SUGGESTING A ROLE FOR REACTIVE OXYGEN METABOLITES IN ISCHEMIC ACUTE RENAL FAILURE

Enhanced generation of reactive oxygen metabolites and xanthine oxidase and increased conversion of xanthine dehydrogenase to oxidase occur in in vitro and in vivo models of injury.

Lipid peroxidation occurs in in vitro and in vivo models of injury, and this can be prevented by scavengers of reactive oxygen metabolites, xanthine oxidase inhibitors, or iron chelators.

Glutathione redox ratio, a parameter of "oxidant stress" decreases during ischemia and markedly increases on reperfusion.

Scavengers of reative oxygen metabolites, antioxidants, xanthine oxidase inhibitors, and iron chelators protect against injury.

A diet deficient in selenium and vitamin E increases susceptibility to injury.

Inhibition of catalase exacerbates injury, and transgenic mice with increased superoxide dismutase activity are less susceptible to injury.

FIGURE 14-25

Evidence suggesting a role for reactive oxygen metabolites in acute renal failure. The increased ROS production results from two major sources: the conversion of hypoxanthine to xanthine by xanthine dehydrogenase and the oxidation of NADH by NADH oxidase(s). During the period of ischemia, oxygen deprivation results in the massive dephosphorylation of adenine nucleotides to hypoxanthine. Normally, hypoxanthine is metabolized by xanthine dehydrogenase which uses NAD^+ rather than oxygen as the acceptor of electrons and does not generate free radicals. However, during ischemia, xanthine dehydrogenase is converted to xanthine oxidase. When oxygen becomes available during reperfusion, the metabolism of hypoxanthine by xanthine oxidase generates superoxide. Conversion of NAD^+ to its reduced form, NADH, and the accumulation of NADH occurs during ischemia. During the reperfusion period, the conversion of NADH back to NAD^+ by NADH oxidase also results in a burst of superoxide production. (*From* Ueda *et al.* [23]; with permission.)

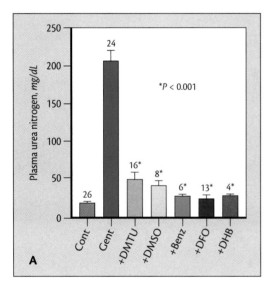

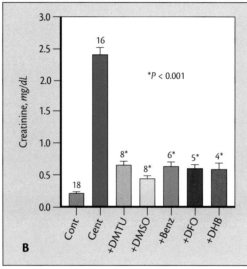

FIGURE 14-26

Effect of different scavengers of reactive oxygen metabolites and iron chelators on, **A**, blood urea nitrogen (BUN) and, **B**, creatinine in gentamicin-induced acute renal failure. The numbers shown above the error bars indicate the number of animals in each group. Benz—sodium benzoate; Cont—control group; DFO—deferoxamine; DHB—2,3 dihydroxybenzoic acid; DMSO—dimethyl sulfoxide; DMTU—dimethylthiourea; Gent—gentamicin group. (*From* Ueda *et al.* [23]; with permission.)

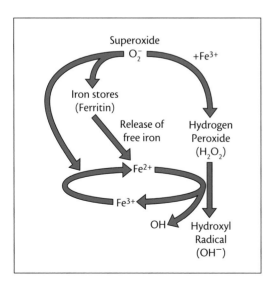

FIGURE 14-27

Production of the hydroxyl radical: the Haber-Weiss reaction. Superoxide is converted to hydrogen peroxide by superoxide dismutase. Superoxide and hydrogen peroxide per se are not highly reactive and cytotoxic. However, hydrogen peroxide can be converted to the highly reactive and injurious hydroxyl radical by an iron-catalyzed reaction that requires the presence of free reduced iron. The availability of free "catalytic iron" is a critical determinant of hydroxyl radical production. In addition to providing a source of hydroxyl radical, superoxide potentiates hydroxyl radical production in two ways: by releasing free iron from iron stores such as ferritin and by reducing ferric iron and recycling the available free iron back to the ferrous form. The heme moiety of hemoglobin, myoglobin, or cytochrome present in normal cells can be oxidized to metheme (Fe^{3+}). The further oxidation of metheme results in the production of an oxyferryl moiety ($Fe^{4+}=O$), which is a long-lived, strong oxidant which likely plays a role in the cellular injury associated with hemoglobinuria and myoglobinuria.

Activated leukocytes produce superoxide and hydrogen peroxide via the activity of a membrane-bound enzyme NADPH oxidase. This superoxide and hydrogen peroxide can be converted to hydroxyl radical via the Haber-Weiss reaction. Also, the enzyme myeloperoxidase, which is specific to leukocytes, converts hydrogen peroxide to another highly reactive and injurious oxidant, hypochlorous acid.

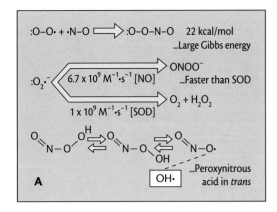

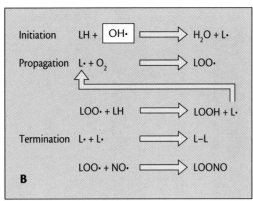

FIGURE 14-28

Cell injury: point of convergence between the reduced oxygen intermediates–generating and reduced nitrogen intermediates–generating pathways, **A**, and mechanisms of lipid peroxidation, **B**.

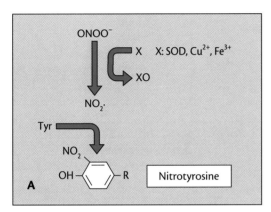

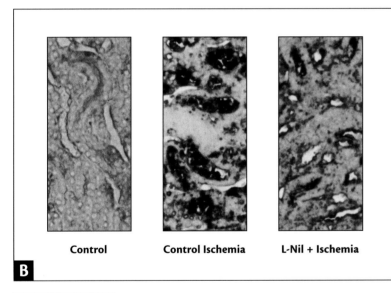

FIGURE 14-29

Detection of peroxynitrite production and lipid peroxidation in ischemic acute renal failure. **A**, Formation of nitrotyrosine as an indicator of ONOO- production. Interactions between reactive oxygen species such as the hydroxyl radical results in injury to the ribose-phosphate backbone of DNA. This results in single- and double-strand breaks. ROS can also cause modification and deletion of individual bases within the DNA molecule. Interaction between reactive oxygen and nitrogen species results in injury to the ribose-phosphate backbone of DNA, nuclear DNA fragmentation (single- and double-strand breaks) and activation of poly-(ADP)-ribose synthase. **B**, Immunohistochemical staining of kidneys with antibodies to nitrotyrosine. **C**, Western blot analysis of nitrotyrosine. **D**, Reactions describing lipid peroxidation and formation of hemiacetal products. The interaction of oxygen radicals with lipid bilayers leads to the removal of hydrogen atoms from the unsaturated fatty acids bound to phospholipid. This

process is called lipid peroxidation. In addition to impairing the structural and functional integrity of cell membranes, lipid peroxidation can lead to a self-perpetuating chain reaction in which additional ROS are generated.

(Continued on next page)

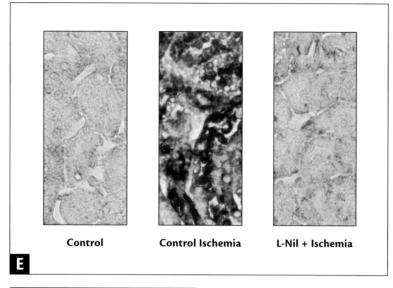

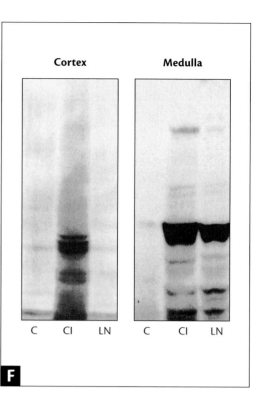

FIGURE 14-29 *(Continued)*

E, Immunohistochemical staining of kidneys with antibodies to HNE–modified proteins. F, Western blot analysis of HNE expression. C—control; CI—central ischemia; LN—ischemia with L-Nil pretreatment (*Courtesy of* E. Noiri, MD.)

Leukocytes in Acute Renal Failure

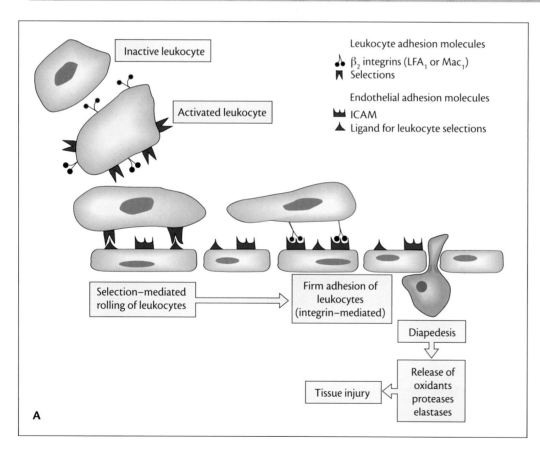

FIGURE 14-30

Role of adhesion molecules in mediating leukocyte attachment to endothelium.
A, The normal inflammatory response is mediated by the release of cytokines that induce leukocyte chemotaxis and activation. The initial interaction of leukocytes with endothelium is mediated by the selectins and their ligands both of which are present on leukocytes and endothelial cells,

(Continued on next page)

B. LEUKOCYTE ADHESION MOLECULES AND THEIR LIGANDS POTENTIALLY IMPORTANT IN ACUTE RENAL FAILURE

Major Families	Cell Distribution
Selectins	
L-selectin	Leukocytes
P-selectin	Endothelial cells
E-selectin	Endothelial cells
Carbohydrate ligands for selectins	
Sulphated polysacharides	Endothelium
Oligosaccharides	Leukocytes
Integrins	
CD11a/CD18	Leukocytes
CD11b/CD18	Leukocytes
Immunoglobulin G–like ligands for integrins	
Intracellular adhesion molecules (ICAM)	Endothelial cells

FIGURE 14-29 (*Continued*)

B. Selectin-mediated leukocyte-endothelial interaction results in the rolling of leukocytes along the endothelium and facilitates the firm adhesion and immobilization of leukocytes. Immobilization of leukocytes to endothelium is mediated by the β_2-integrin adhesion molecules on leukocytes and their ICAM ligands on endothelial cells. Immobilization of leukocytes is necessary for diapedesis of leukocytes between endothelial cells into parenchymal tissue. Leukocytes release proteases, elastases, and reactive oxygen radicals that induce tissue injury. Activated leukocytes also elaborate cytokines such as interleukin 1 and tumor necrosis factor which attract additional leukocytes to the site, causing further injury.

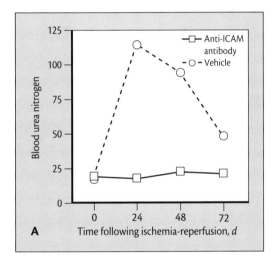
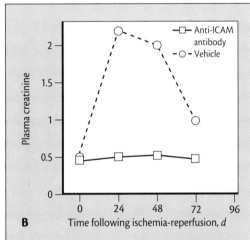

FIGURE 14-31

Neutralizing anti–ICAM antibody ameliorates the course of ischemic renal failure with blood urea nitrogen, **A**, and plasma creatinine, **B**. Rats subjected to 30 minutes of bilateral renal ischemia or a sham-operation were divided into three groups that received either anti-ICAM antibody or its vehicle. Plasma creatinine levels are shown at 24, 48, and 72 hours. ICAM antibody ameliorates the severity of renal failure at all three time points. (*Adapted from* Kelly *et al.* [24]; with permission.)

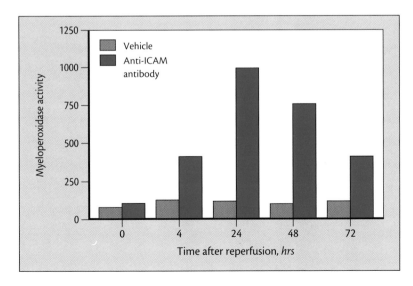

FIGURE 14-32

Neutralizing anti-ICAM-1 antibody reduces myeloperoxidase activity in rat kidneys exposed to 30 minutes of ischemia. Myeloperoxidase is an enzyme specific to leukocytes. Anti-ICAM antibody reduced myeloperoxidase activity (and by inference the number of leukocytes) in renal tissue after 30 minutes of ischemia. (*Adapted from* Kelly *et al.* [24]; with permission.)

Mechanisms of Cell Death: Necrosis and Apoptosis

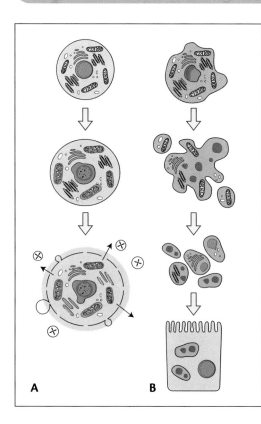

A   **B**

FIGURE 14-33

Apoptosis and necrosis: two distinct morphologic forms of cell death. **A,** Necrosis. Cells undergoing necrosis become swollen and enlarged. The mitochondria become markedly abnormal. The main morphoplogic features of mitochondrial injury include swelling and flattening of the folds of the inner mitochondrial membrane (the christae). The cell plasma membrane loses its integrity and allows the escape of cytosolic contents including lyzosomal proteases that cause injury and inflammation of the surrounding tissues. **B,** Apoptosis. In contrast to necrosis, apoptosis is associated with a progressive decrease in cell size and maintenance of a functionally and structurally intact plasma membrane. The decrease in cell size is due to both a loss of cytosolic volume and a decrease in the size of the nucleus. The most characteristic and specific morphologic feature of apoptosis is condensation of nuclear chromatin. Initially the chromatin condenses against the nuclear membrane. Then the nuclear membrane disappears, and the condensed chromatin fragments into many pieces. The plasma membrane undergoes a process of "budding," which progresses to fragmentation of the cell itself. Multiple plasma membrane–bound fragments of condensed DNA called apoptotic bodies are formed as a result of cell fragmentation. The apoptotic cells and apoptotic bodies are rapidly phagocytosed by neighboring epithelial cells as well as professional phagocytes such as macrophages. The rapid phagocytosis of apoptotic bodies with intact plasma membranes ensures that apoptosis does not cause any surrounding inflammatory reaction.

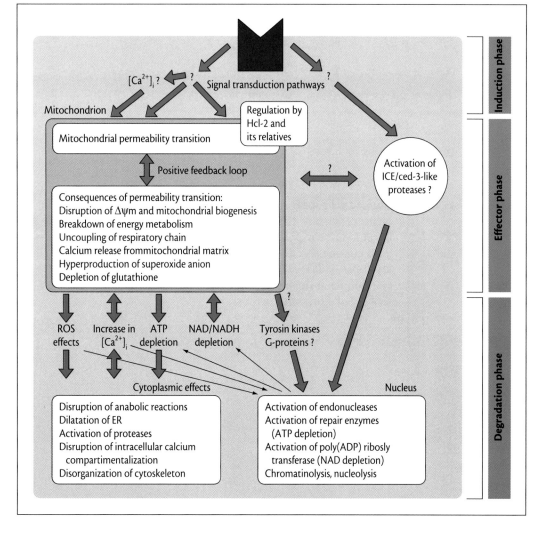

FIGURE 14-34

Hypothetical schema of cellular events triggering apoptotic cell death. (*From* Kroemer *et al.* [25]; with permission.)

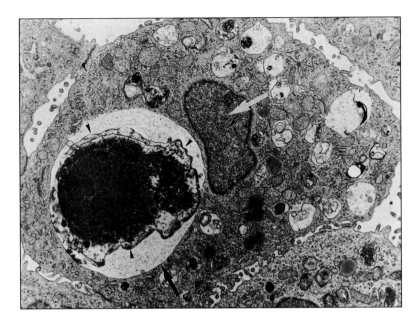

FIGURE 14-35

Phagocytosis of an apoptotic body by a renal tubular epithelial cell. Epithelial cells dying by apoptosis are not only phagocytosed by macrophages and leukocytes but by neighbouring epithelial cells as well. This electron micrograph shows a normal-looking epithelial cell containing an apoptotic body within a lyzosome. The nucleus of an epithelial cell that has ingested the apoptotic body is normal (*white arrow*). The wall of the lyzosome containing the apoptotic body (*black arrow*) is clearly visible. The apoptotic body consists of condensed chromatin surrounded by plasma membrane (*black arrowheads*).

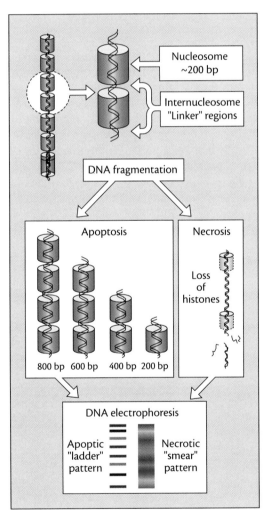

FIGURE 14-36

DNA fragmentation in apoptosis vs necrosis. DNA is made up of nucleosomal units. Each nucleosome of DNA is about 200 base pairs in size and is surrounded by histones. Between nucleosomes are small stretches of DNA that are not surrounded by histones and are called linker regions. During apoptosis, early activation of endonuclease(s) causes double-strand breaks in DNA between nucleosomes. No fragmentation occurs in nucleosomes because the DNA is "protected" by the histones. Because of the size of nucleosomes, the DNA is fragmented during apoptosis into multiples of 200 base pair pieces (*eg*, 200, 400, 600, 800). When the DNA of apoptotic cells is electrophoresed, a characteristic ladder pattern is found.

In contrast, necrosis is associated with the early release of lyzosomal proteases, which cause proteolysis of nuclear histones, leaving "naked" stretches of DNA not protected by histones. Activation of endonucleases during necrosis therefore cause DNA cleavage at multiple sites into double- and single-stranded DNA fragments of varying size. Electrophoresis of DNA from necrotic cells results in a smear pattern.

POTENTIAL CAUSES OF APOPTOSIS IN ACUTE RENAL FAILURE

Loss of survival factors
  Deficiency of renal growth factors (*eg*, IGF-1, EGF, HGF)
  Loss of cell-cell and cell-matrix interactions
Receptor-mediated activators of apoptosis
  Tumor necrosis factor
  Fas/Fas ligand
Cytotoxic events
  Ischemia; hypoxia; anoxia
  Oxidant injury
  Nitric oxide
  Cisplati

FIGURE 14-37

Potential causes of apoptosis in acute renal failure (ARF). The same cytotoxic stimuli that induce necrosis cause apoptosis. The mechanism of cell death induced by a specific injury depends in large part on the severity of the injury. Because most cells require constant external signals, called survival signals, to remain viable, the loss of these survival signals can trigger apoptosis. In ARF, a deficiency of growth factors and loss of cell-substrate adhesion are potential causes of apoptosis. The death pathways induced by engagement of tumour necrosis factor (TNF) with the TNF receptor or Fas with its receptor (Fas ligand) are well known causes of apoptosis in immune cells. TNF and Fas can also induce apoptosis in epithelial cells and may contribute to cell death in ARF.

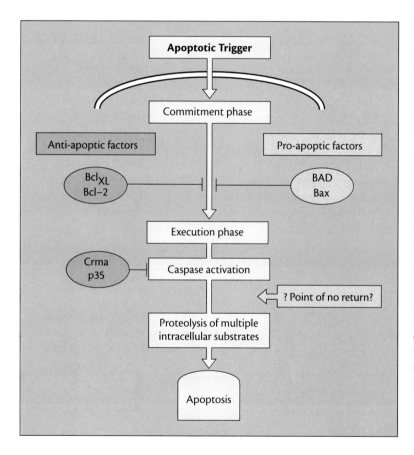

FIGURE 14-38

Apoptosis is mediated by a highly coordinated and genetically programmed pathway. The response to an apoptotic stimulus can be divided into a commitment and execution phases. During the commitment phase the balance between a number of proapoptotic and antiapoptotic mechanisms determine whether the cell survives or dies by apoptosis. The BCL-2 family of proteins consists of at least 12 isoforms, which play important roles in this commitment phase. Some of the BCL-2 family of proteins (*eg*, BCL-2 and BCL-$_{XL}$) protect cells from apoptosis whereas other members of the same family (*eg*, BAD and Bax) serve proapoptotic functions. Apoptosis is executed by a final common pathway mediated by a class of cysteine proteases-caspases. Caspases are proteolytic enzymes present in cells in an inactive form. Once cells are commited to undergo apoptosis, these caspases are activated. Some caspases activate other caspases in a hierarchical fashion resulting in a cascade of caspase activation. Eventually, caspases that target specific substrates within the cell are activated. Some substrates for caspases that have been identified include nuclear membrane components (such as lamin), cytoskeletal elements (such as actin and fodrin) and DNA repair enzymes and transcription elements. The proteolysis of this diverse array of substrates in the cell occurs in a predestined fashion and is responsible for the characteristic morphologic features of apoptosis.

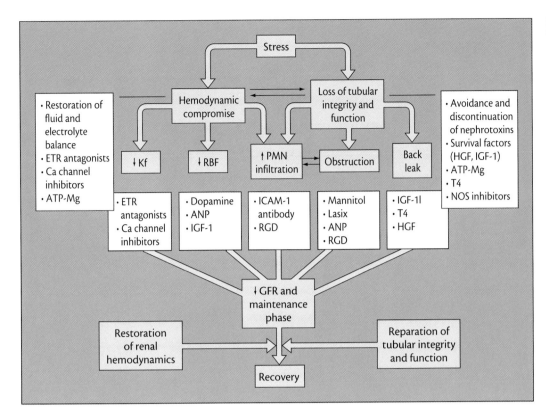

FIGURE 14-39

Therapeutic approaches, both experimental and in clinical use, to prevent and manage acute renal failure based on its pathogenetic mechanisms. ETR—ET receptor; GFR— glomerular filtration rate; HGF—hepatocyte growth factor 1; IGF-1—insulin-like growth factor 1; K_f—glomerular ultrafiltration coefficient; NOS—nitric oxide synthase; PMN— polymorphonuclear leukocytes; RBF—renal blood flow; T4—thyroxine.

References

1. Goligorsky M, Iijima K, Krivenko Y, *et al.*: Role of mesangial cells in macula densa-to-afferent arteriole information transfer. *Clin Exp Pharm Physiol* 1997, 24:527–531.

2. Osswald H, Hermes H, Nabakowski G: Role of adenosine in signal transmission of TGF. *Kidney Int* 1982, 22(Suppl. 12):S136–S142.

3. Miller W, Thomas R, Berne R, Rubio R: Adenosine production in the ischemic kidney. *Circ Res* 1978, 43(3):390–397.

4. Kon V, *et al.*: Glomerular actions of endothelin in vivo. *J Clin Invest* 1989, 83:1762–1767.

5. Gellai M, Jugus M, Fletcher T, *et al.*: Reversal of postischemic acute renal failure with a selective endothelin A receptor antagonist in the rat. *J Clin Invest* 1994, 93:900–906.

6. Fogo, *et al.*: Endothelin receptor antagonism is protective in vivo in acute cyclosporine toxicity. *Kidney Int* 1992, 42:770–774.

7. Conger J: NO in acute renal failure. In: *Nitric Oxide and the Kidney.* Edited by Goligorsky M, Gross S. New York:Chapman and Hall, 1997.

8. Gross S: Nitric oxide synthases and their cofactors. In: *Nitric Oxide and the Kidney.* Edited by Goligorsky M, Gross S. New York:Chapman and Hall, 1997.

9. Reyes A, Karl I, Klahr S: Role of arginine in health and in renal disease. *Am J Physiol* 1994, 267:F331–F346.

10. Kim Y-M, Tseng E, Billiar TR: Role of NO and nitrogen intermediates in regulation of cell functions. In: *Nitric Oxide and the Kidney.* Edited by Goligorsky M, Gross S. New York:Chapman and Hall, 1997.

11. Lieberthal W:Renal ischemia and reperfusion impair endothelium-dependent vascular relaxation. *Am J Physiol* 1989, 256:F894–F900.

12. Yu L, Gengaro P, Niederberger M, *et al.*: Nitric oxide: a mediator in rat tubular hypoxia/reoxygenation injury. *Proc Natl Acad Sci USA* 1994, 91:1691–1695.

13. Noiri E, Peresleni T, Miller F, Goligorsky MS: In vivo targeting of iNOS with oligodeoxynucleotides protects rat kidney against ischemia. *J Clin Invest* 1996, 97:2377–2383.

14. Ling H, Gengaro P, Edelstein C, *et al.*: Injurious isoform of NOS in mouse proximal tubular injury. *Kidney Int*, 1998, 53:1642

15. Agmon Y, *et al.*: Nitric oxide and prostanoids protect the renal outer medulla from radiocontrast toxicity in the rat. *J Clin Invest* 1994, 94:1069–1075.

16. Agmon Y, Brezis M: NO and the medullary circulation. In: *Nitric Oxide and the Kidney*. Edited by Goligorsky M, Gross S. New York:Chapman and Hall, 1997.

17. Goligorsky MS: Cell biology of signal transduction. In: *Hormones, autacoids, and the kidney*. Edited by Goldfarb S, Ziyadeh F. New York:Churchill Livingstone, 1991.

18. Edelstein C, Schrier RW: The role of calcium in cell injury. In: *Acute Renal Failure: New Concepts and Therapeutic Strategies*. Edited by Goligorsky MS, Stein JH. New York:Churchill Livingstone, 1995.

19. Kribben A, Wetzels J, Wieder E, *et al.*:Evidence for a role of cytosolic free calcium in hypoxia-induced proximal tubule injury. *J Clin Invest* 1994, 93:1922.

20. Burke T, Arnold P, Gordon J, Schrier RW: Protective effect of intrarenal calcium channel blockers before or after renal ischemia. *J Clin Invest* 1984, 74:1830.

21. Kashgarian M: Stress proteins induced by injury to epithelial cells. In: *Acute Renal Failure: New Concepts and therapeutic strategies*. Edited by Goligorsky MS, Stein JH. New York:Churchill Livingstone, 1995.

22. *J NIH Research*

23. Ueda N, Walker P, Shah SV: Oxidant stress in acute renal failure. In: *Acute Renal Failure: New Concepts and Therapeutic Strategies*. Edited by Goligorsky MS, Stein JH. New York:Churchill Livingstone, 1995.

24. Kelly KJ, *et al.*: Antibody to anyi-cellular adhesion molecule-1 protects the kidney against ischemic injury. *Proc Natl Acad Sci USA* 1994, 91:812–816.

25. Kroemer G, Petit P, Zamzami N, *et al.*: The biochemistry of programmed cell death. *FASEB J* 1995, 9:1277–1287.

Pathophysiology of Nephrotoxic Acute Renal Failure

Rick G. Schnellmann

Katrina J. Kelly

Humans are exposed intentionally and unintentionally to a variety of diverse chemicals that harm the kidney. As the list of drugs, natural products, industrial chemicals and environmental pollutants that cause nephrotoxicity has increased, it has become clear that chemicals with very diverse chemical structures produce nephrotoxicity. For example, the heavy metal $HgCl_2$, the mycotoxin fumonisin B_1, the immunosuppresant cyclosporin A, and the aminoglycoside antibiotics all produce acute renal failure but are not structurally related. Thus, it is not surprising that the cellular targets within the kidney and the mechanisms of cellular injury vary with different toxicants. Nevertheless, there are similarities between chemical-induced acute tubular injury and ischemia/reperfusion injury.

The tubular cells of the kidney are particularly vulnerable to toxicant-mediated injury due to their disproportionate exposure to circulating chemicals and transport processes that result in high intracellular concentrations. It is generally thought that the parent chemical or a metabolite initiates toxicity through its covalent or noncovalent binding to cellular macromolecules or through their ability to produce reactive oxygen species. In either case the activity of the macromolecule(s) is altered resulting in cell injury. For example, proteins and lipids in the plasma membrane, nucleus, lysosome, mitochondrion and cytosol are all targets of toxicants. If the toxicant causes oxidative stress both lipid peroxidation and protein oxidation have been shown to contribute to cell injury.

In many cases mitochondria are a critical target and the lack of adenosine triphosphate (ATP) leads to cell injury due to the dependence of renal function on aerobic metabolism. The loss of ATP leads to disruption of cellular ion homeostasis with decreased cellular K^+ content, increased Na^+ content and membrane depolarization. Increased cytosolic free Ca^{2+} concentrations can occur in the early or late phase of cell injury and plays a critical role leading to cell death. The increase in Ca^{2+} can activate calcium activated neutral proteases (calpains) that appear to contribute to the cell injury that occurs by a variety of toxicants. During the late phase of cell injury, there is an increase in Cl^- influx, followed by the influx of increasing larger molecules that leads to cell lysis. Two additional enzymes appear to play an important role in cell injury, particularly oxidative injury. Phospholipase A_2 consists of a family of enzymes in which the activity of the cytosolic form increases during oxidative injury and contributes to cell death. Caspases are a family of cysteine proteases that are activated following oxidative injury and contribute to cell death.

Following exposure to a chemical insult those cells sufficiently injured die by one of two mechanisms, apoptosis or oncosis.

Clinically, a vast number of nephrotoxicants can produce a variety of clinical syndromes-acute renal failure, chronic renal failure, nephrotic syndrome, hypertension and renal tubular defects. The evolving understanding of the pathophysiology of toxicant-mediated renal injury has implications for potential therapies and preventive measures. This chapter outlines some of the mechanisms thought to be important in toxicant-mediated renal cell injury and death that leads to the loss of tubular epithelial cells, tubular obstruction, "backleak" of the glomerular filtrate and a decreased glomerular filtration rate. The recovery from the structural and functional damage following chemical exposures is dependent on the repair of sublethally-injured and regeneration of noninjured cells.

Clinical Significance of Toxicant-Mediated Acute Renal Failure

CLINICAL SIGNIFICANCE OF TOXICANT–MEDIATED RENAL FAILURE

Nephrotoxins may account for approximately 50% of all cases of acute and chronic renal failure.

Nephrotoxic renal injury often occurs in conjunction with ischemic acute renal failure.

Acute renal failure may occur in 2% to 5% of hospitalized patients and 10% to 15% of patients in intensive care units.

The mortality of acute renal failure is approximatley 50% which has not changed significantly in the last 40 years.

Radiocontrast media and aminoglycosides are the most common agents associated with nephrotoxic injury in hospitalized patients.

Aminoglycoside nephrotoxicity occurs in 5% to 15% of patients treated with these drugs.

FIGURE 15-1

Clinical significance of toxicant-mediated renal failure.

REASONS FOR THE KIDNEY'S SUSCEPTIBILITY TO TOXICANT INJURY

Receives 25% of the cardiac output

Sensitive to vasoactive compounds

Concentrates toxicants through reabsorptive and secretive processes

Many transporters result in high intracellular concentrations

Large luminal membrane surface area

Large biotransformation capacity

Baseline medullary hypoxia

FIGURE 15-2

Reasons for the kidney's susceptibility to toxicant injury.

FIGURE 15-3

Factors that predispose the kidney to toxicant injury.

FACTORS THAT PREDISPOSE THE KIDNEY TO TOXICANT INJURY

Preexisting renal dysfunction

Dehydration

Diabetes mellitus

Exposure to multiple nephrotoxins

EXOGENOUS AND ENDOGENOUS CHEMICALS THAT CAUSE ACUTE RENAL FAILURE

Antibiotics
  Aminoglycosides (gentamicin, tobramycin,
    amikacin, netilmicin)
  Amphotericin B
  Cephalosporins
  Ciprofloxacin
  Demeclocycline
  Penicillins
  Pentamidine
  Polymixins
  Rifampin
  Sulfonamides
  Tetracycline
  Vancomycin
Chemotherapeutic agents
  Adriamycin
  Cisplatin
  Methotraxate
  Mitomycin C
  Nitrosoureas
    (eg, streptozotocin, lomustine)
Radiocontrast media
  Ionic (eg, diatrizoate, iothalamate)
  Nonionic (eg, metrizamide)

Immunosuppressive agents
  Cyclosporin A
  Tacrolimus (FK 506)
Antiviral agents
  Acyclovir
  Cidovir
  Foscarnet
  Valacyclovir
Heavy metals
  Cadmium
  Gold
  Mercury
  Lead
  Arsenic
  Bismuth
  Uranium
Organic solvents
  Ethylene glycol
  Carbon tetrachloride
  Unleaded gasoline

Vasoactive agents
  Nonsteroidal anti-inflammatory
    drugs (NSAIDs)
  Ibuprofen
  Naproxen
  Indomethacin
  Meclofenemate
  Aspirin
  Piroxicam
  Angiotensin-converting
    enzyme inhibitors
  Captopril
  Enalopril
  Lisinopril
  Angiotensin receptor antagonists
  Losartan

Other drugs
  Acetaminophen
  Halothane
  Methoxyflurane
  Cimetidine
  Hydralazine
  Lithium
  Lovastatin
  Mannitol
  Penicillamine
  Procainamide
  Thiazides
  Lindane
Endogenous compounds
  Myoglobin
  Hemoglobin
  Calcium
  Uric acid
  Oxalate
  Cystine

FIGURE 15-4

Exogenous and endogenous chemicals that cause acute renal failure.

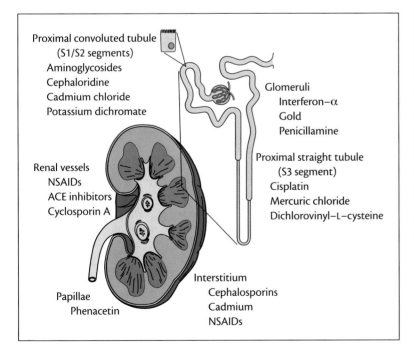

FIGURE 15-5

Nephrotoxicants may act at different sites in the kidney, resulting in altered renal function. The sites of injury by selected nephrotoxicants are shown. Nonsteroidal anti-inflammatory drugs (NSAIDs), angiotensin-converting enzyme (ACE) inhibitors, cyclosporin A, and radiographic contrast media cause vasoconstriction. Gold, interferon-alpha, and penicillamine can alter glomerular function and result in proteinuria and decreased renal function. Many nephrotoxicants damage tubular epithelial cells directly. Aminoglycosides, cephaloridine, cadmium chloride, and potassium dichromate affect the S1 and S2 segments of the proximal tubule, whereas cisplatin, mercuric chloride, and dichlorovinyl-L-cysteine affect the S3 segment of the proximal tubule. Cephalosporins, cadmium chloride, and NSAIDs cause interstitial nephritis whereas phenacetin causes renal papillary necrosis.

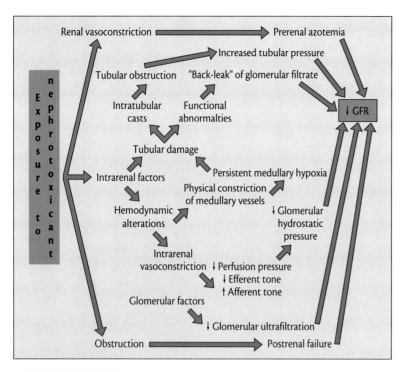

FIGURE 15-6

Mechanisms that contribute to decreased glomerular filtration rate (GFR) in acute renal failure. After exposure to a nephrotoxicant, one or more mechanisms may contribute to a reduction in the GFR. These include renal vasoconstriction resulting in prerenal azotemia (*eg*, cyclosporin A) and obstruction due to precipitation of a drug or endogenous substances within the kidney or collecting ducts (*eg*, methotrexate). Intrarenal factors include direct tubular obstruction and dysfunction resulting in tubular backleak and increased tubular pressure. Alterations in the levels of a variety of vasoactive mediators (*eg*, prostaglandins following treatment with nonsteroidal anti-inflammatory drugs) may result in decreased renal perfusion pressure or efferent arteriolar tone and increased afferent arteriolar tone, resulting in decreased in glomerular hydrostatic pressure. Some nephrotoxicants may decrease glomerular function, leading to proteinuria and decreased renal function.

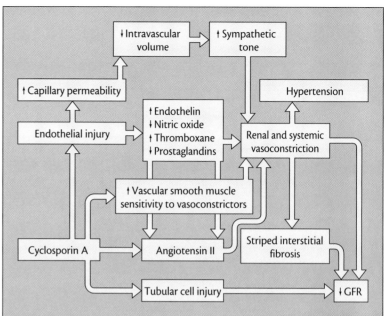

FIGURE 15-7

Renal injury from exposure to cyclosporin A. Cyclosporin A is one example of a toxicant that acts at several sites within the kidney. It can injure both endothelial and tubular cells. Endothelial injury results in increased vascular permeability and hypovolemia, which activates the sympathetic nervous system. Injury to the endothelium also results in increases in endothelin and thromboxane A_2 and decreases in nitric oxide and vasodilatory prostaglandins. Finally, cyclosporin A may increase the sensitivity of the vasculature to vasoconstrictors, activate the renin-angiotensin system, and increase angiotensin II levels. All of these changes lead to vasoconstriction and hypertension. Vasoconstriction in the kidney contributes to the decrease in glomerular filtration rate (GFR), and the histologic changes in the kidney are the result of local ischemia and hypertension.

Renal Cellular Responses to Toxicant Exposures

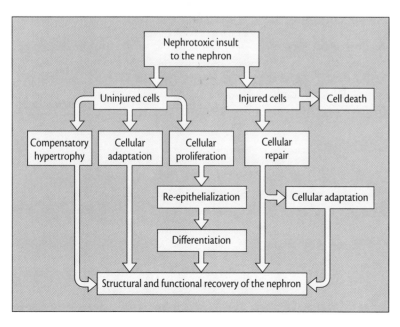

FIGURE 15-8

The nephron's response to a nephrotoxic insult. After a population of cells are exposed to a nephrotoxicant, the cells respond and ultimately the nephron recovers function or, if cell death and loss is extensive, nephron function ceases. Terminally injured cells undergo cell death through oncosis or apoptosis. Cells injured sublethally undergo repair and adaptation (*eg*, stress response) in response to the nephrotoxicant. Cells not injured and adjacent to the injured area may undergo dedifferentiation, proliferation, migration or spreading, and differentiation. Cells that were not injured may also undergo compensatory hypertrophy in response to the cell loss and injury. Finally the uninjured cells may also undergo adaptation in response to nephrotoxicant exposure.

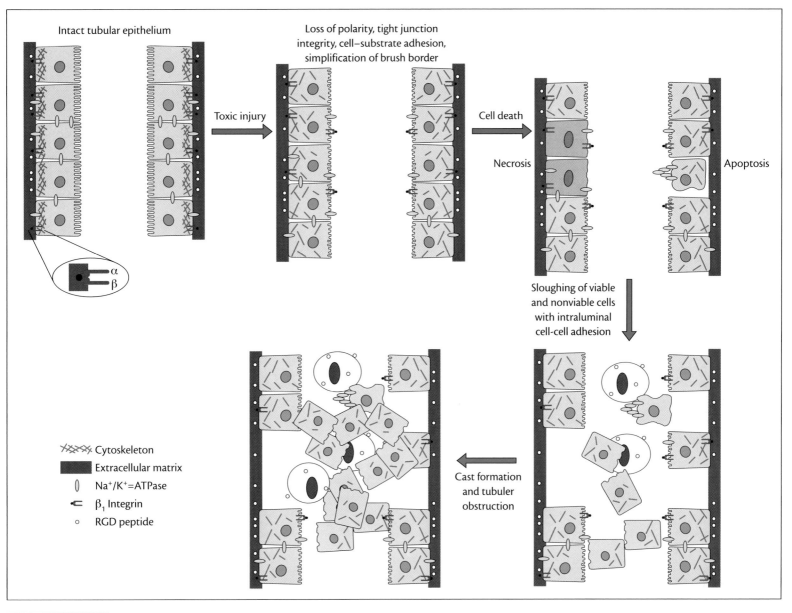

FIGURE 15-9

After injury, alterations can occur in the cytoskeleton and in the normal distribution of membrane proteins such as Na+, K+-ATPase and β_1 integrins in sublethally injured renal tubular cells. These changes result in loss of cell polarity, tight junction integrity, and cell-substrate adhesion. Lethally injured cells undergo oncosis or apoptosis, and both dead and viable cells may be sloughed into the tubular lumen. Adhesion of sloughed cells to other sloughed cells and to cells remaining adherent to the basement membrane may result in cast formation, tubular obstruction, and further compromise the glomerular filtration rate. (*Adapted from* Fish and Molitoris [1], and Gailit *et al.* [2]; with permission.)

FIGURE 15-10

Potential sites where nephrotoxicants can interfere with the structural and functional recovery of nephrons.

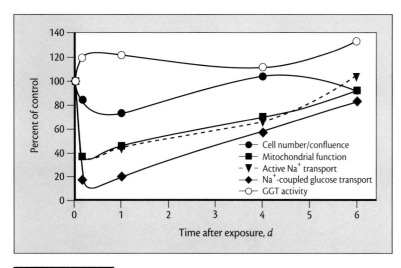

FIGURE 15-11

Inhibition and repair of renal proximal tubule cellular functions after exposure to the model oxidant *t*-butylhydroperoxide. Approximately 25% cell loss and marked inhibition of mitochondrial function active (Na+) transport and Na+-coupled glucose transport occurred 24 hours after oxidant exposure. The activity of the brush border membrane enzyme γ-glutamyl transferase (GGT) was not affected by oxidant exposure. Cell proliferation and migration or spreading was complete by day 4, whereas active Na+ transport and Na+-coupled glucose transport did not return to control levels until day 6. These data suggest that selective physiologic functions are diminished after oxidant injury and that a hierarchy exists in the repair process: migration or spreading followed by cell proliferation forms a monolayer and antedates the repair of physiologic functions. (*Data from* Nowak *et al.* [3].)

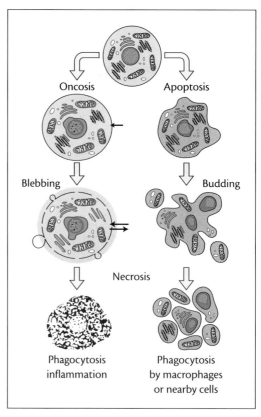

FIGURE 15-12

Apoptosis and oncosis are the two generally recognized forms of cell death. Apoptosis, also known as programmed cell death and cell suicide, is characterized morphologically by cell shrinkage, cell budding forming apoptotic bodies, and phagocytosis by macrophages and nearby cells. In contrast, oncosis, also known as necrosis, necrotic cell death, and cell murder, is characterized morphologically by cell and organelle swelling, plasma membrane blebbing, cell lysis, and inflammation. It has been suggested that cell death characterized by cell swelling and lysis not be called necrosis or necrotic cell death because these terms describe events that occur well after the cell has died and include cell and tissue breakdown and cell debris. (*From* Majno and Joris [4]; with permission.)

Mechanisms of Toxicant-Mediated Cellular Injury

Transport and biotransformation

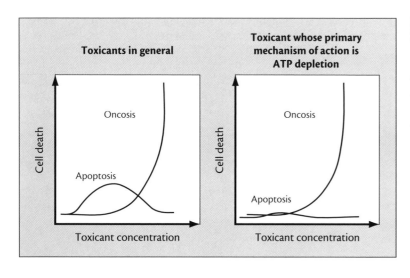

FIGURE 15-13

The general relationship between oncosis and apoptosis after nephrotoxicant exposure. For many toxicants, low concentrations cause primarily apoptosis and oncosis occurs principally at higher concentrations. When the primary mechanism of action of the nephrotoxicant is ATP depletion, oncosis may be the predominant cause of cell death with limited apoptosis occurring.

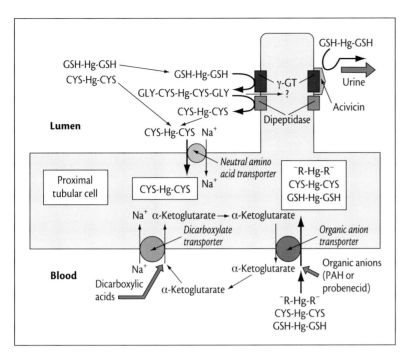

FIGURE 15-14

The importance of cellular transport in mediating toxicity. Proximal tubular uptake of inorganic mercury is thought to be the result of the transport of mercuric conjugates (*eg*, diglutathione mercury conjugate [GSH-Hg-GSH], dicysteine mercuric conjugate [CYS-Hg-CYS]). At the luminal membrane, GSH-Hg-GSH appears to be metabolized by (-glutamyl transferase ((-GT) and a dipeptidase to form CYS-Hg-CYS. The CYS-Hg-CYS may be taken up by an amino acid transporter. At the basolateral membrane, mercuric conjugates appear to be transported by the organic anion transporter. (-Ketoglutarate and the dicarboxylate transporter seem to play important roles in basolateral membrane uptake of mercuric conjugates. Uptake of mercuric-protein conjugates by endocytosis may play a minor role in the uptake of inorganic mercury transport. PAH—*para*-aminohippurate. (*Courtesy of* Dr. R. K. Zalups.)

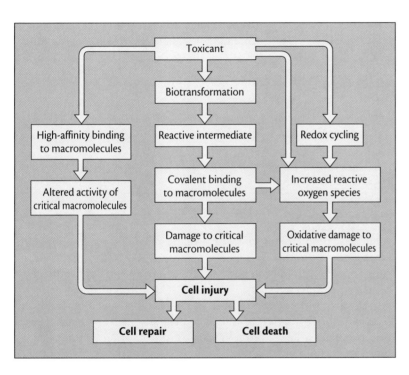

FIGURE 15-15

Covalent and noncovalent binding versus oxidative stress mechanisms of cell injury. Nephrotoxicants are generally thought to produce cell injury and death through one of two mechanisms, either alone or in combination. In some cases the toxicant may have a high affinity for a specific macromolecule or class of macromolecules that results in altered activity (increase or decrease) of these molecules, resulting in cell injury. Alternatively, the parent nephrotoxicant may not be toxic until it is biotransformed into a reactive intermediate that binds covalently to macromolecules and in turn alters their activity, resulting in cell injury. Finally, the toxicant may increase reactive oxygen species in the cells directly, after being biotransformed into a reactive intermediate or through redox cycling. The resulting increase in reactive oxygen species results in oxidative damage and cell injury.

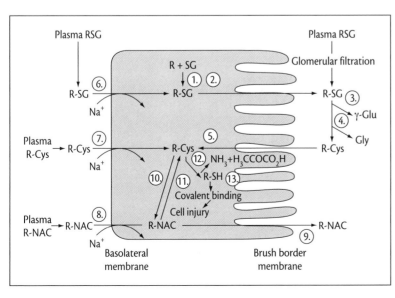

FIGURE 15-16

This figure illustrates the renal proximal tubular uptake, biotransformation, and toxicity of glutathione and cysteine conjugates and mercapturic acids of haloalkanes and haloalkenes (R). 1) Formation of a glutathione conjugate within the renal cell (R-SG). 2) Secretion of the R-SG into the lumen. 3) Removal of the γ-glutamyl residue (γ-Glu) by γ-glutamyl transferase. 4) Removal of the glycinyl residue (Gly) by a dipeptidase. 5) Luminal uptake of the cysteine conjugate (R-Cys). Basolateral membrane uptake of R-SG (6), R-Cys (7), and a mercapturic acid (N-acetyl cysteine conjugate; R-NAC)(8). 9) Secretion of R-NAC into the lumen. 10) Acetylation of R-Cys to form R-NAC. 11) Deacetylation of R-NAC to form R-Cys. 12) Biotransformation of the penultimate nephrotoxic species (R-Cys) by cysteine conjugate β-lyase to a reactive intermediate (R-SH), ammonia, and pyruvate. 13) Binding of the reactive thiol to cellular macromolecules (*eg*, lipids, proteins) and initiation of cell injury. (*Adapted from* Monks and Lau [5]; with permission.)

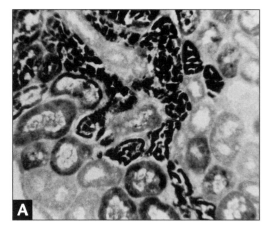
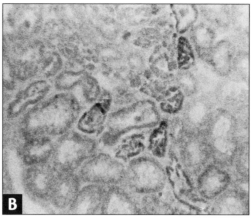

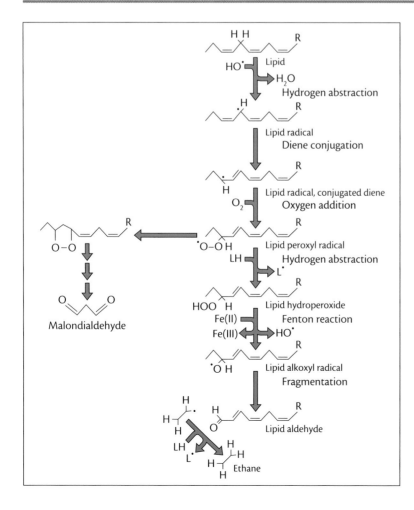

FIGURE 15-17

Covalent binding of a nephrotoxicant metabolite in vivo to rat kidney tissue, localization of binding to the mitochondria, and identification of three proteins that bind to the nephrotoxicant. **A,** Binding of tetrafluoroethyl-L-cysteine (TFEC) metabolites in vivo to rat kidney tissue detected immunohistochemically. Staining was localized to the S3 segments of the proximal tubule, the segment that undergoes necrosis. **B,** Immunoreactivity in untreated rat kidneys. **C,** Isolation and fractionation of renal cortical mitochondria from untreated and TFEC treated rats and immunoblot analysis revealed numerous proteins that bind to the nephrotoxicant (inner-inner membrane, matrix-soluble matrix, outer-outer membrane, inter-intermembrane space). The identity of three of the proteins that bound to the nephrotoxicant: P84, mortalin (HSP70-like); P66, HSP 60; and P42, aspartate aminotransferase. M_r—relative molecular weight. (*From* Hayden *et al.* [6], and Bruschi *et al.* [7]; with permission.)

Lipid peroxidation and mitochondrial dysfunction

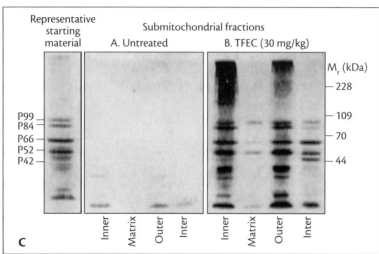

FIGURE 15-18

A simplified scheme of lipid peroxidation. The first step, hydrogen abstraction from the lipid by a radical (*eg,* hydroxyl), results in the formation of a lipid radical. Rearrangement of the lipid radical results in conjugated diene formation. The addition of oxygen results in a lipid peroxyl radical. Additional hydrogen abstraction results in the formation of a lipid hydroperoxide. The Fenton reaction produces a lipid alkoxyl radical and lipid fragmentation, resulting in lipid aldehydes and ethane. Alternatively, the lipid peroxyl radical can undergo a series of reactions that result in the formation of malondialdehyde.

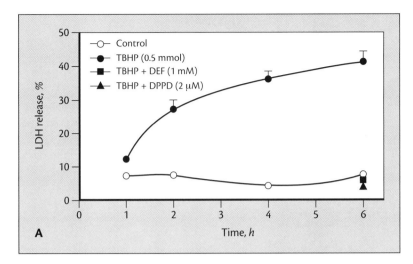

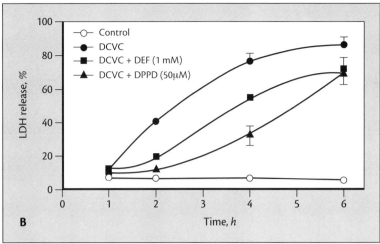

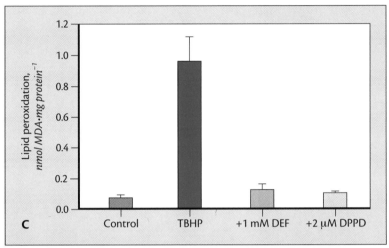

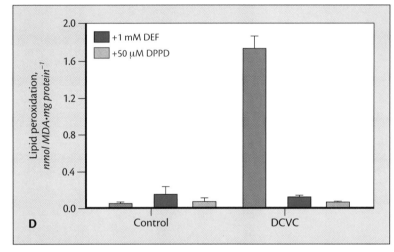

FIGURE 15-19

A–D, Similarities and differences between oxidant-induced and halocarbon-cysteine conjugate–induced renal proximal tubular lipid peroxidation and cell death. The model oxidant *t*-butylhydroperoxide (TBHP) and the halocarbon-cysteine conjugate dichlorovinyl-L-cysteine (DCVC) caused extensive lipid peroxidation after 1 hour of exposure and cell death (lactate dehydrogenase (LDH) release) over 6-hours' exposure. The iron chelator deferoxamine (DEF) and the antioxidant N,N'-diphenyl-1, 4-phenylenediamine (DPPD) completely blocked both the lipid peroxidation and cell death caused by TBHP. In contrast, while DEF and DPPD completely blocked the lipid peroxidation caused by DCVC, cell death was only delayed. These results suggest that the iron-mediated oxidative stress caused by TBHP is responsible for the observed toxicity, whereas the iron-mediated oxidative stress caused by DCVC accelerates cell death. One reason that cells die in the absence of iron-mediated oxidative stress is that DCVC causes marked mitochondrial dysfunction. (*Data from* Groves *et al.* [8], and Schellmann [9].)

ALTERATION OF RENAL TUBULAR CELL ENERGETICS AFTER EXPOSURE TO TOXICANTS

Decreased oxygen delivery secondary to vasoconstriction

Inhibition of mitochondrial respiration

Increased tubular cell oxygen consumption

FIGURE 15-20

Mechanisms by which nephrotoxicants can alter renal tubular cell energetics.

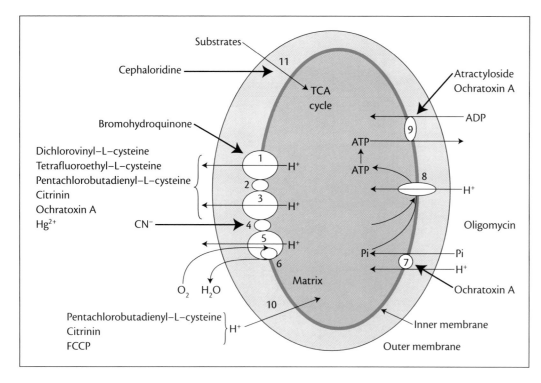

FIGURE 15-21

Some of the mitochondrial targets of nephrotoxicants: 1) nicotinamide adenine dinucleotide (NADH) dehydrogenase; 2) succinate dehydrogenase; 3) coenzyme Q–cytochrome C reductase; 4) cytochrome C; 5) cytochrome C oxidase; 6) cytochrome Aa_3; 7) H^+-Pi contransporter; 8) F_0F_1-ATPase; 9) adenine triphosphate/diphosphate (ATP/ADP) translocase; 10) protonophore (uncoupler); 11) substrate transporters.

Disruption of ion homeostasis

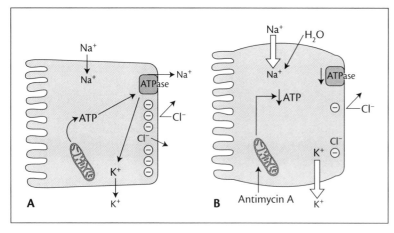

FIGURE 15-22

Early ion movements after mitochondrial dysfunction. **A,** A control renal proximal tubular cell. Within minutes of mitochondrial inhibition (*eg,* by antimycin A), ATP levels drop, resulting in inhibition of the Na^+, K^+-ATPase. **B,** Consequently, Na^+ influx, K^+ efflux, membrane depolarization, and a limited degree of cell swelling occur.

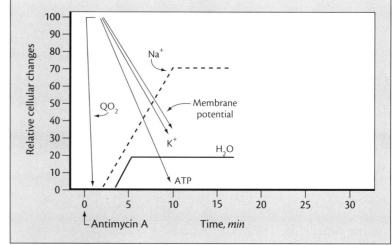

FIGURE 15-23

A graphic of the phenomena diagrammed in Figure 15-22.

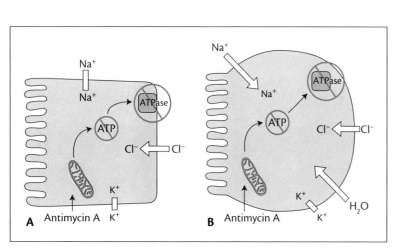

FIGURE 15-24

The late ion movements after mitochondrial dysfunction that leads to cell death/lysis. **A,** Cl^- influx occurs as a distinct step subsequent to Na^+ influx and K^+ efflux. **B,** Following Cl^- influx, additional Na^+ and water influx occur resulting in terminal cell swelling. Ultimately cell lysis occurs.

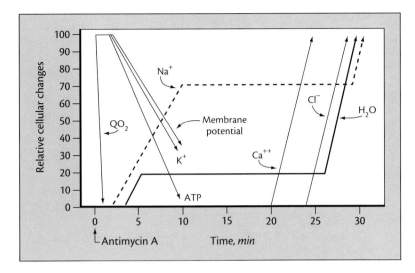

FIGURE 15-25

A graph of the phenomena depicted in Figures 15-22 through 15-24, illustrating the complete temporal sequence of events following mitochondrial dysfunction. QO_2—oxygen consumption.

Disregulation of regulatory enzymes

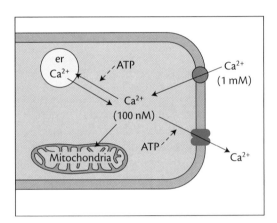

FIGURE 15-26

A simplified schematic drawing of the regulation of cytosolic free Ca^{2+}.

BIOCHEMICAL CHARACTERISTICS OF CALPAIN

Endopeptidase

Heterodimer: 80-kD catalytic subunit, 30-kD regulatory subunit

—Calpain and μ-calpain are ubiquitously distributed cytosolic isozymes

—Calpain and μ-calpain have identical regulatory subunits but distinctive catalytic subunits

—Calpain requires a higher concentration of Ca^{2+} for activation than μ-calpain

Phospholipids reduce the Ca^{2+} requirement

Substrates: cytoskeletal and membrane proteins and enzymes

FIGURE 15-27

Biochemical characteristics of calpain.

FIGURE 15-28

Calpain translocation. Proposed pathways of calpain activation and translocation. Both calpain subunits may undergo calcium (Ca^{2+})-mediated autolysis within the cytosol and hydrolyze cytosolic substrates. Calpains may also undergo Ca^{2+}-mediated translocation to the membrane, Ca^{2+}-mediated, phospholipid-facilitated autolysis and hydrolyze membrane-associated substrates. The autolyzed calpains may be released from the membrane and hydrolyze cytosolic substrates. (*From* Suzuki and Ohno [10], and Suzuki *et al*. [11]; with permission.)

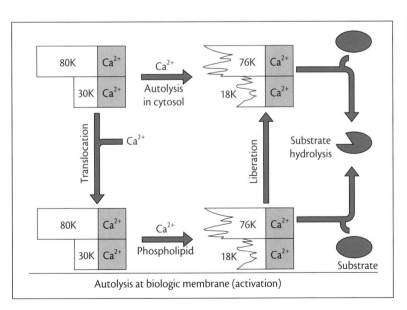

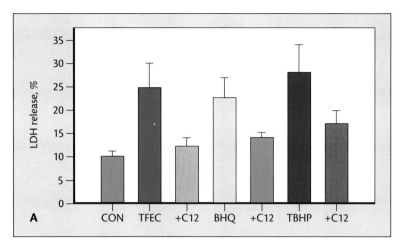
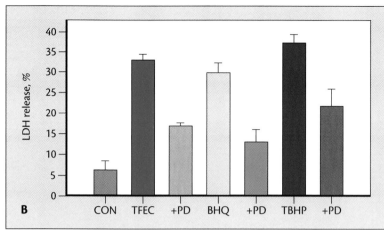

FIGURE 15-29

A, B, Dissimilar types of calpain inhibitors block renal proximal tubular toxicity of many agents. Renal proximal tubular suspensions were pretreated with the calpain inhibitor 2 (CI2) or PD150606 (PD). CI2 is an irreversible inhibitor of calpains that binds to the active site of the enzyme. PD150606 is a reversible inhibitor of calpains that binds to the calcium (Ca^{2+})-binding domain on the enzyme. The toxicants used were the haloalkane cysteine conjugate tetrafluoroethyl-L-cysteine (TFEC), the alkylating quinone bromohydroquinone (BHQ), and the model oxidant *t*-butylhydroperoxide (TBHP). The release of lactate dehydrogenase (LDH) was used as a marker of cell death. CON—control. (*From* Waters *et al.* [12]; with permission.)

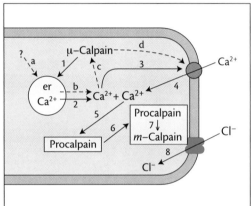

FIGURE 15-30

One potential pathway in which calcium (Ca^{2+}) and calpains play a role in renal proximal tubule cell death. These events are subsequent to mitochondrial inhibition and ATP depletion. 1) μ-Calpain releases endoplasmic reticulum (er) Ca^{2+} stores. 2) Release of er Ca^{2+} stores increases cytosolic free Ca^{2+} concentrations. 3) The increase in cytosolic free Ca^{2+} concentration mediates extracellular Ca^{2+} entry. (This may also occur as a direct result of er Ca^{2+} depletion.) 4) The influx of extracellular Ca^{2+} further increases cytosolic free Ca^{2+} concentrations. 5) This initiates the translocation of nonactivated *m*-calpain to the plasma membrane (6). 7) At the plasma membrane nonactivated *m*-calpain is autolyzed and hydrolyzes a membrane-associated substrate. 8) Either directly or indirectly, hydrolysis of the membrane-associated substrate results in influx of extracellular chloride ions (Cl⁻). The influx of extracellular Cl⁻ triggers terminal cell swelling. *Steps a–d* represent an alternate pathway that results in extracellular Ca^{2+} entry. (*Data from* Waters *et al.* [12,13,14].)

FIGURE 15-31

Biochemical characteristics of several identified phospholipase A_2s.

PROPERTIES OF PHOSPHOLIPASE A₂ GROUP

Characteristics	Secretory	Cytosolic	Ca^{2+}-Independent	
Localization	Secreted	Cytosolic	Cytosolic	Membrane
Molecular mass	~14 kDa	~85 kDa	~40 kDa	unknown
Arachidonate preference	–	+	+	+
Ca^{2+} required	mM	(M	None	None
Ca^{2+} role	Catalysis	Memb. Assoc.	None	None

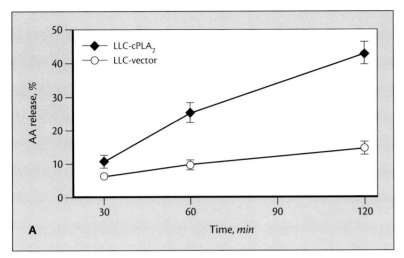

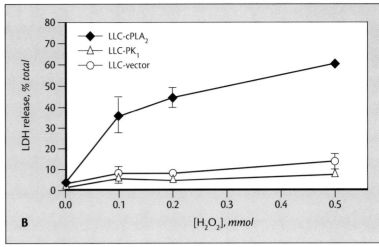

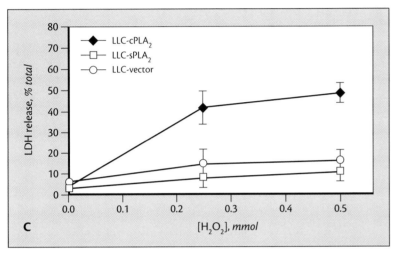

FIGURE 15-32

The importance of the cytosolic phospholipase A_2 in oxidant injury. **A,** Time-dependent release of arachidonic acid (AA) from LLC-PK$_1$ cells exposed to hydrogen peroxide (0.5 mM). **B** and **C,** The concentration-dependent effects of hydrogen peroxide on LLC-PK$_1$ cell death (using lactate dehydrogenase [LDH] release as marker) after 3 hours' exposure. Cells were transfected with 1) the cytosolic PLA$_2$ (LLC-cPLA$_2$), 2) the secretory PLA$_2$ (LLC-sPLA$_2$), 3) vector (LLC-vector), or 4) were not transfected (LLC-PK$_1$). Cells transfected with cytosolic PLA$_2$ exhibited greater AA release and cell death in response to oxidant exposure than cells transfected with the vector or secretory PLA$_2$ or not transfected. These results suggest that activation of cytosolic PLA$_2$ during oxidant injury contributes to cell injury and death. (*From* Sapirstein *et al.* [15]; with permission.)

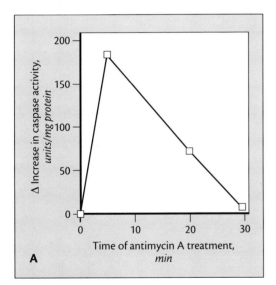

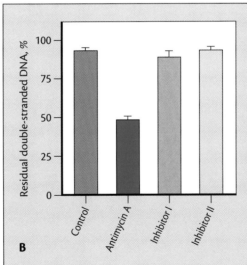

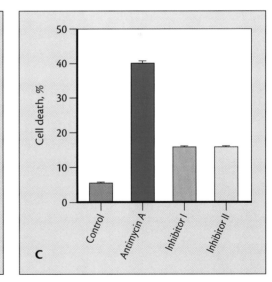

FIGURE 15-33

Potential role of caspases in cell death in LLC-PK$_1$ cells exposed to antimycin A. **A,** Time-dependent effects of antimycin A treatment on caspase activity in LLC-PK$_1$ cells. **B, C,** The effect of two capase inhibitors on antimycin A–induced DNA damage and cell death, respectively. Antimycin A is an inhibitor of mitochondrial electron transport.

Inhibitor 1 is IL-1β converting enzyme inhibitor 1 (YVAD-CHO) and inhibitor II is CPP32/apopain inhibitor (DEVD-CHO). These results suggest that caspases are activated after mitochondrial inhibition and that caspases may contribute to antimycin A–induced DNA damage and cell death. (*From* Kaushal *et al.* [16]; with permission.)

References

1. Fish EM, Molitoris BA: Alterations in epithelial polarity and the pathogenesis of disease states. *N Engl J Med* 1994, 330:1580.

2. Gailit J, Colfesh D, Rabiner I, *et al.*: Redistribution and dysfunction of integrins in cultured renal epithelial cells exposed to oxidative stress. *Am J Physiol* 1993, 264:F149.

3. Nowak G, Aleo MD, Morgan JA, Schnellmann RG: Recovery of cellular functions following oxidant injury. *Am J Physiol* 1998, 274:F509.

4. Majno G, Joris I: Apoptosis, oncosis and necrosis. *Am J Pathol* 1995, 146:3.

5. Monks TJ, Lau SS: Renal transport processes and glutathione conjugate–mediated nephrotoxicity. *Drug Metab Dispos* 1987, 15:437.

6. Hayden PJ, Ichimura T, McCann DJ, *et al.*: Detection of cysteine conjugate metabolite adduct formation with specific mitochondrial proteins using antibodies raised against halothane metabolite adducts. *J Biol Chem* 1991, 266:18415.

7. Bruschi SA, West KA, Crabb JW, *et al.*: Mitochondrial HSP60 (P1 protein) and a HSP70-like protein (mortalin) are major targets for modification during S-(1,1,2,2-tetrafluoroethyl)-L-cysteine–induced nephrotoxicity. *J Biol Chem* 1993, 268:23157.

8. Groves CE, Lock EA, Schnellmann RG: Role of lipid peroxidation in renal proximal tubule cell death induced by haloalkene cysteine conjugates. *Toxicol Appl Pharmacol* 1991, 107:54.

9. Schnellmann RG: Pathophysiology of nephrotoxic cell injury. In *Diseases of the Kidney*. Edited by Schrier RW, Gottschalk CW. Boston:Little Brown; 1997:1049.

10. Suzuki K, Ohno S: Calcium activated neutral protease: Structure-function relationship and functional implications. *Cell Structure Function* 1990, 15:1.

11. Suzuki K, Sorimachi H, Yoshizawa T, *et al.*: Calpain: Novel family members, activation, and physiologic function. *Biol Chem Hoppe-Seyler* 1995, 376:523.

12. Waters SL, Sarang SS, Wang KKW, Schnellmann RG: Calpains mediate calcium and chloride influx during the late phase of cell injury. *J Pharmacol Exp Ther* 1997, 283:1177.

13. Waters SL, Wong JK, Schnellmann RG: Depletion of endoplasmic reticulum calcium stores protects against hypoxia- and mitochondrial inhibitor–induced cellular injury and death. *Biochem Biophys Res Commun* 1997, 240:57.

14. Waters SL, Miller GW, Aleo MD, Schnellmann RG: Neurosteroid inhibition of cell death. *Am J Physiol* 1997, 273:F869.

15. Sapirstein A, Spech RA, Witzgall R, Bonventre JV: Cytosolic phospholipase A_2 (PLA_2), but not secretory PLA_2, potentiates hydrogen peroxide cytotoxicity in kidney epithelial cells. *J Biol Chem* 1996, 271:21505.

16. Kaushal GP, Ueda N, Shah SV: Role of caspases (ICE/CED3 proteases) in DNA damage and cell death in response to a mitochondrial inhibitor, antimycin A. *Kidney Int* 1997, 52:438.

Acute Renal Failure: Cellular Features of Injury and Repair

Kevin T. Bush
Hiroyuki Sakurai
Tatsuo Tsukamoto
Sanjay K. Nigam

A lthough ischemic acute renal failure (ARF) is likely the result of many different factors, much tubule injury can be traced back to a number of specific lesions that occur at the cellular level in ischemic polarized epithelial cells. At the onset of an ischemic insult, rapid and dramatic biochemical changes in the cellular environment occur, most notably perturbation of the intracellular levels of ATP and free calcium and increases in the levels of free radicals, which lead to alterations in structural and functional cellular components characteristic of renal epithelial cells [1–7]. These alterations include a loss of tight junction integrity, disruption of actin-based microfilaments, and loss of the apical basolateral polarity of epithelial cells. The result is loss of normal renal cell function [7–12].

After acute renal ischemia, the recovery of renal tubule function is critically dependent on reestablishment of the permeability barrier, which is crucial to proper functioning of epithelial tissues such as renal tubules. After ischemic injury the formation of a functional permeability barrier, and thus of functional renal tubules, is critically dependent on the establishment of functional tight junctions. The tight junction is an apically oriented structure that functions as both the "fence" that separates apical and basolateral plasma membrane domains and the major paracellular permeability barrier (gate). It is not yet clear how the kidney restores tight junction structure and function after ischemic injury. In fact, tight junction assembly under normal physiological conditions remains ill-understood; however, utilization of the "calcium switch" model with cultured renal epithelial cells has helped to elucidate some of the critical features of tight junction bioassembly. In this model for tight junction reassembly, signaling events involving G proteins, protein kinase C, and calcium appear necessary for the reestablishment of tight junctions [13–19]. Tight junction injury and recovery, like that which occurs after ischemia and reperfusion, has similarly been modeled by subjecting cultured renal epithelial cells to ATP depletion ("chemical anoxia") followed by repletion. While there are many similarities to the calcium switch, biochemical studies have recently revealed major differences, for example, in the way tight junction proteins interact with the cytoskeleton [12]. Thus, important insights into the basic and applied biology of tight junctions are likely to be forthcoming from further analysis of the ATP depletion-repletion model. Nevertheless, it is likely that, as in the calcium switch model, tight junction reassembly is regulated by classical signaling pathways that might potentially be pharmacologically modulated to enhance recovery after ischemic insults.

More prolonged insults can lead to greater, but still sublethal, injury. Key cellular proteins begin to break down. Many of these (*eg*, the tight junction protein, occludin, and the adherens junction protein, E-cadherin) are membrane proteins. Matrix proteins and their integrin receptors may need to be resynthesized, along with growth factors and cytokines, all of which pass through the endoplasmic reticulum (ER). The rate-limiting events in the biosynthesis and assembly of these proteins occur in the ER and are catalyzed by a set of ER-specific molecular chaperones, some of which are homologs of the cytosolic heat-shock proteins [20]. The levels of mRNAs for these proteins may increase 10-fold or more in the ischemic kidney, to keep up with the cellular need to synthesize and transport these new membrane proteins, as well as secreted ones.

If the ischemic insult is sufficiently severe, cell death and/or detachment leads to loss of cells from the epithelium lining the kidney tubules. To recover from such a severe insult, cell regeneration, differentiation, and possibly morphogenesis, are necessary. To a limited extent, the recovery of kidney tubule function after such a severe ischemic insult can be viewed as a recapitulation of various steps in renal development. Cells must proliferate and differentiate, and, in fact, activation of growth factor–mediated signaling pathways (some of the same ones involved in kidney development) appears necessary to ameliorate renal recovery after acute ischemic injury [21–30].

The Ischemic Epithelial Cell

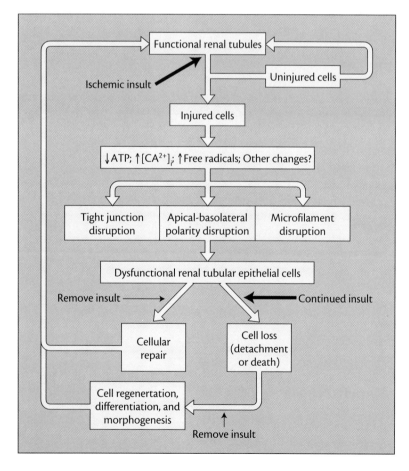

FIGURE 16-1

Ischemic acute renal failure (ARF). Flow chart illustrates the cellular basis of ischemic ARF. As described above, renal tubule epithelial cells undergo a variety of biochemical and structural changes in response to ischemic insult. If the duration of the insult is sufficiently short, these alterations are readily reversible, but if the insult continues it ultimately leads to cell detachment and/or cell death. Interestingly, unlike other organs in which ischemic injury often leads to permanent cell loss, a kidney severely damaged by ischemia can regenerate and replace lost epithelial cells to restore renal tubular function virtually completely, although it remains unclear how this happens.

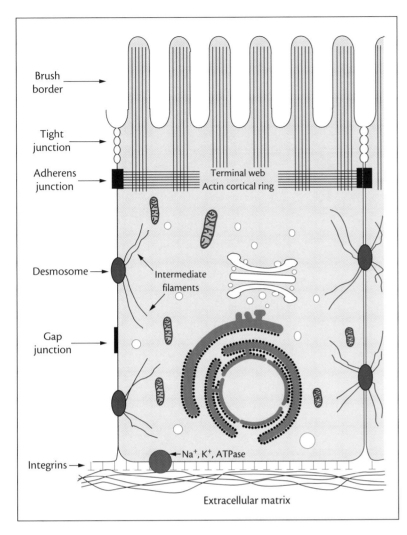

FIGURE 16-2

Typical renal epithelial cell. Diagram of a typical renal epithelial cell. Sublethal injury to polarized epithelial cells leads to multiple lesions, including loss of the permeability barrier and apical-basolateral polarity [7–12]. To recover, cells must reestablish intercellular junctions and repolarize to form distinct apical and basolateral domains characteristic of functional renal epithelial cells. These junctions include those necessary for maintaining the permeability barrier (ie, tight junctions), maintaining cell-cell contact (ie, adherens junctions and desmosomes), and those involved in cell-cell communication (ie, gap junctions). In addition, the cell must establish and maintain contact with the basement membrane through its integrin receptors. Thus, to understand how kidney cells recover from sublethal ischemic injury it is necessary to understand how renal epithelial cells form these junctions. Furthermore, after lethal injury to tubule cells new cells may have to replace those lost during the ischemic insult, and these new cells must differentiate into epithelial cells to restore proper function to the tubules.

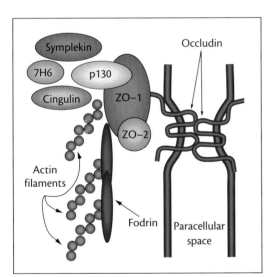

FIGURE 16-3

The tight junction. The tight junction, the most apical component of the junctional complex of epithelial cells, serves two main functions in epithelial cells: 1) It separates the apical and basolateral plasma membrane domains of the cells, allowing for vectorial transport of ions and molecules; 2) it provides the major framework for the paracellular permeability barrier, allowing for generation of chemical and electrical gradients [31]. These functions are critically important to the proper functioning of renal tubules. The tight junction is comprised of a number of proteins (cytoplasmic and transmembrane) that interact with a similar group of proteins between adjacent cells to form the permeability barrier [16, 32–37]. These proteins include the transmembrane protein occludin [35, 38] and the cytosolic proteins zonula occludens 1 (ZO-1), ZO-2 [36], p130, [39], cingulin [33, 40], 7H6 antigen [34] and symplekin [41], although other as yet unidentified components likely exist. The tight junction also appears to interact with the actin-based cytoskeleton, probably in part through ZO-1–fodrin interactions.

Reassembly of the Permeability Barrier

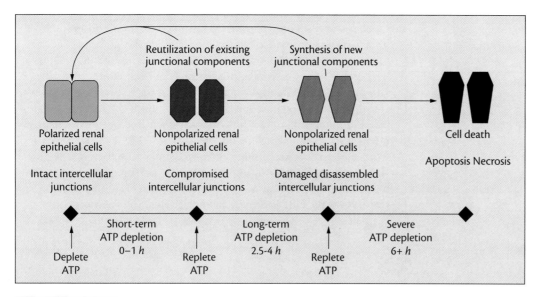

FIGURE 16-4

Cell culture models of tight junction disruption and reassembly. The disruption of the permeability barrier, mediated by the tight junction, is a key lesion in the pathogenesis of tubular dysfunction after ischemia and reperfusion. Cell culture models employing ATP depletion and repletion protocols are a commonly used approach for understanding the molecular

mechanisms underlying tight junction dysfunction in ischemia and how tight junction integrity recovers after the insult [6, 12, 42]. After short-term ATP depletion (1 hour or less) in Madin-Darby canine kidney cells, although some new synthesis probably occurs, by and large it appears that reassembly of the tight junction can proceed with existing (disassembled) components after ATP repletion. This model of short-term ATP depletion-repletion is probably most relevant to transient sublethal ischemic injury of renal tubule cells. However, in a model of longterm ATP depletion (2.5 to 4 hours), that probably is most relevant to prolonged ischemic (though still sublethal) insult to the renal tubule, it is likely that reestablishment of the permeability barrier (and thus of tubule function) depends on the production (message and protein) and bioassembly of new tight junction components. Many of these components (membrane proteins) are assembled in the endoplasmic reticulum.

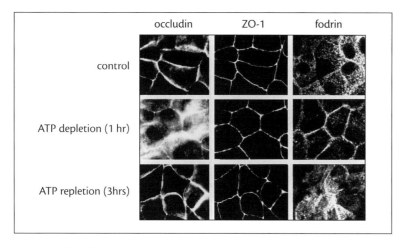

FIGURE 16-5

Immunofluorescent localization of proteins of the tight junction after ATP depletion and repletion. The cytosolic protein zonula

occludens 1 (ZO-1), and the transmembrane protein occludin are integral components of the tight junction that are intimately associated at the apical border of epithelial cells. This is demonstrated here by indirect immunofluorescent localization of these two proteins in normal kidney epithelial cells. After 1 hour of ATP depletion this association appears to change, occludin can be found in the cell interior, whereas ZO-1 remains at the apical border of the plasma membrane. Interestingly, the intracellular distribution of the actin-cytoskeletal–associated protein fodrin also changes after ATP depletion. Fodrin moves from a random, intracellular distribution and appears to become co-localized with ZO-1 at the apical border of the plasma membrane. These changes are completely reversible after ATP repletion. These findings suggest that disruption of the permeability barrier could be due, at least in part, to altered association of ZO-1 with occludin. In addition, the apparent co-localization of ZO-1 and fodrin at the level of the tight junction suggests that ZO-1 is becoming intimately associated with the cytoskeleton.

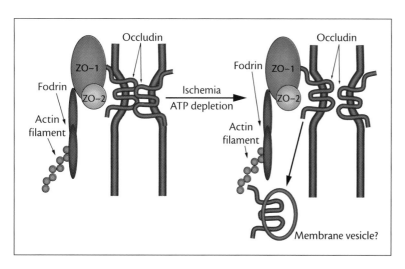

FIGURE 16-6

ATP depletion causes disruption of tight junctions. Diagram of the changes induced in tight junction structure by ATP depletion. ATP depletion causes the cytoplasmic tight junction proteins zonula occludens 1 (ZO-1) and ZO-2 to form large insoluble complexes, probably in association with the cytoskeletal protein fodrin [12], though aggregation may also be significant. Furthermore, occludin, the transmembrane protein of the tight junction, becomes localized to the cell interior, probably in membrane vesicles. These kinds of studies have begun to provide insight into the biochemical basis of tight junction disruption after ATP depletion, although how the tight junction reassembles during recovery of epithelial cells from ischemic injury remains unclear.

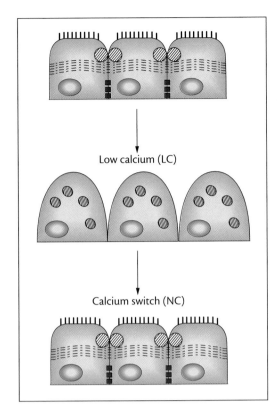

FIGURE 16-7

Madin-Darby canine kidney (MDCK) cell calcium switch. Insight into the molecular mechanisms involved in the assembly of tight junctions (that may be at least partly applicable to the ischemia-reperfusion setting) has been gained from the MDCK cell calcium switch model [43]. MDCK cells plated on a permeable support form a monolayer with all the characteristics of a tight, polarized transporting epithelium. Exposing such cell monolayers to conditions of low extracellular calcium (less than $5\mu M$) causes the cells to lose cell-cell contact and to "round up." Upon switching back to normal calcium media (1.8 mM), the cells reestablish cell-cell contact, intercellular junctions, and apical-basolateral polarity. These events are accompanied by profound changes in cell shape and reorganization of the actin cytoskeleton. (*From* Denker and Nigam [19]; with permission)

Low calcium (LC)

Calcium switch (NC)

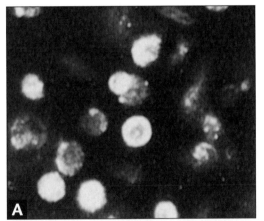
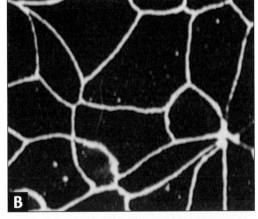
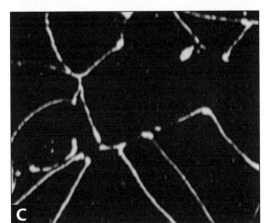
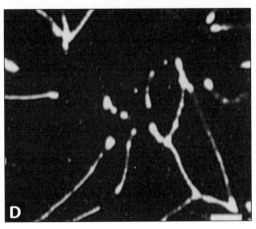

FIGURE 16-8

Protein kinase C (PKC) is important for tight junction assembly. Immunofluorescent localization of the tight junction protein zonula occludens 1 (ZO-1) during the Madin-Darby canine kidney (MDCK) cell calcium switch. In low-calcium media MDCK cells are round and have little cell-cell contact. Under these conditions, ZO-1 is found in the cell interior and has little, if any, membrane staining, **A**. After 2 hours incubation in normal calcium media, MDCK cells undergo significant changes in cell shape and make extensive cell-cell contact along the lateral portions of the plasma membrane. **B**, Here, ZO-1 has redistributed to areas of cell-cell contact with little apparent intracellular staining. This process is blocked by treatment with either 500 nM calphostin C, **C**, or $25\mu M$ H7, **D**, inhibitors of PKC. These results suggest that PKC plays a role in regulating tight junction assembly. Similar studies have demonstrated roles for a number of other signaling molecules, including calcium and G proteins, in the assembly of tight junctions [12, 13, 16–19, 37, 44–46]. An analogous set of signaling events is likely responsible for tight junction reassembly after ischemia. (*From* Stuart and Nigam [16]; with permission.)

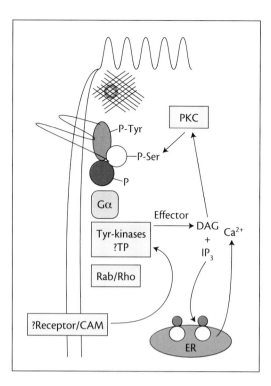

FIGURE 16-9

Signalling molecules that may be involved in tight junction assembly. Model of the potential signaling events involved in tight junction assembly. Tight junction assembly probably depends on a complex interplay of several signaling molecules, including protein kinase C (PKC), calcium (Ca^{2+}), heterotrimeric G proteins, small guanodine triphosphatases (Rab/Rho), and tyrosine kinases [13–16, 18, 37, 44–53]. Although it is not clear how this process is initiated, it depends on cell-cell contact and involves wide-scale changes in levels of intracellular free calcium. Receptor/CAM—cell adhesion molecule; DAG—diacylglycerol; ER—endoplasmic reticulum; Gα—alpha subunit of GTP-binding protein; IP3—inositol trisphosphate. (*From* Denker and Nigam [19]; with permission.)

The Endoplasmic Reticulum Stress Response in Ischemia _____

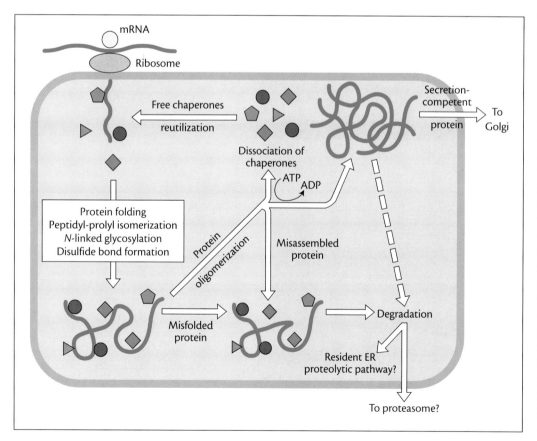

FIGURE 16-10

Protein processing in the endoplasmic reticulum (ER). To recover from serious injury, cells must synthesize and assemble new membrane (tight junction proteins) and secreted (growth factors) proteins. The ER is the initial site of synthesis of all membrane and secreted proteins. As a protein is translocated into the lumen of the ER it begins to interact with a group of resident ER proteins called molecular chaperones [20, 54–57]. Molecular chaperones bind transiently to and interact with these nascent polypeptides as they fold, assemble, and oligomerize [20, 54, 58]. Upon successful completion of folding or assembly, the molecular chaperones and the secretion-competent protein part company via a reaction that requires ATP hydrolysis, and the chaperones are ready for another round of protein folding [20, 59–61]. If a protein is recognized as being misfolded or misassembled it is retained within the ER via stable association with the molecular chaperones and is ultimately targeted for degradation [62]. Interestingly, some of the more characteristic features of epithelial ischemia include loss of cellular functions mediated by proteins that are folded and assembled in the ER (*ie*, cell adhesion molecules, integrins, tight junctional proteins, transporters). This suggests that proper functioning of the protein-folding machinery of the ER could be critically important to the ability of epithelial cells to withstand and recover from ischemic insult. ADP—adenosine diphosphate.

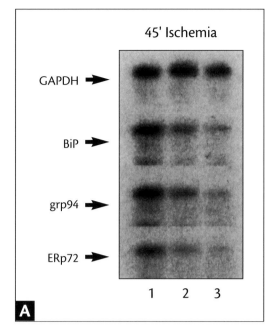

45' Ischemia

GAPDH

BiP

grp94

ERp72

1 2 3

A

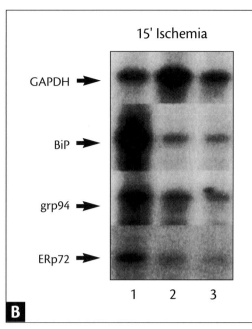

15' Ischemia

GAPDH

BiP

grp94

ERp72

1 2 3

B

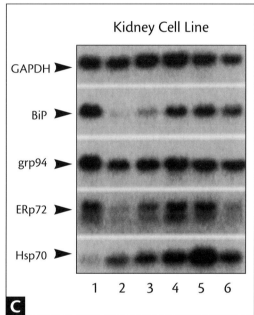

Kidney Cell Line

GAPDH

BiP

grp94

ERp72

Hsp70

1 2 3 4 5 6

C

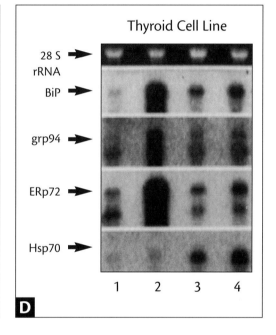

Thyroid Cell Line

28 S
rRNA

BiP

grp94

ERp72

Hsp70

1 2 3 4

D

FIGURE 16-11

Ischemia upregulates endoplasmic reticulum (ER) molecular chaperones. Molecular chaperones of the ER are believed to function normally to prevent inappropriate intra- or intermolecular interactions during the folding and assembly of proteins [20, 54]. However, ER molecular chaperones are also part of the "quality control" apparatus involved in the recognition, retention, and degradation of proteins that fail to fold or assemble properly as they transit the ER [20, 54]. In fact, the messages encoding the ER molecular chaperones are known to increase in response to intraorganelle accumulation of such malfolded proteins [11, 20, 54, 55]. Here, Northern blot analysis of total RNA from either whole kidney or cultured epithelial cells demonstrates that ischemia or ATP depletion induces the mRNAs that encode the ER molecular chaperones, including immunoglobulin binding protein (BiP), 94 kDa glucose regulated protein (grp94), and 72 kDa endoplasmic reticulum protein (Erp72) [11]. This suggests not only that ischemia or ATP depletion causes the accumulation of malfolded proteins in the ER but that a major effect of ischemia and ATP depletion could be perturbation of the "folding environment" of the ER and disruption of protein processing. GAPDH—glyceraldehyde-3-phosphate dehydrogenase; Hsp70—70 kDa heat-shock protein. (*From* Kuznetsov *et al.* [11]; with permission.)

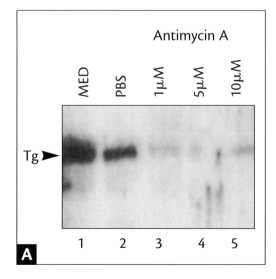

Antimycin A

MED PBS 1μM 5μM 10μM

Tg

1 2 3 4 5

A

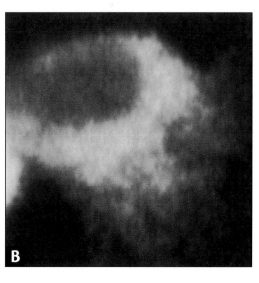

B

FIGURE 16-12

ATP depletion perturbs normal endoplasmic reticulum (ER) function. Because ATP and a proper redox environment are necessary for folding and assembly [20, 54, 63, 64] and ATP depletion alters ATP levels and the redox environment, the secretion of proteins is perturbed under these conditions. Here, Western blot analysis of the culture media from thyroid epithelial cells subjected to ATP depletion (*ie*, treatment with antimycin A, an inhibitor of oxidative phosphorylation) illustrates this point. **A,** Treatment with as little as 1μM antimycin A for 1 hour completely blocks the secretion of thyroglobulin (Tg) from these cells.

(*Continued on next page*)

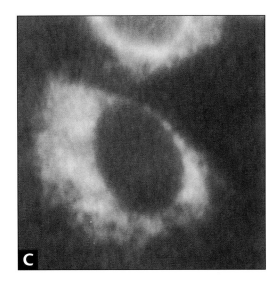

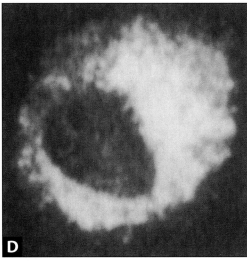

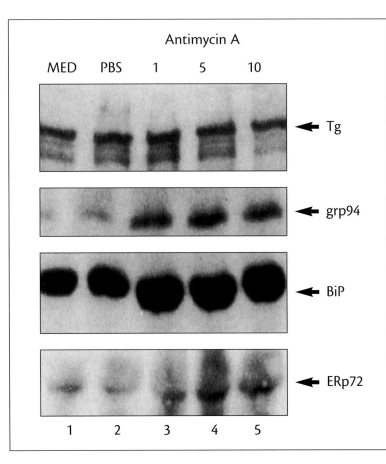

FIGURE 16-12 (*Continued*)

B–D, Moreover, indirect immunofluorescence with antithyroglobulin antibody demonstrates that the nonsecreted protein is trapped almost entirely in the ER. Together with data from Northern blot analysis, this suggests that perturbation of ER function and disruption of the secretory pathway is likely to be a key cellular lesion in ischemia [11]. MED—control media; PBS—phosphate-buffered saline. (*From* Kuznetsov *et al.* [11]; with permission.)

FIGURE 16-13

ATP depletion increases the stability of chaperone-folding polypeptide interactions in the endoplasmic reticulum (ER). Immunoglobulin binding protein (BiP), and perhaps other ER molecular chaperones, associate with nascent polypeptides as they are folded and assembled in ER [20, 54, 56, 57, 65–73]. The dissociation of these proteins requires hydrolysis of ATP [69]. Thus, when levels of ATP drop, BiP should not dissociate from the secretory proteins and the normally transient interaction should become more stable. Here, the associations of ER molecular chaperones with a model ER secretory protein is examined by Western blot analysis of thyroglobulin (Tg) immunoprecipitates from thyroid cells subjected to ATP depletion. After treatment with antimycin A, there is an increase in the amounts of ER molecular chaperones (BiP, grp94 and ERP72) which co-immunoprecipitate with antithyroglobulin antibody [11], suggesting that ATP depletion causes stabilization of the interactions between molecular chaperones and secretory proteins folded and assembled in the ER. Moreover, because a number of proteins critical to the proper functioning of polarized epithelial cells (*ie*, occludin, E-cadherin, Na-K-ATPase) are folded and assembled in the ER, this suggests that recovery from ischemic injury is likely to depend, at least in part, on the ability of the cell to rescue the protein-folding and -assembly apparatus of the ER. Control media (MED) and phosphate buffered saline (PBS)—no ATP depletion; 1, 5, 10μM antimycin A—ATP-depleting conditions. (*From* Kuznetsov *et al.* [11]; with permission.)

Growth Factors and Morphogenesis

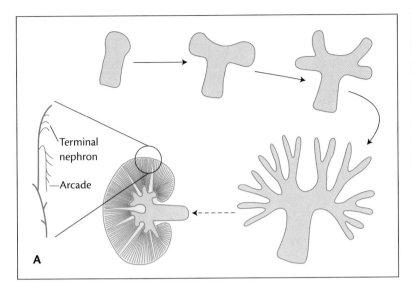

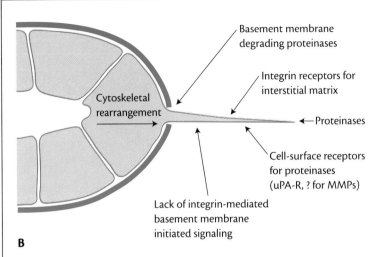

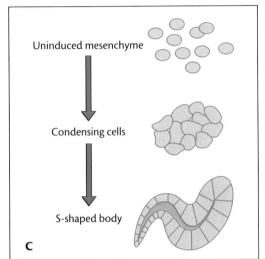

FIGURE 16-14

Kidney morphogenesis. Schematics demonstrate the development of the ureteric bud and metanephric mesenchyme during kidney organogenesis. During embryogenesis, mutual inductive events between the metanephric mesenchyme and the ureteric bud give rise to primordial structures that differentiate and fuse to form functional nephrons [74-76]. Although the process has been described morphologically, the nature and identity of molecules involved in the signaling and regulation of these events remain unclear. **A**, Diagram of branching tubulogenesis of the ureteric bud during kidney organogenesis. The ureteric bud is induced by the metanephric mesenchyme to branch and elongate to form the urinary collecting system [74-76]. **B**, Model of cellular events involved in ureteric bud branching. To branch and elongate, the ureteric bud must digest its way through its own basement membrane, a highly complicated complex of extracellular matrix proteins. It is believed that this is accomplished by cellular projections, "invadopodia," which allow for localized sites of proteolytic activity at their tips [77-81]. **C**, Mesenchymal cell compaction. The metanephric mesenchyme not only induces ureteric bud branching but is also induced by the ureteric bud to epithelialize and differentiate into the proximal through distal tubule [74–76]. (*From* Stuart and Nigam [80] and Stuart *et al*. [81]; with permission.)

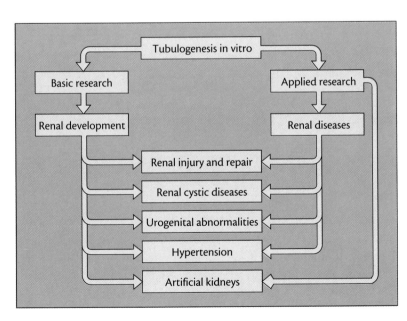

FIGURE 16-15

Potential of in vitro tubulogenesis research. Flow chart indicates relevance of in vitro models of kidney epithelial cell branching tubulogenesis to basic and applied areas of kidney research. While results from such studies provide critical insight into kidney development, this model system might also contribute to the elucidation of mechanisms involved in kidney injury and repair for a number of diseases, including tubular epithelial cell regeneration secondary to acute renal failure. Moreover, these models of branching tubulogenesis could lead to therapies that utilize tubular engineering as artificial renal replacement therapy [82].

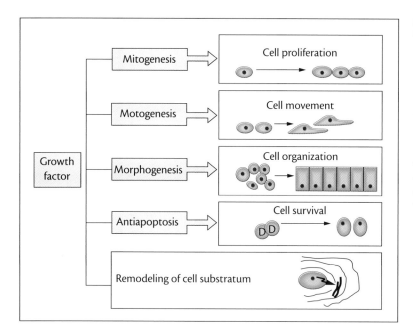

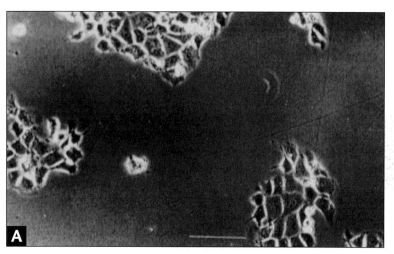

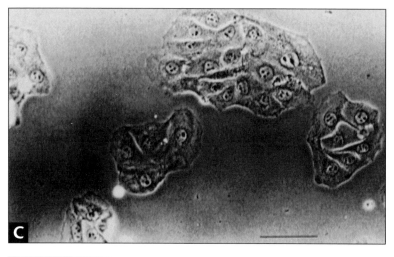

FIGURE 16-16

Cellular response to growth factors. Schematic representation of the pleiotrophic effects of growth factors, which share several properties and are believed to be important in the development and morphogenesis of organs and tissues, such as those of the kidney. Among these properties are the ability to regulate or activate numerous cellular signaling responses, including proliferation (mitogenesis), motility (motogenesis), and differentiation (morphogenesis). These characteristics allow growth factors to play critical roles in a number of complex biological functions, including embryogenesis, angiogenesis, tissue regeneration, and malignant transformation [83].

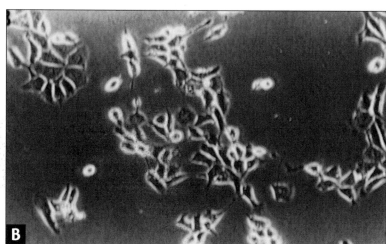

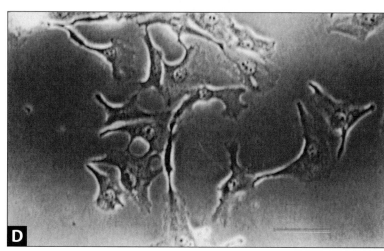

FIGURE 16-17

Motogenic effect of growth factors—hepatocyte growth factor (HGF) induces cell "scattering." During development or regeneration the recruitment of cells to areas of new growth is vital. Growth factors have the ability to induce cell movement. Here, subconfluent monolayers of either Madin-Darby canine kidney (MDCK) **C, D,** or murine inner medullary collecting duct (mIMCD) **A, B,** cells were grown for 24 hours in the absence, **A, C,** or presence **B, D,** of 20 ng/mL HGF. Treatment of either type of cultured renal epithelial cell with HGF induced the dissociation of islands of cells into individual cells. This phenomenon is referred to as scattering. HGF was originally identified as *scatter factor*, based on its ability to induce the scattering of MDCK cells [83]. Now, it is known that HGF and its receptor, the transmembrane tyrosine kinase *c-met*, play important roles in development, regeneration, and carcinogenesis [83]. (*From* Cantley *et al.* [84]; with permission.)

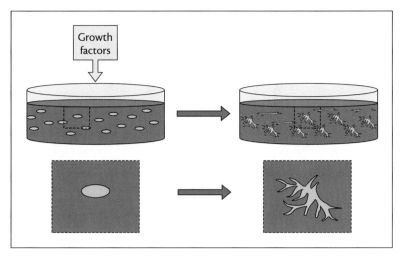

FIGURE 16-18

Three-dimensional extracellular matrix gel tubulogenesis model. Model of the three-dimensional gel culture system used to study

the branching and tubulogenesis of renal epithelial cells. Analyzing the role of single factors (*ie*, extracellular matrix, growth factors, cell-signaling processes) involved in ureteric bud branching tubulogenesis in the context of the developing embryonic kidney is an extremely daunting task, but a number of model systems have been devised that allow for such investigation [77, 79, 85]. The simplest model exploits the ability of isolated kidney epithelial cells suspended in gels composed of extracellular matrix proteins to form branching tubular structures in response to growth factors. For example, Madin-Darby canine kidney (MDCK) cells suspended in gels of type I collagen undergo branching tubulogenesis reminiscent of ureteric bud branching morphogenesis in vivo [77, 79]. Although the results obtained from such studies in vitro might not correlate directly with events in vivo, this simple, straightforward system allows one to easily manipulate individual components (*eg*, growth factors, extracellular matrix components) involved in the generation of branching epithelial tubules and has provided crucial insights into the potential roles that these various factors play in epithelial cell branching morphogenesis [77, 79, 84–87].

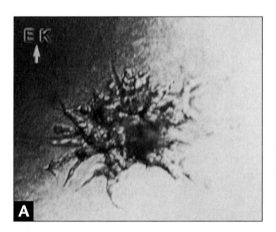

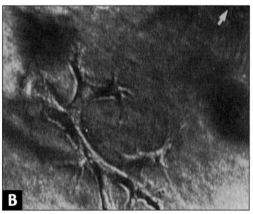

FIGURE 16-19 ∘

An example of the branching tubulogenesis of renal epithelial cells cultured in three-dimensional extracellular matrix gels. Microdissected mouse embryonic kidneys (11.5 to 12.5 days) were cocultured with **A**, murine inner medullary collecting duct

(mIMCD) or, **B**, Madin-Darby canine kidney (MDCK) cells suspended in gels of rat-tail collagen (type I). Embryonic kidneys (EK) induced the formation of branching tubular structures in both mIMCD and MDCK cells after 48 hours of incubation at 37°C. EKs produce a number of growth factors, including hepatocyte growth factor, transforming growth factor-alpha, insulin-like growth factor, and transforming growth factor–β, which have been shown to effect tubulogenic activity [86–93]. Interestingly, many of these same growth factors have been shown to be effective in the recovery of renal function after acute ischemic insult [21–30]. (*From* Barros *et al.* [87]; with permission.)

FIGURE 16-20

Development of cell lines derived from embryonic kidney. Flow chart of the establishment of ureteric bud and metanephric mesenchymal cell lines from day 11.5 mouse embryo. Although the results obtained from the analysis of kidney epithelial cells— Madin-Darby canine kidney (MDCK) or murine inner medullary collecting duct (mIMCD) seeded in three-dimensional extracellular matrix gels has been invaluable in furthering our understanding of the mechanisms of epithelial cell branching tubulogenesis, questions can be raised about the applicability to embryonic development of results using cells derived from terminally differentiated adult kidney epithelial cells [94]. Therefore, kidney epithelial cell lines have been established that appear to be derived from the ureteric bud and metanephric mesenchyme of the developing embryonic kidney of SV-40 transgenic mice [94, 95]. These mice have been used to establish a variety of "immortal" cell lines.

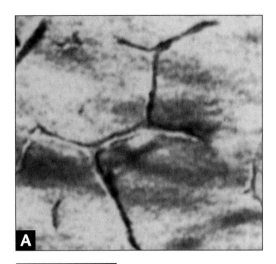
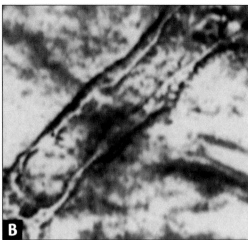
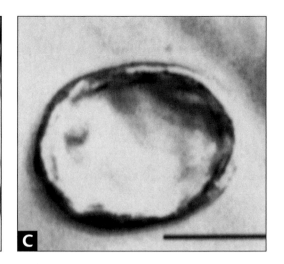

FIGURE 16-21

Ureteric bud cells undergo branching tubulogenesis in three-dimensional extracellular matrix gels. Cell line derived from ureteric bud (UB) and metanephric mesenchyme from day 11.5 mouse embryonic kidney undergo branching tubulogenesis in three-dimensional extracellular matrix gels. Here, UB cells have been induced to form branching tubular structures in response to "conditioned" media collected from the culture of metanephric mesenchymal cells. During normal kidney morphogenesis, these two embryonic cell types undergo a mutually inductive process that ultimately leads to the formation of functional nephrons [74–76]. This model system illustrates this process, ureteric bud cells being induced by factors secreted from metanephric mesenchymal cells. Thus, this system could represent the simplest in vitro model with the greatest relevance to early kidney development [94]. **A,** UB cells grown for 1 week in the presence of conditioned media collected from cells cultured from the metanephric mesenchyme. Note the formation of multicellular cords. **B,** After 2 weeks' growth under the same conditions, UB cells have formed more substantial tubules, now with clear lumens. **C,** Interestingly, after 2 weeks of culture in a three-dimensional gel composed entirely of growth factor–reduced Matrigel, ureteric bud cells have not formed cords or tubules, only multicellular cysts. Thus, changing the matrix composition can alter the morphology from tubules to cysts, indicating that this model might also be relevant to renal cystic disease, much of which is of developmental origin. (*From* Sakurai *et al.* [94]; with permission.)

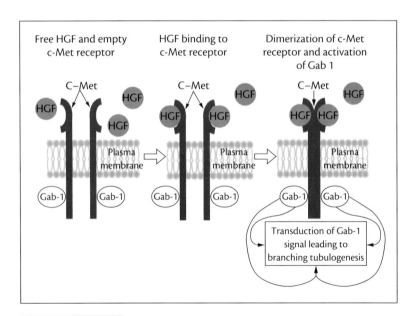
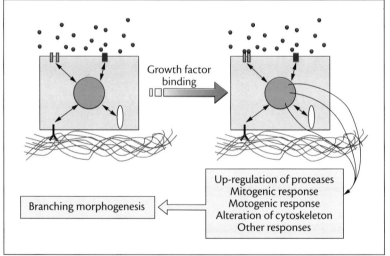

FIGURE 16-22

Signalling pathway of hepatocyte growth factor action. Diagram of the proposed intracellular signaling pathway involved in hepatocyte growth factor (HGF)–mediated tubulogenesis. Although HGF is perhaps the best-characterized of the growth factors involved in epithelial cell-branching tubulogenesis, very little of its mechanism of action is understood. However, recent evidence has shown that the HGF receptor (c-Met) is associated with Gab-1, a docking protein believed to be involved in signal transduction [96]. Thus, on binding to c-Met, HGF activates Gab-1–mediated signal transduction, which, by an unknown mechanism, affects changes in cell shape and cell movement or cell-cell–cell-matrix interactions. Ultimately, these alterations lead to epithelial cell–branching tubulogenesis.

FIGURE 16-23

Mechanism of growth factor action. Proposed model for the generalized response of epithelial cells to growth factors, which the depends on their environment. Epithelial cells constantly monitor their surrounding environment via extracellular receptors (*ie,* integrin receptors) and respond accordingly to growth factor stimulation. If the cells are in the appropriate environment, growth factor binding induces cellular responses necessary for branching tubulogenesis. There are increases in the levels of extracellular proteinases and of structural and functional changes in the cytoarchitecture that enable the cells to form branching tubule structures.

GROWTH FACTORS IN DEVELOPMENTAL AND RENAL RECOVERY

Growth Factor	Expression Following Renal Ischemia	Effect of Exogenous Administration	Branching/Tubulogenic Activity
HGF	Increased [97]	Enhanced recovery [103]	Facilatory [109,110]
EGF	Unclear [98,99]	Enhanced recovery [104,105]	Facilatory [111]
HB-EGF	Increased [100]	Undetermined	Facilatory [111]
TGF-α	Unclear	Enhanced recovery [106]	Facilatory [111]
IGF	Increased [101]	Enhanced recovery [107,108]	Facilatory [112,113]
KGF	Increased [102]	Undetermined	Undetermined
bFGF	Undetermined	Undetermined	Facilatory [112]
GDNF	Undetermined	Undetermined	Facilatory [114]
TGF-β	Increased† [98]	Undetermined	Inhibitory for branching [115]
PDGF	Increased† [98]	Undetermined	No effect [112]

*Increase in endogenous biologically active EGF probably from preformed sources; increase in EGF-receptor mRNA

†Chemoattractants for macrophages and monocytes (important source of growth promoting factors)

FIGURE 16-24

Growth factors in development and renal recovery. This table describes the roles of different growth factors in renal injury or in branching tubulogenesis. A large variety of growth factors have been tested for their ability either to mediate ureteric branching tubulogenesis or to affect recovery of kidney tubules after ischemic or other injury. Interestingly, growth factors that facilitate branching tubulogenesis in vitro also enhance the recovery of injured renal tubules.

References

1. Zager RA, Gmur DJ, Bredl CR, *et al.*: Regional responses within the kidney to ischemia: Assessment of adenine nucleotide and catabolite profiles. *Biochim Biophys Acta* 1990, 1035:29–36.

2. Hays SR: Ischemic acute renal failure. *Am J Med Sci* 1992, 304:93–108.

3. Toback FG: Regeneration after acute tubular necrosis. *Kidney Int* 1992, 41:226–246.

4. Liu S, Humes HD: Cellular and molecular aspects of renal repair in acute renal failure. *Curr Opin Nephrol Hypertension* 1993, 2:618–624.

5. Doctor RB, Bennett V, Mandel LJ: Degradation of spectrin and ankyrin in the ischemic rat kidney. *Am J Physiol* 1993, 264:C1003–C1013.

6. Doctor RB, Bacallao R, Mandel LJ: Method for recovering ATP content and mitochondrial function after chemical anoxia in renal cell cultures. *Am J Physiol* 1994, 266:C1803–C1811.

7. Edelstein CL, Ling H, Schrier RW: The nature of renal cell injury. *Kidney Int* 1997, 51:1341–1351.

8. Fish EM, Molitoris BA: Alterations in epithelial polarity and the pathogenesis of disease states. *N Engl J Med* 1994, 330:1580–1587.

9. Mandel LJ, Bacallao R, Zampighi G: Uncoupling of the molecular 'fence' and paracellular 'gate' functions in epithelial tight junctions. *Nature* 1993, 361:552–555.

10. Goligorsky MS, Lieberthal W, Racusen L, Simon EE: Integrin receptors in renal tubular epithelium: New insights into pathophysiology of acute renal failure. *Am J Physiol* 1993, 264:F1–F8.

11. Kuznetsov G, Bush KT, Zhang PL, Nigam SK: Perturbations in maturation of secretory proteins and their association with endoplasmic reticulum chaperones in a cell culture model for epithelial ischemia. *Proc Natl Acad Sci USA* 1996, 93:8584–8589.

12. Tsukamoto T, Nigam SK: Tight junction proteins become insoluble, form large complexes and associate with fodrin in an ATP depletion model for reversible junction disassembly. *J Biol Chem* 1997, 272:16133–16139.

13. Nigam SK, Denisenko N, Rodriguez-Boulan E, Citi S: The role of phosphorylation in development of tight junctions in cultured renal epithelial (MDCK) cells. *Biochem Biophys Res Commun* 1991, 181:548–553.

14. Nigam SK, Rodriguez-Boulan E, Silver RB: Changes in intracellular calcium during the development of epithelial polarity and junctions. *Proc Natl Acad Sci USA* 1992, 89:6162–6166.

15. Stuart RO, Sun A, Panichas M, *et al.*: Critical role for intracellular calcium in tight junction biogenesis. *J Cellular Physiology* 1994, 159:423–433.

16. Stuart RO, Nigam SK: Regulated assembly of tight junctions by protein kinase C. *Proc Natl Acad Sci USA* 1995, 92:6072–6076.

17. Stuart RO, Sun A, Bush KT, Nigam SK: Dependence of epithelial intercellular junction biogenesis on thapsigargin-sensitive intracellular calcium stores. *J Biol Chem* 1996, 271:13636–13641.

18. Denker BM, Saha C, Khawaja S, Nigam SK: Involvement of a heterotrimeric G protein α subunit in tight junction biogenesis. *J Biol Chem* 1996, 271:25750–25753.

19. Denker BM, Nigam SK: Molecular structure and assembly of the tight junction. *Am J Physiol* 1998, 274:F1–F9.

20. Gething M-J, Sambrook J: Protein folding in the cell. *Nature* 1992, 355:33–45.

21. Humes HD, Cielinski DA, Coimbra T, *et al.*: Epidermal growth factor enhances renal tubule cell regeneration and repair and accelerates the recovery of renal function in postischemic acute renal failure. *J Clin Invest* 1989, 84:1757–1761.

22. Humes HD, Beals TF, Cieslinski DA, *et al.*: Effects of transforming growth factor–beta, transforming growth factor-alpha, and other growth factors on renal proximal tubule cells. *Lab Invest* 1991, 64:538–545.

23. Miller SB, Martin DR, Kissane J, Hammerman MR: Insulin-like growth factor I accelerates recovery from ischemic acute tubular necrosis in the rat. *Proc Natl Acad Sci USA* 1992, 89:11876–11880.

24. Border W, Noble N: Transforming growth factor beta in tissue fibrosis. *N Engl J Med* 1994, 331:1286–1292.

25. Kawaida K, Matsumoto K, Shimazu H, Nakamura T: Hepatocyte growth factor prevents acute renal failure and accelerates renal regeneration in mice. *Proc Natl Acad Sci USA* 1994, 91:4357–4361.

26. Miller S, Martin D, Kissane J, Hammerman M: Hepatocyte growth factor accelerates recovery from acute ischemic renal injury in rats. *Am J Physiol* 1994, 266:F129–F134.

27. Miller S, Martin D, Kissane J, Hammerman M: Rat models for clinical use of insulin-like growth factor I in acute renal failure. *Am J Physiol* 1994, 266:F949–F956.

28. Noiri E, Romanov V, Forest T, *et al.*: Pathophysiology of renal tubular obstruction: Therapeutic role of synthetic RGD peptides in acute renal failure. *Kidney Int* 1995, 48:1375–1385.

29. Rahman SN, Butt AR, DuBose TD, *et al.*: Differential clinical effects of anaritide atrial natiuretic peptide (ANP) in oliguric and non-oliguric ATN. *J Am Soc Nephrol* 1995, 6:474.

30. Franklin S, Moulton M, Hammerman MR, Miller SB: Sustained improvement of renal function and amelioration of symptoms in patients with chronic renal failure (CRF) treated with insulin-like growth factor I (IGF-I). *J Am Soc Nephrol* 1995, 6:387.

31. Farquhar M, Palade GE: Junctional complexes in various epithelia. *J Cell Biol* 1963, 17:375–412.

32. Anderson JM, Itallie CMV: Tight junctions and the molecular basis for regulation of paracellular permeability. *Am J Physiol* 1995, 269:G467–G475.

33. Citi S, Sabanay H, Jakes R, *et al.*: Cingulin, a new peripheral component of tight junctions. *Nature* 1988, 333:272–276.

34. Zhong Y, Saitoh T, Minase T, *et al.*: Monoclonal antibody 7H6 reacts with a novel tight junction–associated protein distinct from ZO-1, cingulin and ZO-2. *J Cell Biol* 1993, 120:477–483.

35. Furuse M, Hirose T, Itoh M, *et al.*: Occludin: A novel integral membrane protein localizing at tight junctions. *J Cell Biol* 1993, 123:1777–1788.

36. Jesaitis LA, Goodenough DA: Molecular characterization and tissue distribution of ZO-2, a tight junction protein homologous to ZO-1 and *Drosophila* discs–large tumor suppressor protein. *J Cell Biol* 1994, 124:949–961.

37. Balda MS, Gonzalez-Mariscal L, Matter K, *et al.*: Assembly of the tight junction: The role of diacylglycerol. *J Cell Biol* 1993, 123:293–302.

38. Furuse M, Itoh M, Hirase T, *et al.*: Direct association of occludin with ZO-1 and its possible involvement in the localization of occludin at tight junctions. *J Cell Biol* 1994, 127:1617–1626.

39. Balda M, Whitney J, Flores C, *et al.*: Functional dissociation of paracellular permeability and transepithelial resistance and disruption of the apical-basolateral intramembrane diffusion barrier by expression of a mutant tight junction protein. *J Cell Biol* 1996, 134:1031–1049.

40. Citi S, Sabanay H, Kendrick-Jones J, Geiger B: Cingulin: Characterization and localization. *J Cell Sci* 1989, 93:107–122.

41. Keon BH, Schafer S, Kuhn C, *et al.*: Symplekin, a novel type of tight junction plaque protein. *J Cell Biol* 1996, 134:1003–1018.

42. Canfield PE, Geerdes AM, Molitoris BA: Effect of reversible ATP depletion on tight-junction integrity in LLC-PK1 cells. *Am J Physiol* 1991, 261:F1038–F1045.

43. Rodriguez-Boulan E, Nelson WJ: Morphogenesis of the polarized epithelial cell phenotype. *Science* 1989, 245:718–725.

44. Balda MS, Gonzalez-Mariscal L, Contreras RG, *et al.*: Assembly and sealing of tight junctions: Possible participation of G-proteins, phospholipase C, protein kinase C and calmodulin. *J Membrane Biol* 1991, 122:193–202.

45. de Almeida JB, Holtzman EJ, Peters P, *et al.*: Targeting of chimeric G-alpha-i proteins to specific membrane domains. *J Cell Sci* 1994, 107:507–515.

46. Dodane V, Kachar B: Identification of isoforms of G proteins and PKC that colocalize with tight junctions. *J Membrane Biol* 1996, 149:199–209.

47. Tsukita S, Oishi K, Akiyama T, *et al.*: Specific proto-oncogenic tyrosine kinase of src family are enriched in cell-to-cell adherens junctions where the level of tyrosine phosphorylation is elevated. *J Cell Biol* 1991, 113:867–879.

48. Citi S: Protein kinase inhibitors prevent junction dissociation induced by low extracellular calcium in MDCK epithelial cells. *J Cell Biol* 1992, 117:169–178.

49. Reynolds AB, Daniel J, McCrea PD, *et al.*: Identification of a new catenin: The tyrosine kinase substrate pl20cas associates with E-cadherin complexes. *Molec Cell Biol* 1994, 14:8333–8342.

50. Weber E, Berta G, Tousson A, *et al.*: Expression and polarized targeting of a Rab3 isoform in epithelial cells. *J Cell Biol* 1994, 125:583–594.

51. Zahraoui A, Joberty G, Arpin M, *et al.*: A small rab GTPase is distributed in cytoplasmic vesicles in non-polarized cells but colocalizes with the tight junction marker ZO-1 in polarized epithelial cells. *J Cell Biol* 1994, 124:101–115.

52. Citi S, Denisenko N: Phosphorylation of the tight junction protein cingulin and the effects of protein kinase inhibitors and activators in MDCK epithelial cells. *J Cell Sci* 1995, 108:2917–2926.

53. Nilsson M, Fagman H, Ericson LE: Ca2+-dependent and Ca2+-independent regulation of the thyroid epithelial junction complex by protein kinases. *Exp Cell Res* 1996, 225:1–11.

54. Braakman I, Helenius J, Helenius A: Role of ATP and disulphide bonds during protein folding in the endoplasmic reticulum. *Nature* 1992, 356:260–262.

55. Bush KT, Hendrickson BA, Nigam SK: Induction of the FK506–binding protein, FKBP13, under conditions which misfold proteins in the endoplasmic reticulum. *Biochem J* 1994, 303:705–708.

56. Kuznetsov G, Chen LB, Nigam SK: Several endoplasmic reticulum stress proteins, including ERp72, interact with thyroglobulin during its matulation. *J Biol Chem* 1994, 269:22990–22995.

57. Nigam SK, Goldberg AL, Ho S, *et al.*: A set of ER proteins with properties of molecular chaperones includes calcium binding proteins and members of the thioredoxin superfamily. *J Biol Chem* 1994, 269:1744–1749.

58. Knittler MR, Haas IG: Interaction of BIP with newly synthesized immunoglobulin light chain molecules: cycles of sequential binding and release. *EMBO J* 1992, 11:1573–1581.

59. Pelham H: Speculations on the functions of the major heat shock and glucose regulated proteins. *Cell* 1986, 46:959–961.

60. Pelham HR: Heat shock and the sorting of luminal ER proteins. *Embo J* 1989, 8:3171–3176.

61. Ellis R, Van Der Vies S: Molecular chaperones. *Annu Rev Biochem* 1991, 60:321–347.

62. Fra A, Sitia R: The endoplasmic reticulum as a site of protein degradation. *Subcell Biochem* 1993, 21:143–168.

63. Hwang C, Sinskey A, Lodish H: Oxidized redox state of glutathione in the endoplasmic reticulum. *Science* 1992, 257:1496–1502.

64. Gaut J, Hendershot L: The modification and assembly of proteins in the endoplasmic reticulum. *Curr Opin Cell Biol* 1993, 5:589–595.

65. Bole DG, Hendershot LM, Kearny JF: Posttranslational association of immunoglobulin heavy chain binding protein with nascent heavy chains in nonsecreting and secreting hybridomas. *J Cell Biol* 1986, 102:1558–1566.

66. Gething MJ, McCammon K, Sambrook J: Expression of wild-type and mutant forms of influenza hemagglutinin: The role of folding in intracellular transport. *Cell* 1986, 46:939–950.

67. Dorner AJ, Bole DG, Kaufman RJ: The relationship of N-linked glycosylation and heavy chain–binding protein association with the secretion of glycoproteins. *J Cell Biol* 1987, 105:2665–2674.

68. Ng DT, Randall RE, Lamb RA: Intracellular maturation and transport of the SV5 type II glycoprotein hemagglutinin-neuraminidase: Specific and transient association with GRP78-BiP in the endoplasmic reticulum and extensive internalization from the cell surface. *J Cell Biol* 1989, 109:3273–3289.

69. Rothman JE: Polypeptide chain binding proteins: catalysts of protein folding and related processes in cells. *Cell* 1989, 59:591–601.

70. Blount P, Merlie JP: BIP associates with newly synthesized subunits of the mouse muscle nicotinic receptor. *J Cell Biol* 1991, 113:1125–1132.

71. Melnick J, Aviel S, Argon Y: The endoplasmic reticulum stress protein GRP94, in addition to BiP, associates with unassembled immunoglobulin chains. *J Biol Chem* 1992, 267:21303–21306.

72. Pind S, Riordan J, Williams D: Participation of the endoplasmic reticulum chaperone calnexin (p88, IP90) in the biogenesis of the cystic fibrosis transmembrane conductance regulator. *J Biol Chem* 1994, 269:12784–12788.

73. Kuznetsov G, Chen L, Nigam S: Multiple molecular chaperones complex with misfolded large oligomeric glycoproteins in the endoplasmic reticulum. *J Biol Chem* 1997, 272:3057–3063.

74. Saxen L: *Organogenesis of the Kidney*. Cambridge: Cambridge University Press; 1987.

75. Brenner BM: Determinants of epithelial differentiation during early nephrogenesis. *J Am Soc Nephrol* 1990, 1:127–139.

76. Nigam SK, Aperia A, Brenner BM: Development and maturation of the kidney. In *The Kidney*. Edited by Brenner BM. Philadelphia: WB Saunders; 1996.

77. Montesano R, Schaller G, Orci L: Induction of epithelial tubular morphogenesis in vitro by fibroblast-derived soluble factors. *Cell* 1991, 66:697–711.

78. Montesano R, Matsumoto K, Nakamura T, Orci L: Identification of a fibroblast-derived epithelial morphogen as hepatocyte growth factor. *Cell* 1991, 67:901–908.

79. Santos OFP, Nigam SK: HGF-induced tubulogenesis and branching of epithelial cells is modulated by extracellular matrix and TGF-β. *Dev Biol* 1993, 160:293–302.

80. Stuart RO, Barros EJG, Ribeiro E, Nigam SK: Epithelial tubulogenesis through branching morphogenesis: Relevance to collecting system development. *J Am Soc Nephrol* 1995, 6:1151–1159.

81. Stuart RO, Nigam SK: Development of the tubular nephron. *Semin Nephrol* 1995, 15:315–326.

82. Sakurai H, Nigam SK: In vitro branching tubulogenesis: Implications for developmental and cystic disorders, nephron number, renal repair and nephron engineering. *Kidney Int* 1998, 54:14–26.

83. Matsumoto K, Nakamura T: Emerging multipotent aspects of hepatocyte growth factor. *J Biochem* 1996, 119:591–600.

84. Cantley LG, Barros EJG, Gandhi M, *et al.*: Regulation of mitogenesis, motogenesis, and tubulogenesis by hepatocyte growth factor in renal collecting duct cells. *Am J Phisiol* 1994, 267:F271–F280.

85. Perantoni AO, Williams CL, Lewellyn AL: Growth and branching morphogenesis of rat collecting duct anlagen in the absence of metanephric mesenchyme. *Differentiation* 1991, 48:107–113.

86. Santos OF, Barros EJ, Yang X-M, *et al.*: Involvement of hepatocyte growth factor in kidney development. *Dev Biol* 1994, 163:525–529.

87. Barros EJG, Santos OF, Matsumoto K, *et al.*: Differential tubulogenic and branching morphogenetic activities of growth factors: Implications for epithelial tissue development. *Proc Natl Acad Sci USA* 1995, 92:4412–4416.

88. Rogers S, Ryan G, Hammerman MR: Insulin-like growth factors I and II are produced in metanephros and are required for growth and development in vitro. *J Cell Biol* 1991, 113:1447–1453.

89. Rogers SA, Ryan G, Hammerman MR: Metanephric transforming growth factor alpha is required for renal organogenesis in vitro. *Am J Physiol* 1992, 262:F533–F539.

90. Liu Z, Wada J, Alvares K, *et al.*: Distribution and relevance of insulin-like growth factor I receptor in metanephric development. *Kidney Int* 1993, 44:1242–1250.

91. Liu J, Baker J, Perkins A, *et al.*: Mice carrying null mutations of the genes encoding insulin-like growth factor I (IGF-1) and type I IGF receptor (IGF1R). *Cell* 1993, 75:59–72.

92. Sakurai H, Tsukamoto T, Kjelsberg C, *et al.*: EGF receptor ligands are a large fraction of in vitro branching morphogens secreted by embryonic kidney. *Am J Physiol* 1997, 273:F463–F472.

93. Sakurai H, Nigam SK: TGF-β selectively inhibits branching morphogenesis but not tubulogenesis. *Am J Physiol* 1997, 272:F139–F146.

94. Sakurai H, Barros EJ, Tsukamoto T, *et al.*: An in vitro tubulogenesis system using cell lines derived from the embryonic kidney shows dependence on multiple soluble growth factors. *Proc Natl Acad Sci USA* 1997, 94:6279–6284.

95. Barasch J, Pressler L, Connor J, Malik A: A ureteric bud cell line induces nephrogenesis in two steps by two distinct signals. *Am J Physiol* 1996, 271:F50–F61.

96. Weidner K, Di Cesare S, Sachs M, *et al.*: Interaction between Gab1 and the c-Met receptor tyrosine kinase is responsible for epithelial morphogenesis. *Nature* 1996, 384:173–176.

97. Igawa T, Matsumoto K, Kanda S, *et al.*: Hepatocyte growth factor may function as a renotropic factor for regeneration in rats with acute renal injury. *Am J Physiol* 1993, 265:F61–F69.

98. Schaudies RP, Johnson JP: Increased soluble EGF after ischemia is accompanied by a decrease in membrane-associated precursors. *Am J Physiol* 1993, 264:F523–F531.

99. Salido EC, Lakshmanan J, Fisher DA, *et al.*: Expression of epidermal growth factor in the rat kidney. An immunocytochemical and in situ hybridization study. *Histochemistry* 1991, 96:65–72.

100. Homma T, Sakai M, Cheng HF, *et al.*: Induction of heparin-binding epidermal growth factor-like growth factor mRNA in rat kidney after acute injury. *J Clin Invest* 1995, 96:1018–1025.

101. Metejka GL, Jennische E: IGF-I binding and IGF-I mRNA expression in the post-ischemic regenerating rat kidney. *Kidney Int* 1992, 42:1113–1123.

102. Ichimura T, Finch PW, Zhang G, *et al.*: Induction of FGF-7 after kidney damage: a possible paracrine mechanism for tubule repair. *Am J Physiol* 1996, 271:F967–F976.

103. Kawaida K, Matsumoto K, Shimazu H, Nakamura T: Hepatocyte growth factor prevents acute renal failure and accelerates renal regeneration in mice. *Proc Natl Acad Sci USA* 1994, 91:4357–4361.

104. Humes HD, Cielski DA, Coimbra T, *et al.*: Epidermal growth factor enhances renal tubule cell regeneration and repair and accelerates the recovery of renal function in postischemic acute renal failure. *J Clin Invest* 1989, 84:1757–1761.

105. Coimbra T, Cielinski DA, Humes HD: Epidermal growth factor accelerates renal repair in mercuric chloride nephrotoxicity. *Am J Physiol* 1990, 259:F438–F443.

106. Reiss R, Cielinski DA, Humes HD: *Kidney Int* 1990, 37:1515–1521.

107. Miller SB, Martin DR, Kissane J, Hammerman MR: Insulin-like growth factor I accelerates recovery from ischemic acute tubular necrosis in the rat. *Proc Natl Acad Sci USA* 1992, 89:11876–11880.

108. Rabkin R, Sorenson A, Mortensen D, Clark R: *J Am Soc Nephrol* 1992, 3:713.

109. Montesano R, Schaller G, Orci L: Induction of epithelial tubular morphogenesis in vitro by fibroblast-derived soluable factors. *Cell* 1991, 66:697–711.

110. Santos OFP, Nigam SK: Modulation of HGF-induced tubulogenesis and branching by multiple phosphorylation mechanisms. *Dev Biol* 1993, 159:535–548.

111. Sakurai H, Tsukamoto T, Kjelsberg CA, *et al.*: EGF receptor ligands are a large fraction of in vitro branching morphogens secreted by embryonic kidney. *Am J Physiol* 1997, 273:F463–F472.

112. Sakurai H, Barros EJG, Tsukamoto T, *et al.*: An in vitro tubulogenesis system using cell lines derived from the embrionic kidney shows dependence on multiple soluble growth factors. *Proc Natl Acad Sci USA* 1997, 94:6297–6284.

113. Rogers SA, Ryan G, Hammerman MR: *Cell Biol* 113:1447–1453.

114. Vega QC, Worby CA, Lechner MS, *et al.*: Glial cell line-derived neurotrophic factor activates the receptor tyrosine kinase RET and promotes kidney morphogenesis. *Proc Natl Acad Sci USA* 1996, 93:10657–10661.

115. Sakurai H, Nigam SK: Transforming growth factor-beta selectively inhibits branching morphogenesis but not tubulogenesis. *Am J Physiol* 1997, 272:F139–F146.

Molecular Responses and Growth Factors

Steven B. Miller
Babu J. Padanilam

T he kidney possesses a remarkable capacity for restoring its structure and functional ability following an ischemic or toxic insult. It is unique as a solid organ in its ability to suffer an injury of such magnitude that the organ can fail for weeks and yet recover full function. Studying the natural regenerative process after an acute renal insult has provided new insights into the pathogenesis of acute renal failure (ARF) and possible new therapies. These therapies may limit the extent of injury or even accelerate the regenerative process and improve outcomes for patients suffering with ARF. In this chapter we illustrate some of the molecular responses of the kidney to an acute insult and demonstrate the effects of therapy with growth factors in the setting of experimental models of ARF. We conclude by demonstrating strategies that will provide future insights into the molecular response of the kidney to injury.

The regions of the nephron most susceptible to ischemic injury are the distal segment (S_3) of the proximal tubule and the medullary thick ascending limb of the loop of Henle. Following injury, there is loss of the epithelial lining as epithelial cells lose their integrin-mediated attachment to basement membranes and are sloughed into the lumen. An intense regenerative process follows. Normally quiescent renal tubule cells increase their nucleic acid synthesis and undergo mitosis. It is theorized that surviving cells situated close to or within the denuded area dedifferentiate and enter mitotic cycles. These cells then redifferentiate until nephron segment integrity is restored. The molecular basis that regulates this process is poorly-understood. After an injury, there is a spectrum of cell damage that is dependent on the type and severity of the insult. If the intensity of the insult is limited, cells become dysfunctional but survive. More severe injury results in detachment of cells from the tubule basement membranes, resulting in necrosis. Still other cells have no apparent damage and may proliferate to reepithelialize the damaged nephron segments. Thus, several

CHAPTER

17

different processes are required to achieve structural and functional integrity of the kidney after a toxic or ischemic insult: 1) uninjured cells must proliferate and reepithelialize damaged nephron segments; 2) nonlethally damaged cells must recover; and 3) some damaged cells may actually die—not as a result of the initial insult but through a process of programmed cell death known as apoptosis. Figure 17-1 provides a schematic representation of the renal response to an ischemic or toxic injury.

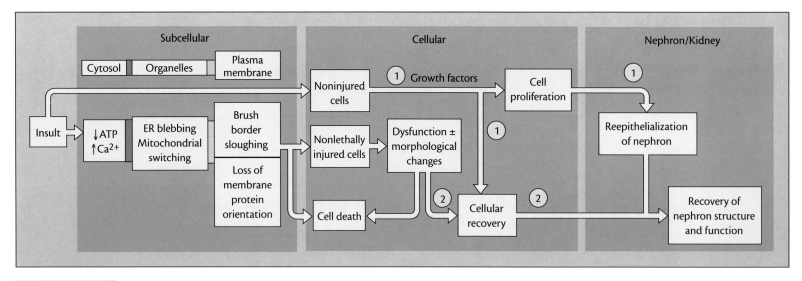

FIGURE 17-1

Schematic representation of some of the events pursuant to a renal insult and epithelial cell repair. **Subcellular;** Initial events include a decrease in cellular ATP and an increase in intracellular free calcium. There is blebbing of the endoplasmic reticulum with mitochondrial swelling and dysfunction. The brush border of the proximal tubules is sloughed into the tubule lumen, and there is redistribution of membrane proteins with the loss of cellular polarity. **Cellular;** At a cellular level this results in three populations of tubule cells, depending on the severity of the insult. Some cells are intact and are poised to participate in the proliferative process (*Pathway 1*). Growth factors participate by stimulating cells to undergo mitosis. Nonlethally injured cells have the potential to follow one of two pathways. In the appropriate setting, perhaps stimulated by growth factors, these cells may recover with restoration of cellular integrity and function (*Pathway 2*); however, if the injury is significant the cell may still die, but through a process of programmed cell death or apoptosis. The third population of cells are those with severe injury that undergo necrotic cell death. **Nephron/Kidney;** With the reepithelialization of damaged nephron segments and cellular recovery of structural and functional integrity, renal function is restored. (*Modified from* Toback [1]; with permission.)

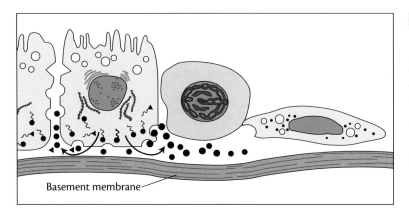

FIGURE 17-2

Growth regulation after an acute insult in regenerating renal tubule epithelial cells. Under the influence of growth-stimulating factors the damaged renal tubule epithelium is capable of regenerating with restoration of tubule integrity and function. The growth factors may be 1) produced by the tubule epithelium itself and act locally in an autocrine, juxtacrine or paracrine manner; 2) produced by surrounding cells to work in a paracrine manner; or 3) presented to the regenerating area via the circulation mediated by an endocrine mechanism. Cells at the edge of an injured nephron segment are illustrated on the left. These cells proliferate in response to the growth-stimulating factors. The middle cell is in the process of dividing and the cell on the right is migrating into the area of injury. (*Adapted from* Toback [1]; with permission.)

Growth Factors in Acute Renal Failure

GROWTH FACTORS IN ACUTE RENAL FAILURE

EGF	HGF
Ischemic and toxic	Ischemic and toxic
	Established ARF
IGF-I	
Ischemic and toxic	
Pretreatment and established ARF	

ARF—acute renal failure; EGF—epidermal growth factor; HGF—hepatocyte growth factor; IGF-I—insulin-like growth factor.

FIGURE 17-3

At least three growth factors have now been demonstrated to be useful as therapeutic agents in animal models of acute renal failure (ARF). These include epidermal growth factor (EGF), insulin-like growth factor I (IGF-I) and hepatocyte growth factor (HGF). All have efficacy in ischemia models and in a variety of toxic models of ARF. In addition, both IGF-I and HGF are beneficial when therapy is delayed and ARF is "established" after an ischemic insult. IGF-I has the additional advantage in that it also ameliorates the course of renal failure when given prophylactically before an acute ischemic insult.

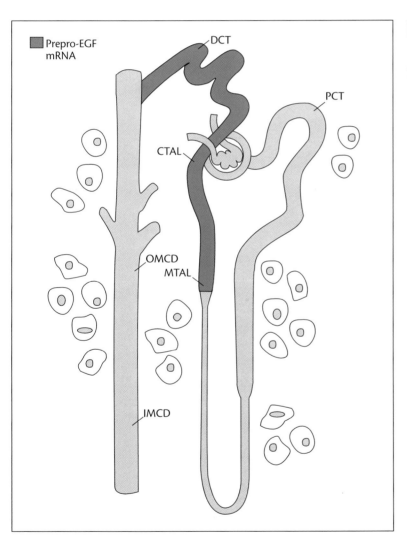

FIGURE 17-4

Expression of messenger RNA (mRNA) for prepro–epidermal growth factor (EGF) in kidney. This schematic depicts the localization of mRNA for prepro-EGF under basal states in kidney. Prepro-EGF mRNA is localized to the medullary thick ascending limbs (MTAL) and distal convoluted tubules (DCT). Immunohistochemical studies demonstrate that under basal conditions the peptide is located on the luminal membrane with the active peptide actually residing within the tubule lumen. It is speculated that, during pathologic states, preformed EGF is either transported or routed to the basolateral membrane or can enter the interstitium via backleak. After a toxic or ischemic insult, expression of EGF is rapidly suppressed and can remain low for a long time. Likewise, total renal content and renal excretion of EGF decreases. CTAL—cortical thick ascending limb; IMCD—inner medullary collecting duct; OMCD—outer medullary collecting duct; and PCT—proximal convoluted tubule.

GROWTH FACTOR PRODUCTION

EGF	IGF-I
Submandibular salivary glands	Liver
Kidney	Lung
Others	Kidney
	Heart
HGF	Muscle
Liver	Other organs
Spleen	
Kidney	
Lung	
Other organs	

FIGURE 17-5

Production of epidermal growth factor (EGF), insulin-like growth factor (IGF-I), and hepatocyte growth factor (HGF) by various tissues. EGF, IGF-I, and HGF have all been demonstrated to improve outcomes in various animal models of acute renal failure (ARF). All three growth-promoting factors are produced in the kidneys and in a variety of other organs. The local production is probably most important for recovery from an acute renal insult. The influence of production in other organs in the setting of ARF has yet to be determined. This chapter deals primarily with local production and actions of EGF, IGF-I, and HGF.

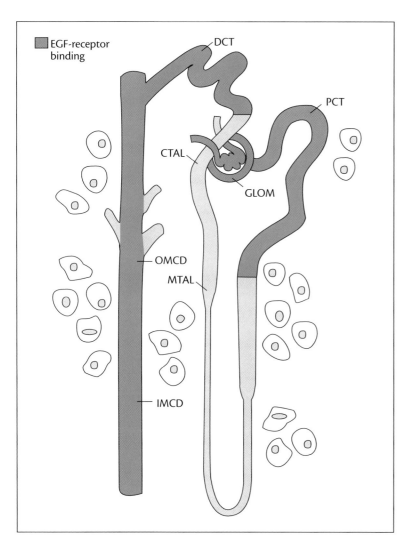

EGF-receptor binding

FIGURE 17-6

Receptor binding for epidermal growth factor (EGF). EGF binding in kidney under basal conditions is extensive. The most significant specific binding occurs in the proximal convoluted (PCT) and proximal straight tubules. There is also significant EGF binding in the glomeruli (GLOM), distal convoluted tubules (DCT), and the entire collecting duct (OMCD, IMCD). After an ischemic renal insult, EGF receptor numbers increase. This change in the renal EGF system may be responsible for the beneficial effect of exogenously administered EGF is the setting of acute renal failure. CTAL—cortical thick ascending loop.

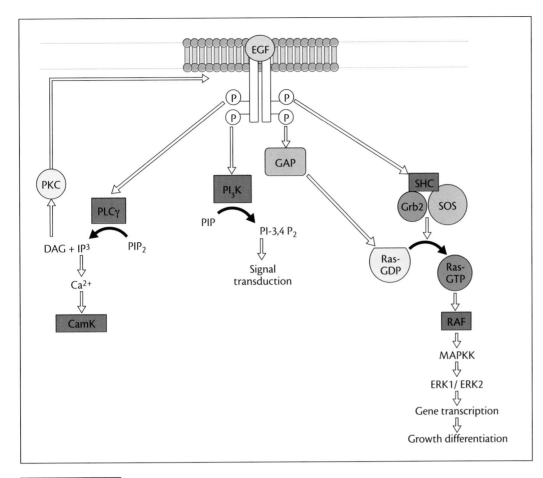

FIGURE 17-7

Epidermal growth factor (EGF)–mediated signal transduction pathways. The EGF receptor triggers the phospholipase C-gamma (PLC-gamma), phosphatidylinositol-3 kinase (PI₃K), and mitogen-activated protein kinase (MAPK) signal transduction pathways described in the text that follows.

Growth factors exert their downstream effects through their plasma membrane–bound protein tyrosine kinase (PTK) receptors. All known PTK receptors are found to have four major domains: 1) a glycosylated extracellular ligand-binding domain; 2) a transmembrane domain that anchors the receptor to the plasma membrane; 3) an intracellular tyrosine kinase domain; and 4) regulatory domains for the PTK activity. Upon ligand binding, the receptors dimerize and autophosphorylate, which leads to a cascade of intracellular events resulting in cellular proliferation, differentiation, and survival.

The tyrosine phosphorylated residues in the cytoplasmic domain of PTK are of utmost importance for its interactions with cytoplasmic proteins involved in EGF–mediated signal transduction pathways. The interactions of cytoplasmic proteins are governed by specific domains termed Src homology type 2 (SH2) and type 3 (SH3) domains. The SH2 domain is a conserved 100–amino acid sequence initially characterized in the PTK-Src and binds to tyrosine phosphorylated motifs in proteins; the SH3 domain binds to their targets through proline-rich sequences. SH2 domains have been found in a multitude of signal transducers and docking proteins such as growth factor receptor–bound protein 2 (Grb2), phophatidylinositol-3 kinase (p85-PI₃K), phospholipase C-gamma (PLC-gamma), guanosine triphosphatase (GTPase)–activating protein of ras (ras-GAP), and signal transducer and activator of transcription 3 (STAT-3).

Upon ligand binding and phosphorylation of PTKs, SH2–domain containing proteins interact with the receptor kinase domain. PLC-gamma on interaction with the PTK, becomes phosphorylated and catalyzes the turnover of phosphatidylinositol (PIP₂) to two other second messengers, inositol triphosphate (IP₃) and diacylglycerol (DAG).

DAG activates protein kinase C; IP₃ raises the intracellular calcium (Ca²⁺) levels by inducing its release from intracellular stores. Ca²⁺ is involved in the activation of the calmodulin-dependent CAM-kinase, which is a serine/threonine kinase.

A more important signal transduction pathway activated by PTKs concerns the ras pathway. The ras cycle is connected to activated receptors via the adapter protein Grb2 and the guanosine diphosphate-guanosine triphosphate exchange factor Sos (son of sevenless). GDP-ras, upon phosphorylation, is converted to its activated form, GTP-ras. The activated ras activates another Ser/Thr kinase called raf-1, which in turn activates another kinase, the mitogen activated protein kinase kinase (MAPKK). MAPKK activates the serine/threonine kinases, and extracellular signal-regulated kinases Erk1 and 2. Activation of Erk1/2 leads to translocation into the nucleus, where it phosphorylates key transcription factors such as Elk-1, and c-myc. Phosphorylated Elk-1 associates with serum response factor (SRF) and activates transcription of c-fos. The protein products of c-fos and c-jun function cooperatively as components of the mammalian transcription factor AP-1. AP-1 binds to specific DNA sequences in putative promoter sequences of target genes and regulates gene transcription. Similarly, c-myc forms a heterodimer with another immediate early gene max and regulates transcription.

The expression of c-fos, c-jun, and Egr-1 is found to be upregulated after ischemic renal injury. Immunohistochemical analysis showed the spatial expression of c-fos and Egr-1 to be in thick ascending limbs, where cells are undergoing minimal proliferation as compared with the S3 segments of the proximal tubules. This may suggest that the expression of immediate early genes after ischemic injury is not associated with cell proliferation.

Several mechanisms control the specificity of RTK signaling: 1) the specific ligand-receptor interaction; 2) the repertoire of substrates and signaling molecules associated with the activated RTK; 3) the existence of tissue-specific signaling molecules; and 4) the apparent strength and persistence of the biochemical signal. Interplay of these factors can determine whether a given ligand-receptor interaction lead to events such as growth, differentiation, scatter or survival.

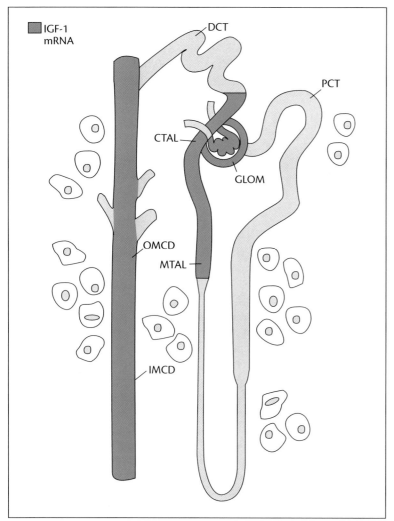

FIGURE 17-8

Expression of mRNA for insulin-like growth factor I (IGF-I). Under basal conditions, a variety of nephron segments can produce IGF-I. Glomeruli (GLOM), medullary and cortical thick ascending limbs (MTAL/CTAL), and collecting ducts (OMCD, IMCD) are all reported to produce IGF-I. Within hours of an acute ischemic renal insult, the expression of IGF-I decreases; however, 2 to 3 days after the insult, when there is intense regeneration, there is an increase in the expression of IGF-I in the regenerative cells. In addition, extratubule cells, predominantly macrophages, express IGF-I in the regenerative period. This suggests that IGF-I works by both autocrine and paracrine mechanisms during the regenerative process. DCT/PCT—distal/proximal convoluted tubule.

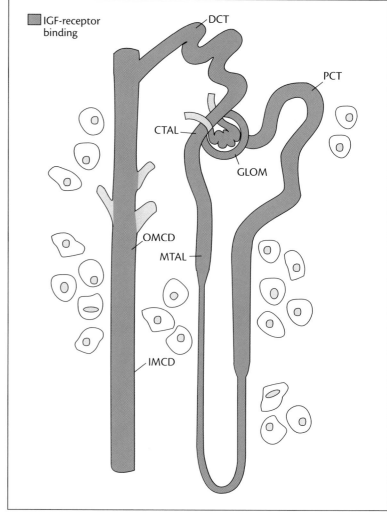

FIGURE 17-9

Receptor binding for insulin-like growth factor I (IGF-I). IGF-I binding sites are conspicuous throughout the normal kidney. Binding is higher in the structures of the inner medulla than in the cortex. After an acute ischemic insult, there is a marked increase in IGF-I binding throughout the kidney. The increase appears to be greatest in the regenerative zones, which include structures of the cortex and outer medulla. These findings suggest an important trophic effect of IGF-I in the setting of acute renal injury. CTAL/MTAL—cortical/medullary thick ascending loop; DCT/PCT—distal/proximal convoluted tubule; GLOM—glomerulus; OMCD/IMCD—outer/inner medullary collecting duct.

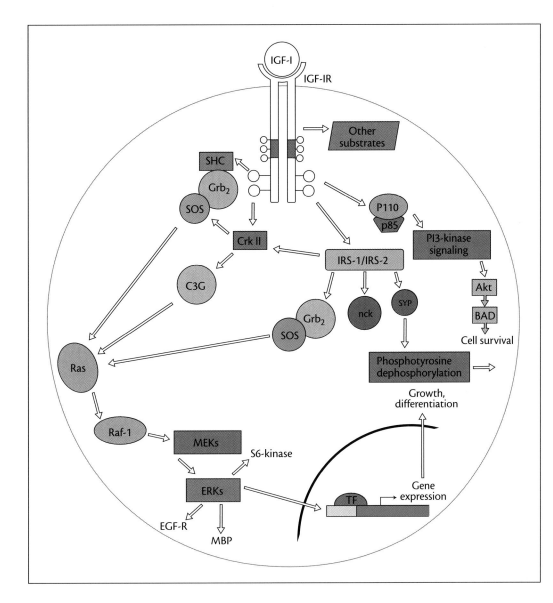

FIGURE 17-10

Diagram of intracellular signaling pathways mediated by the insulin-like growth factor I (IGF-IR) receptor. IGF-IR when bound to IGF-I undergoes autophosphorylation on its tyrosine residues. This enhances its intrinsic tyrosine kinase activity and phosphorylates multiple substrates, including insulin receptor substrate 1 (IRS-1), IRS-2, and Src homology/collagen (SHC). IRS-1 upon phosphorylation associates with the p85 subunit of the PI3-kinase (PI3K) and phosphorylates PI3-kinase. PI3K upon phosphorylation converts phosphoinositide-3 phosphate (PI-3P) into PI-3,4-P2, which in turn activates a serine-thronine kinase Akt (protein kinase B). Activated Akt kinase phosphorylates the proapoptotic factor Bad on a serine residue, resulting in its dissociation from B-cell lymphoma-X (Bcl-X_L) . The released Bcl-X_L is then capable of suppressing cell death pathways that involve the activity of apoptosis protease activating factor (Apaf-1), cytochrome C, and caspases. A number of growth factors, including platelet-derived growth factor (PDGF) and IGF 1 promotes cell survival. Activation of the PI3K cascade is one of the mechanisms by which growth factors mediate cell survival. Phosphorylated IRS-1 also associates with growth factor receptor bound protein 2 (Grb2), which bind son of sevenless (Sos) and activates the ras-raf-mitogen activated protein (ras/raf-MAP) kinase cascade. SHC also binds Grb2/Sos and activates the ras/raf-MAP kinase cascade. Other substrates for IGF-I are phosphotyrosine phosphatases and SH_2 domain containing tyrosine phosphatase (Syp). Figure 17-7 has details on the other signaling pathways in this figure. MBP—myelin basic protein; nck—an adaptor protein composed of SH2 and SH3 domains; TF—transcription factor.

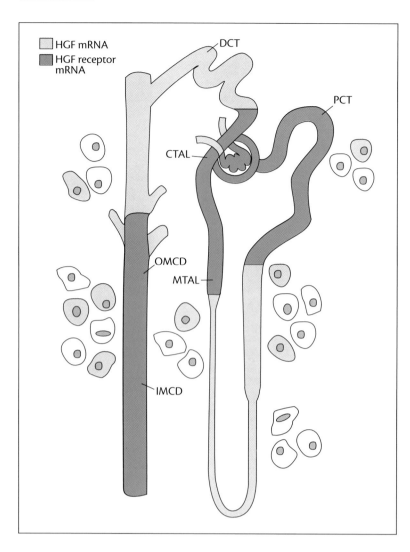

HGF mRNA
HGF receptor mRNA

DCT
PCT
CTAL
OMCD
MTAL
IMCD

FIGURE 17-11

Expression of hepatocyte growth factor (HGF) mRNA and HGF receptor mRNA in kidney. While the liver is the major source of circulating HGF, the kidney also produces this growth-promoting peptide. Experiments utilizing in situ hybridization, immunohisto-chemistry, and reverse transcription–polymerase chain reaction (RT-PCR) have demonstrated HGF production by interstitial cells but not by any nephron segment. Presumably, these interstitial cells are macrophages and endothelial cells. Importantly, HGF expression in kidney actually increases within hours of an ischemic or toxic insult. This expression peaks within 6 to 12 hours and is followed a short time later by an increase in HGF bioactivity. HGF thus seems to act as a renotrophic factor, partic-ipating in regeneration via a paracrine mechanism; however, its expression is also rapidly induced in spleen and lung in animal models of acute renal injury. Reported levels of circulating HGF in patients with acute renal failure suggest that an endocrine mechanism may also be operational.

The receptor for HGF is the c-met proto-oncogene product. Receptor binding has been demonstrated in kidney in a variety of sites, including the proximal convoluted (PCT) and straight tubules, medullary and cortical thick ascending limbs (MTAL, CTAL), and in the outer and inner medullary collecting ducts (OMCD, IMCD). As with HGF peptide production, expression of c-met mRNA is induced by acute renal injury.

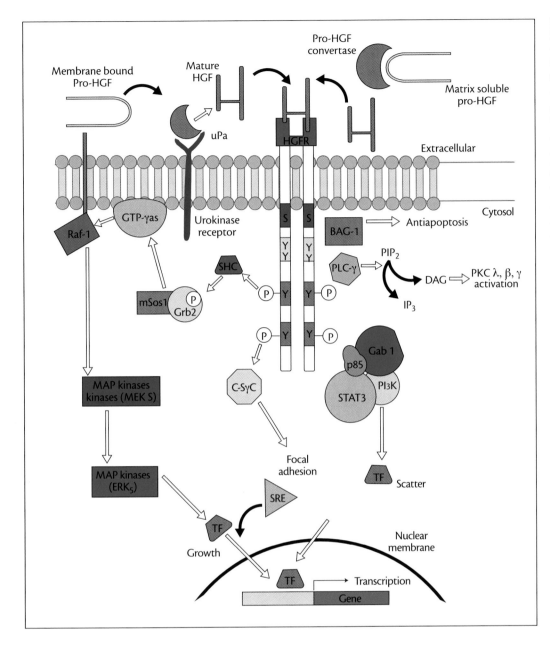

FIGURE 17-12

Model of hepatocyte growth factor (HGF)/c-met signal transduction. In the extracellular space, single-chain precursors of HGF bound to the proteoglycans at the cell surface are converted to the active form by urokinase plasminogen activator (uPA), while the matrix soluble precursor is processed by a serum derived pro-HGF convertase. HGF, upon binding to its receptor c-met, induces its dimerization as well as autophosphorylation of tyrosine residues. The phosphorylated residue binds to various adaptors and signal transducers such as growth factor receptor bound protein-2 (Grb2), p85-PI3 kinase, phospholipase C-gamma (PLC-gamma), signal transducer and activator of transcription-3 (STAT-3) and Src homology/collagen (SHC) via Src homology 2 (SH2) domains and triggers various signal transduction pathways. A common theme among tyrosine kinase receptors is that phosphorylation of different specific tyrosine residues determines which intracellular transducer will bind the receptor and be activated. In the case of HGF receptor, phosphorylation of a single multifunctional site triggers a pleiotropic response involving multiple signal transducers. The synchronous activation of several signaling pathways is essential to conferring the distinct invasive growth ability of the HGF receptor. HGF functions as a scattering (dissociation/motility) factor for epithelial cells, and this ability seems to be mediated through the activation of STAT-3.

Phosphorylation of adhesion complex regulatory proteins such as ZO-1, beta-catenin, and focal adhesion kinase (FAK) may occur via activation of c-src. Another Bcl_2 interacting protein termed BAG-1 mediates the antiapoptotic signal of HGF receptor by a mechanism of receptor association independent from tyrosine residues.

DETERMINANT MECHANISMS FOR OUTCOMES OF ACUTE RENAL FAILURE

Mitogenic	Anabolic
Morphogenic	Alter leukocyte function
Cell migration	Alter inflammatory process
Hemodynamic	Apoptosis
Cytoprotective	Others

FIGURE 17-13

Mechanisms by which growth factors may possibly alter outcomes of acute renal failure (ARF). Epidermal growth factor, insulin-like growth factor, and hepatocyte growth factor (HGF) have all been demonstrated to improve outcomes when administered in the setting of experimental ARF. While the results are the same, the respective mechanisms of actions of each of these growth factors are probably quite different. Many investigators have examined individual growth factors for a variety of properties that may be beneficial in the setting of ARF. This table lists several of the properties examined to date. Suffice it to say that the mechanisms by which the individual growth factors alter the course of experimental ARF is still unknown.

ACTIONS OF GROWTH FACTORS IN ACUTE RENAL FAILURE

Actions	IGF-I	EGF	HGF
Protein	↓/↑	↑/↓	↑
mRNA	↓/↑	↓	↑
Receptiors	↑	↑	↑
Vascular	↑	↓	↔
Anabolic	↑	↔	↔
Mitogenic	↑	↑↑↑	↑↑↑
Apoptosis	↓	↓↓	↓↓

FIGURE 17-14

Selected actions of growth factors in the setting of acute renal failure (ARF). After an acute renal injury, a spectrum of molecular responses occur involving the local expression of growth factors and their receptors. In addition, there is considerable variation in the mechanisms by which the growth factors are beneficial for ARF. After an acute renal insult there is an initial decrease in both insulin-like growth factor (IGF-I) peptide and mRNA, which recovers over several days but only after the regenerative process is under way. The pattern with epidermal growth factor (EGF) is different in that a transient increase in available mature peptide from cleavage of preformed EGF is followed by a pronounced and prolonged decrease in both peptide and message. Both peptide and message for hepatocyte growth factor (HGF) are transiently increased in kidney after a toxic or an ischemic insult. The receptors for all three growth factors are increased after injury, which may be crucial to the response to exogenous administration.

The mechanism by which the different growth factors act in the setting of acute renal injury is quite variable. IGF-I is known to increase renal blood flow and glomerular filtration rate in both normal animals and those with acute renal injury. To the other extreme, EGF is a vasoconstrictor and HGF is vasoneutral. IGF-I has an additional advantage in that it has anabolic properties, and ARF is an extremely catabolic state. Neither EGF nor HGF seems to affect nutritional parameters. Finally, both EGF and HGF are potent mitogens for renal proximal tubule cells, the nephron segment is most often damaged by ischemic acute renal injury, whereas IGF-I is only a modest mitogen. Likewise, both EGF and HGF appear to be more effective than IGF-I at inhibiting apoptosis in the setting of acute renal injury, but it is not clear whether this is an advantage or a disadvantage.

Clinical Use of Growth Factors in Acute Renal Failure

RATIONALE FOR INSULIN-LIKE GROWTH FACTOR I (IGF-I) IN ACUTE RENAL FAILURE

Receptors are present on proximal tubules
Regulates proximal tubule metabolism and transport
Increases renal plasma flow and glomerular filtration rates
Mitogenic for proximal tubule cells
Enhanced expression after acute renal injury
Anabolic

FIGURE 17-15

Rationale for the use of insulin-like growth factor IGF-I in the setting of acute renal failure (ARF). Of the growth factors that have been demonstrated to improve outcomes after acute renal injury, the most progress has been made with IGF-I. From this table, it is evident that IGF-I has a broad spectrum of activities, which makes it a logical choice for treatment of ARF. An agent that increased renal plasma flow and glomerular filtration rate and was mitogenic for proximal tubule cells and anabolic would address several features of ARF.

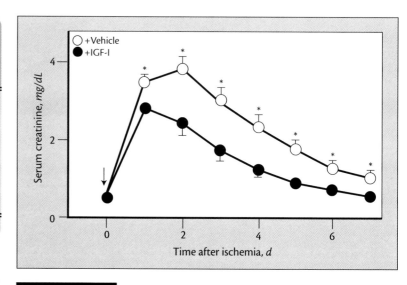

FIGURE 17-16

Serial serum creatinine values in rats with ischemic acute renal failure (ARF) treated with insulin-like growth factor (IGF-I) or vehicle. This is the original animal experiment that demonstrated a benefit from IGF-I in the setting of ARF. In this study, IGF-I was administered beginning 30 minutes after the ischemic insult (*arrow*). Data are expressed as mean ± standard error. Significant differences between groups are indicated by asterisks.

This experiment has been reproduced, with variations, by several groups, with similar findings. IGF-I has now been demonstrated to be beneficial when administered prophylactically before an ischemic injury and when started as late as 24 hours after reperfusion when injury is established. It has also been reported to improve outcomes for a variety of toxic injuries and is beneficial in a model of renal transplantation with delayed graft function and in cyclosporine-induced acute renal insufficiency. (*From* Miller *et al.* [2]; with permission.)

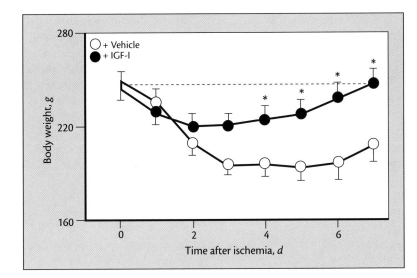

FIGURE 17-17

Body weights of rats with ischemic acute renal failure (ARF) treated with insulin-like growth factor (IGF-I) or vehicle. Unlike epidermal growth factor or hepatocyte growth factor (HGF), IGF-I is anabolic even in the setting of acute renal injury. These data are from the experiment described in Figure 17-16. As the data in this figure demonstrate, ARF is a highly catabolic state: vehicle-treated animals experience 15% weight reduction. Animals that received IGF-I experienced only a 5% reduction in body weight and were back to baseline by 7 days. Data are expressed as mean ± standard error. Significant differences between groups are indicated by asterisks. (*From* Miller *et al.* [2]; with permission.)

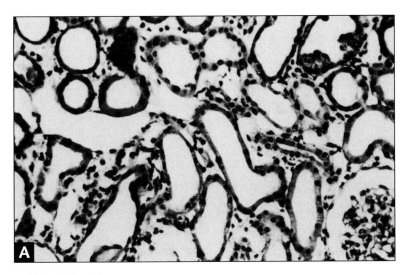
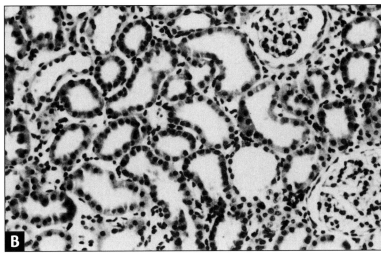

FIGURE 17-18

Photomicrograph of kidneys from rats with acute renal failure (ARF) treated with insulin-like growth factor (IGF-I) or vehicle. These photomicrographs are of histologic sections stained with hematoxylin and eosin originating from kidneys of rats that received vehicle or IGF 1 after ischemic renal injury. Kidneys were obtained 7 days after the insult. There is evidence of considerable residual injury in the kidney from the vehicle-treated rat (**A**): dilation and simplification of tubules, interstitial calcifications, and papillary proliferations the tubule lumen of proximal tubules. The kidney obtained from the IGF-I–treated rat (**B**) appears almost normal, showing evidence of regeneration and restoration of normal renal architecture. In this experiment the histologic appearance of kidneys from the IGF-I–treated animals was statistically better than that of the vehicle-treated controls, as determined by a pathologist blinded to therapy. (*From* Miller *et al.* [2]; with permission.)

THERAPEUTIC TRIALS OF INSULIN-LIKE GROWTH FACTOR I IN HUMANS

Growth hormone–resistant short stature
  Laron-type dwarfism

Anabolic agent in catabolic states
  AIDS (Protein wasting malnutrition)
  Burns
  Corticosteroid therapy
  Postoperative state

Insulin-dependent and non–insulin-dependent diabetes mellitus
Acute renal failure
Chronic renal failure

FIGURE 17-19

Reported therapeutic trials of insulin-like growth factor (IGF-I) in humans. Based on the compelling animal data and the fact that there are clearly identified disease states involving both

over- and underexpression of IGF-I, this is the first growth factor that has been used in clinical trials for kidney disease. Listed above are a variety of studies of the effects of IGF-I in humans. This peptide has now been examined in several published studies of both acute and chronic renal failure. Additional studies are currently in progress.

In the area of acute renal failure there are now two reported trials of IGF-I. In the initial study IGF-I or placebo was administered to patients undergoing surgery involving the suprarenal aorta or the renal arteries. This group was selected as it best simulated the work that had been reported in animal trials of ischemic acute renal injury. Fifty-four patients were randomized in a double-blind, placebo-controlled trial of IGF-I to prevent the acute decline in renal function frequently associated with this type of surgery. The primary end-point in this study was the incidence of renal dysfunction, defined as a reduction of the glomerular filtration rate as compared with a preoperative baseline, at each of three measurements obtained during the 3 postoperative days. Modern surgical techniques have decreased the incidence of acute renal failure to such a low level, even in this high-risk group, so as to make it impractical to perform a single center trial with enough power to obtain differences in clinically important end-points. Thus, this trial was intended only to offer "proof of concept" that IGF-I is useful for patients with acute renal injuries.

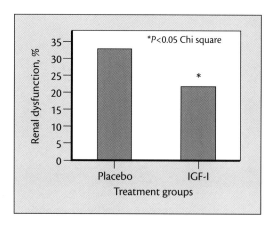

FIGURE 17-20

Incidence of postoperative renal dysfunction treated with insulin (IGF-I) or placebo. IGF-I significantly reduced the incidence of postoperative renal dysfunction in these high-risk patients. Renal dysfunction occurred in 33% of those who received placebo but in only 22% of patients treated with IGF-I. The groups were well-matched with respect to age, sex, type of operation, ischemia time, and baseline renal function as defined by serum creatinine or glomerular filtration rate. The IGF-I was tolerated well: no side effects were attributed to the drug. Secondary end-points such as discharge, serum creatinine, length of hospitalization, length of stay in the intensive care unit, or duration of intubation were not significantly different between the two groups. (*Adapted from* Franklin, *et al.* [3]; with permission.)

LACK OF EFFECT OF RECOMBINANT HUMAN IGF-I IN PATIENTS WITH ARF*

Multicenter, double-blind, randomized, placebo-controlled
ARF secondary to surgery, trauma, hypertensive nephropathy, sepsis, or drugs
Treated within the first 6 days for 14 days
Evaluated renal function and mortality

*No difference between the groups were observed in final values or changes in values for glomerular filtration rates, urine volumes, or mortality at 14 or 28 days.
ARF—acute renal failure; IGF-I—insulin-like growth factor.

FIGURE 17-21

Summary of an abstract describing the trial of insulin-like growth factor (IGF-I) in the treatment of patients with established acute renal failure (ARF). Based on the accumulated animal and human data, a multicenter, double-blind, randomized, placebo-controlled trial was performed to examine the effects of IGF-I in patients with established ARF. Enrolled patients had ARF of a wide variety of causes, including surgery, trauma, hypertension, sepsis, and nephrotoxic injury. Approximately 75 patients were enrolled, treatment being initiated within 6 days of the renal insult. Renal function was evaluated by iodothalimate clearance. Unfortunately, at an interim analysis (the study was originally designed to enroll 150 patients) there was no difference in renal function or survival between the groups. The investigators recognized several potential problems with the trial, including the severity of many patients' illnesses, the variety of causes of the renal injury, and delay in initiating therapy [4].

ADVANTAGES OF IGF-I

Well-tolerated

Safe in short-term studies

Experience with diseases of overexpression and underexpression

Did not worsen outcomes

IGF-I—insulin-like growth factor.

FIGURE 17-22

Advantages of insulin-like growth factor (IGF-I) in the treatment of acute renal failure. The limited data obtained to date on the use of IGF-I for acute renal failure demonstrate that the peptide is well-tolerated and may be useful in selected patient populations. Additional human trials are ongoing including use in the settings of renal transplantation and chronic renal failure.

GROWTH FACTOR LIMITATIONS IN ACUTE RENAL FAILURE

Lack of basic knowledge of the pathophysiology of ARF

No screening system for compounds to treat ARF

Animal models may not be relevant

Animal studies have not predicted results in human trials

Difficulty of identifying appropriate target populations

ARF—acute renal failure.

FIGURE 17-23

Limitations in the use of growth factors to treat acute renal failure (ARF). The disappointing results of several recent clinical trials of ARF therapy reflect the fact that our understanding of its pathophysiology is still limited. Screening compounds using animal models may be irrelevant. Most laboratories use relatively young animals, even though ARF frequently affects older humans, whose organ regenerative capacity may be limited. In addition, our laboratory models are usually based on a single insult, whereas many of our patients suffer repeated or multiple insults. Until we gain a better understanding of the basic pathogenic mechanisms of ARF, studies in human patients are likely to be frustrating.

Future Directions

MOLECULAR RESPONSE TO RENAL ISCHEMIC/REPERFUSION INJURY

Genes	1 Hour	1 Day	2 Days	5 Days	References
Transcription factors					
c-jun	↑	↔			Bardella *et al.* [5]
c-fos	↑	↔			Ouellette *et al.* [6]
Egr-1	↑	↔			Bonventre *et al.* [7]
Kid 1	↔	↓	↓	↓	Witzgall *et al.* [8]
Cytokines					
JE	↑	↑	↑	↑	Safirstein *et al.* [9]
KC	↑	↔			"
IL-2				↑	Goes *et al.* [10]
IL-10		↑		↑	"
IFN-γ				↑	"
GM-CSF		↑		↑	"
MIP-2	↑	↑			Singh *et al.* [11]
IL-6	↑	↑			"
IL-11	↑	↑			"
LIF	↑	↑			"
PTHrP	↑	↑	↔	↔	Soifer *et al.* [12]
Endothelin 1	↑ (6 h)	↑	↑		Firth and Ratcliffe [13]
Endothelin 3	↓ (6 h)	↓	↓		"

(Table continued on next page)

FIGURE 17-24

A list of genes whose expression is induced at various time points by ischemic renal injury. The molecular response of the kidney to an ischemic insult is complex and is the subject of investigations by several laboratories.

(Continued on next page)

MOLECULAR RESPONSE TO RENAL ISCHEMIC/REPERFUSION INJURY (Continued)

Genes	1 Hour	1 Day	2 Days	5 Days	References
Cell cycle markers					
PCNA			↑	↑	Witzgall et al. [14]
Vimentin			↑	↑	"
Apoptosis					
Clusterin	↑	↑	↑		Witzgall et al. [14]
Bcl2	↔	↑	↑	↔	Basile et al. [15]
Bax	↔	↑	↑	↑	"
Growth factors and receptors					
IGF-I			↑	↑	Matejka et al. [16]
HGF	↑ (6 h)	↔	↔		Ishibashi et al. [17]
HGF-R (c-met)	↑ (6 h)	↔	↔		"
EGF	↓	↓	↓	↓	Safirstein et al. [18]
TGF-β1		↑	↑	↑	Basile et al. [19]
Signal transduction					
RACK1		↑	↑	↑	Padanilam et al. [20]
PKC-α		↑			La Porta and Comolli [21]
SAPK	↑	↔	↔	↔	Pombo et al. [22]
c-ros		↑			Safirstein et al. [23]
Heat shock proteins					
HSP-32 (heme oxygenase-1)		↑	↔		Raju et al. [24]
HSP-70	↑	↔			Van Why et al. [25]
HSP-72	↑	↑	↑		"
ECM Components					
Osteopontin		↑	↑	↑	Padanilam et al. [26]
Laminin		↓	↓	↑	Walker [27]
Fibronectin	↑	↑	↑	↑	"
Collagen type IV		↔	↔	↔	"
Others					
Na+-K+-ATPase	↓	↓			Van Why et al. [28]
H-K-ATPase	↑	↔			Wang et al. [29]
Na/H exchanger (NHE3)	↓	↓			"
Tamm Horsfall protein	↔	↓	↓		Safirstein et al. [18]
Annexin I (p35)			↑		McKanna et al. [30]
PLA2	↑				Nakamura et al. [31]
Calcyclin		↑	↑	↑	Lewington et al. [32]

FIGURE 17-24 (Continued)

Several genes have already been identified to be induced or down-regulated after ischemia and reperfusion. This table lists genes whose expression is altered as a result of ischemic injury. It is not clear at present if the varied expression of these genes plays a role in cell injury, survival, or proliferation.

IDENTIFICATION OF DIFFERENTIALLY EXPRESSED GENES

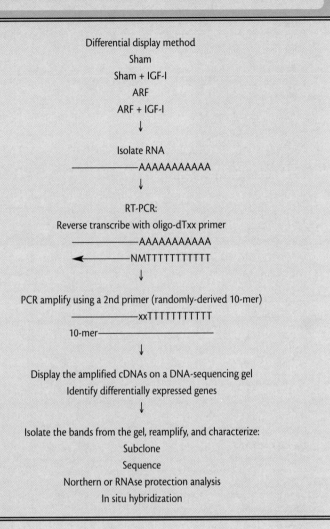

Differential display method

Sham

Sham + IGF-I

ARF

ARF + IGF-I

↓

Isolate RNA

————————AAAAAAAAAA

↓

RT-PCR:

Reverse transcribe with oligo-dTxx primer

————————AAAAAAAAAA

◄————NMTTTTTTTTTTT

↓

PCR amplify using a 2nd primer (randomly-derived 10-mer)

————————xxTTTTTTTTTTT

10-mer————————

↓

Display the amplified cDNAs on a DNA-sequencing gel

Identify differentially expressed genes

↓

Isolate the bands from the gel, reamplify, and characterize:

Subclone

Sequence

Northern or RNAse protection analysis

In situ hybridization

FIGURE 17-25

Schematic representation of differential display. In a complex organ like the kidney, ischemic renal injury triggers altered expression of various cell factors and vascular components. Depending on the severity of the insult, expression of these genes can vary in individual cells, leading to their death, survival, or proliferation. A better understanding of the various factors and the signal transduction pathways transduced by them that contribute to cell death can lead to development of therapeutic strategies to interfere with the process of cell death. Similarly, identification of factors that are involved in initiating cell migration, dedifferentiation, and proliferation may lead to therapy aimed at accelerating the regeneration program. To identify the various factors involved in cell injury and regeneration, powerful methods for identification and cloning of differentially expressed genes are critical. One such method that has been used extensively by several laboratories is the differential display polymerase chain reaction (DD-PCR).

In this schematic, mRNA is derived from kidneys of sham-operated (controls) and ischemia-injured rats, some pretreated with insulin-like growth factor (IGF-I). The mRNAs are reverse transcribed using an anchored deoxy thymidine-oligonucleotide (oligo-dT) primer (*Example*: dT[12]-MX, where M represent G, A, or C, and X represents one of the four nucleotides). An anchored primer limits the reverse transcription to a subset of mRNAs. The first strand cDNA is then PCR amplified using an arbitrary 10 nucleotide-oligomer primer and the anchored primer. The PCR reaction is performed in the presence of radioactive or fluorescence-labeled nucleotides, so that the amplified fragments can be displayed on a sequencing gel. Bands of interest can be excised from the gel and used for further characterization. ARF—acute renal failure.

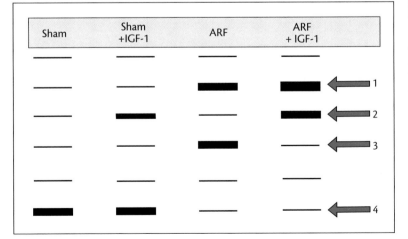

FIGURE 17-26

Schematic representation of a differential display gel in which mRNA from kidneys is reverse-transcribed and polymerase chain reaction (PCR) amplified (*see* Figure 17-25). The PCR amplification is conducted in the presence of radioactive nucleotides. The cDNA fragments corresponding to the 3' end of the mRNA species are displayed by running them on a sequencing gel, followed by autoradiography. The arrows show bands corresponding to mRNA transcripts that are expressed differentially 1) in response to insulin-like growth factor (IGF-I) treatment and induction of ischemic injury; 2) in an IGF-I–dependent manner; 3) in response to induction of ischemic injury; and 4) to genes that are down-regulated after induction of ischemic injury. ARF—acute renal failure.

References

1. Toback GF: Regeneration after acute tubular necrosis. *Kidney Int* 1992, 41:226–246.

2. Miller SB, Martin DR, Kissane J, Hammerman, MR: Insulin-like growth factor I accelerates recovery from ischemic acute tubular necrosis in the rat. *Proc Natl Acad Sci USA* 1992, 89:11876–11880.

3. Franklin SC, Moulton M, Sicard GA, *et al.*: Insulin-like growth factor I preserves renal function postoperatively. *Am J Physiol* 1997, 272:F257–F259.

4. Kopple JD, Hirschberg R, Guler H-P, *et al.*: Lack of effect of recombinant human insulin-like growth factor I (IGF-I) in patients with acute renal failure (ARF). *J Amer Soc Nephro* 1996, 7:1375.

5. Bardella L, Comolli R: Differential expression of c-jun, c-fos and hsp 70 mRNAs after folic acid and ischemia reperfusion injury: effect of antioxidant treatment. *Exp Nephrol* 1994, 2:158–165.

6. Ouellette AJ, *et al.*: Expression of two "immediate early" genes, Egr-1 and c-fos, in response to renal ischemia and during compensatory renal hypertrophy in mice. *J Clin Invest* 1990, 85:766–771.

7. Bonventre JV, *et al.*: Localization of the protein product of the immediate early growth response gene, Egr-1, in the kidney after ischemia and reperfusion. *Cell Regulation* 1991, 2:251–60.

8. Witzgall R, *et al.*: Kid-1, a putative renal transcription factor: regulation during ontogeny and in response to ischemia and toxic injury. *Mol Cell Biol* 1993, 13:1933–1942.

9. Safirstein R, *et al.*: Expression of cytokine-like genes JE and KC is increased during renal ischemia. *Amer J Physiol* 1991, 261:F1095–F1101.

10. Goes N, *et al.*: Ischemic acute tubular necrosis induces an extensive local cytokine response. Evidence for induction of interferon-gamma, transforming growth factor-beta 1, granulocyte-macrophage colony–stimulating factor, interleukin-2, and interleukin-10. *Transplantation* 1995, 59:565–572.

11. Singh AK, *et al.*: Prominent and sustained upregulation of MIP-2 and gp130 signaling cytokines in murine renal ischemic-reperfusion injury. *J Am Soc Nephrol* 1997, 8:595A.

12. Soifer NE, *et al.*: Expression of parathyroid hormone–related protein in the rat glomerulus and tubule during recovery from renal ischemia. *J Clin Invest* 1993, 92:2850–2857.

13. Firth JD, Ratcliffe PJ: Organ distribution of the three rat endothelin messenger RNAs and the effects of ischemia on renal gene expression. *J Clin Invest* 1992, 90:1023–1031.

14. Witzgall R, *et al.*: Localization of proliferating cell nuclear antigen, vimentin, c-Fos, and clusterin in the postischemic kidney. Evidence for a heterogeneous genetic response among nephron segments, and a large pool of mitotically active and dedifferentiated cells. *J Clin Invest* 1994, 93:2175–2188.

15. Basile DP, Liapis H, Hammerman MR: Expression of bcl-2 and bax in regenerating rat renal tubules following ischemic injury. *Am J Physiol* 1997, 272:F640–F647.

16. Matejka GL, Jennische E: IGF-I binding and IGF-1 mRNA expression in the post-ischemic regenerating rat kidney. *Kidney Int* 1992, 42(5):1113–1123.

17. Ishibashi K, *et al.*: Expressions of receptor for hepatocyte growth factor in kidney after unilateral nephrectomy and renal injury. *Biochem Biophys Res Commun* 1993, 187:1454–1459.

18. Safirstein R, *et al.*: Changes in gene expression after temporary renal ischemia. *Kidney Int* 1990, 37:1515–1521.

19. Basile DP, *et al.*: Increased transforming growth factor-beta 1 expression in regenerating rat renal tubules following ischemic injury. *Amer J Physiol* 1996, 270:F500–F509.

20. Padanilam BJ, Hammerman MR: Ischemia-induced receptor for activated C kinase (RACK1) expression in rat kidneys. *Amer J Physiol* 1997, 272:F160–F166.

21. Pombo CM, *et al.*: The stress-activated protein kinases are major c-Jun amino-terminal kinases activated by ischemia and reperfusion. *J Biol Chem* 1994, 269:26546–26551.

22. Safirstein R: Gene expression in nephrotoxic and ischemic acute renal failure [editorial]. *J Am Soc Nephrol* 1994, 4:1387–1395.

23. Safirstein R, Zelent AZ, Price PM: Reduced renal prepro-epidermal growth factor mRNA and decreased EGF excretion in ARF. *Kid Int* 1989, 36:810–815.

24. Raju VS, Maines, MD: Renal ischemia/reperfusion up-regulates heme oxygenase-1 (HSP32) expression and increases cGMP in rat heart. *J Pharmacol Exp Ther* 1996, 277:1814–1822.

25. Van Why SK, *et al.*: Induction and intracellular localization of HSP-72 after renal ischemia. *Am J Physiol* 1992, 263:F769–F775.

26. Padanilam BJ, Martin DR, Hammerman MR: Insulin-like growth factor I–enhanced renal expression of osteopontin after acute ischemic injury in rats. *Endocrinology* 1996, 137:2133–2140.

27. Walker PD: Alterations in renal tubular extracellular matrix components after ischemia-reperfusion injury to the kidney. *Lab Invest* 1994, 70:339–345.

28. Van Why SK, *et al.*: Expression and molecular regulation of Na+-K+-ATPase after renal ischemia. *Am J Physiol* 1994, 267:F75–F85.

29. Wang Z, *et al.*: Ischemic-reperfusion injury in the kidney: overexpression of colonic H+-K+-ATPase and suppression of NHE-3. *Kidney Int* 1997, 51:1106–1115.

30. McKanna JA, *et al.*: Localization of p35 (annexin I, lipocortin I) in normal adult rat kidney and during recovery from ischemia. *J Cell Physiol* 1992, 153:467–76.

31. Nakamura H, *et al.*: Subcellular characteristics of phospholipase A2 activity in the rat kidney. Enhanced cytosolic, mitochondrial, and microsomal phospholipase A2 enzymatic activity after renal ischemia and reperfusion. *J Clin Invest* 1991, 87:1810–1818.

32. Lewington AJP, Padanilam BJ, Hammerman MR: Induction of calcyclin after ischemic injury to rat kidney. *Am J Physiol* 1997, 273(42):F380–F385.

Nutrition and Metabolism in Acute Renal Failure

Wilfred Druml

Adequate nutritional support is necessary to maintain protein stores and to correct pre-existing or disease-related deficits in lean body mass. The objectives for nutritional support for patients with acute renal failure (ARF) are not much different from those with other catabolic conditions. The principles of nutritional support for ARF, however, differ from those for patients with chronic renal failure (CRF), because diets or infusions that satisfy minimal requirements in CRF are not necessarily sufficient for patients with ARF.

In patients with ARF modern nutritional therapy must include a tailored regimen designed to provide substrate requirements with various degrees of stress and hypercatabolism. If nutrition is provided to a patient with ARF the composition of the dietary program must be specifically designed because there are complex metabolic abnormalities that affect not only water, electrolyte, and acid-base-balance but also carbohydrate, lipid, and protein and amino acid utilization.

In patients with ARF the main determinants of nutrient requirements (and outcome) are not renal dysfunction per se but the degree of hypercatabolism caused by the disease associated with ARF, the nutritional state, and the type and frequency of dialysis therapy. Pre-existing or hospital-acquired malnutrition has been identified as an important contributor to the persisting high mortality in critically ill persons.

Thus, with modern nutritional support requirements must be met for all nutrients necessary for preservation of lean body mass, immunocompetence, and wound healing for a patient who has acquired ARF—in may instances among other complications. At the same time the specific metabolic alterations and demands in ARF and the impaired excretory renal function must be respected to limit uremic toxicity.

In this chapter the multiple metabolic alterations associated with ARF are reviewed, methods for estimating nutrient requirements are discussed and, current concepts for the type and composition of nutritional programs are summarized. This information is relevant for designing nutritional support in an individual patient with ARF.

CHAPTER

18

NUTRITION IN ACUTE RENAL FAILURE

Goals

Preservation of lean body mass

Stimulation of wound healing and reparatory functions

Stimulation of immunocompetence

Acceleration of renal recovery (?)

But not (in contrast to stable CRF)

Minimization of uremic toxicity (perform hemodialysis and CRRT as required)

Retardation of progression of renal failure

Thus, provision of optimal but not minimal amounts of substrates

FIGURE 18-1

Nutritional goals in patients with acute renal failure (ARF). The goals of nutritional intervention in ARF differ from those in patients with chronic renal failure (CRF): One should not provide a minimal intake of nutrients (to minimize uremic toxicity or to retard progression of renal failure, as recommended for CRF) but rather an optimal amount of nutrients should be provided for correction and prevention of nutrient deficiencies and for stimulation of immunocompetence and wound healing in the mostly hypercatabolic patients with ARF [1].

METABOLIC PERTURBATIONS IN ACUTE RENAL FAILURE

Determined by	Plus
Renal dysfunction (acute uremic state)	Specific effects of renal replacement therapy
Underlying illness	
The acute disease state, such as systemic inflammatory response syndrome (SIRS)	Nonspecific effects of extracorporeal circulation (bioincompatibility)
Associated complications (such as infections)	

FIGURE 18-2

Metabolic perturbations in acute renal failure (ARF). In most instances ARF is a complication of sepsis, trauma, or multiple organ failure, so it is difficult to ascribe specific metabolic alterations to ARF. Metabolic derangements will be determined by the acute uremic state plus the underlying disease process or by complications such as severe infections and organ dysfunctions and, last but not least by the type and frequency of renal replacement therapy [1, 2].

Nevertheless, ARF does not affect only water, electrolyte, and acid base metabolism: it induces a global change of the metabolic environment with specific alterations in protein and amino acid, carbohydrate, and lipid metabolism [2].

Metabolic Alterations in Acute Renal Failure

Energy metabolism

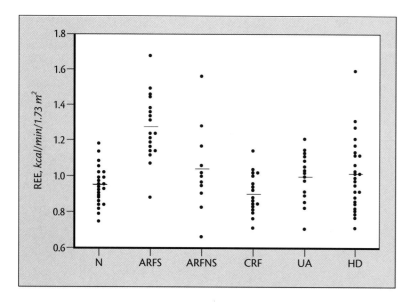

FIGURE 18-3

Energy metabolism in acute renal failure (ARF). In experimental animals ARF decreases oxygen consumption even when hypothermia and acidosis are corrected (uremic hypometabolism) [3]. In contrast, in the clinical setting oxygen consumption of patients with various form of renal failure is remarkably little changed [4]. In subjects with chronic renal failure (CRF), advanced uremia (UA), patients on regular hemodialysis therapy (HD) but also in patients with uncomplicated ARF (ARFNS) resting energy expenditure (REE) was comparable to that seen in controls (N). However, in patients with ARF and sepsis (ARFS) REE is increased by approximately 20%.

Thus, energy expenditure of patients with ARF is more determined by the underlying disease than acute uremic state and taken together these data indicate that when uremia is well-controlled by hemodialysis or hemofiltration there is little if any change in energy metabolism in ARF. In contrast to many other acute disease processes ARF might rather decrease than increase REE because in multiple organ dysfunction syndrome oxygen consumption was significantly higher in patients without impairment of renal function than in those with ARF [5]. (*From* Schneeweiss [4]; with permission.)

ESTIMATION OF ENERGY REQUIREMENTS

Calculation of resting energy expenditure (REE) (Harris Benedict equation):

Males: $66.47 \div (13.75 \times BW) \div (5 \times height) - (6.76 \times age)$

Females: $655.1 \div (9.56 \times BW) \div (1.85 \times height) - (4.67 \times age)$

The average REE is approximately 25 kcal/kg BW/day

Stress factors to correct calculated energy requirement for hypermetabolism:

Postoperative (no complications) 1.0

Long bone fracture 1.15–1.30

Cancer 1.10–1.30

Peritonitis/sepsis 1.20–1.30

Severe infection/polytrauma 1.20–1.40

Burns (= approxim. REE + % burned body surface area) 1.20–2.00

Corrected energy requirements (kcal/d) = REE $\times$ stress factor

FIGURE 18-4

Estimation of energy requirements. Energy requirements of patients with acute renal failure (ARF) have been grossly over-estimated in the past and energy intakes of more than 50 kcal/kg of body weight (BW) per day (*ie*, about 100% above resting energy expenditure (REE) haven been advocated [6]. Adverse effects of overfeeding have been extensively documented during the last decades, and it should be noted that energy intake must not exceed the actual energy consumption. Energy requirements can be calculated with sufficient accuracy by standard formulas such as the Harris Benedict equation. Calculated REE should be multiplied with a stress factor to correct for hypermetabolic disease; however, even in hypercatabolic conditions such as sepsis or multiple organ dysfunction syndrome, energy requirements rarely exceed 1.3 times calculated REE [1].

Protein metabolism

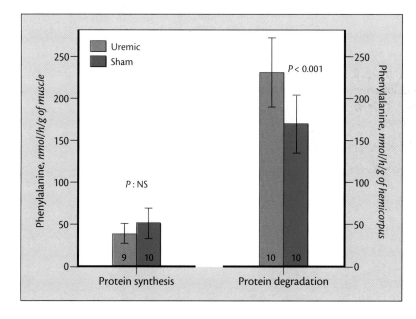

FIGURE 18-5

Protein metabolism in acute renal failure (ARF): activation of protein catabolism. Protein synthesis and degradation rates in acutely uremic and sham-operated rats. The hallmark of metabolic alterations in ARF is activation of protein catabolism with excessive release of amino acids from skeletal muscle and sustained negative nitrogen balance [7, 8]. Not only is protein breakdown accelerated, but there also is defective muscle utilization of amino acids for protein synthesis. In muscle, the maximal rate of insulin-stimulated protein synthesis is depressed by ARF and protein degradation is increased, even in the presence of insulin [9]. (*From* [8]; with permission.)

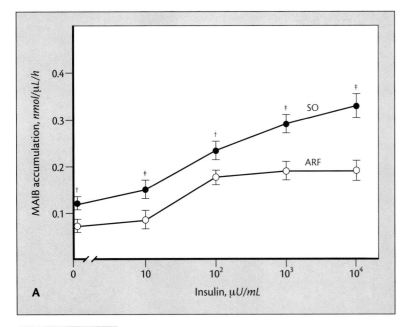

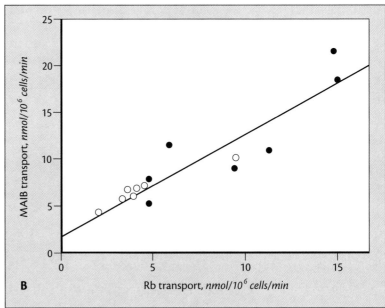

FIGURE 18-6

Protein metabolism in acute renal failure (ARF): impairment of cellular amino acid transport. **A,** Amino acid transport into skeletal muscle is impaired in ARF [10]. Transmembranous uptake of the amino acid analogue methyl-amino-isobutyrate (MAIB) is reduced in uremic tissue in response to insulin (muscle tissue from uremic animals, *black circles*, and from sham-operated animals, *open circles*, respectively). Thus, insulin responsiveness is reduced in ARF tissue, but, as can be seen from the parallel shift of the curves, insulin sensitivity is maintained (*see also* Fig. 18-14). This abnormality can be linked both to insulin resistance and to a generalized defect in ion transport in uremia; both the activity and receptor density of the sodium pump are abnormal in adipose cells and muscle tissue [11]. **B,** The impairment of rubidium uptake (Rb) as a measure of Na-K-ATPase activity is tightly correlated to the reduction in amino acid transport. (*From* [10,11]; with permission.)

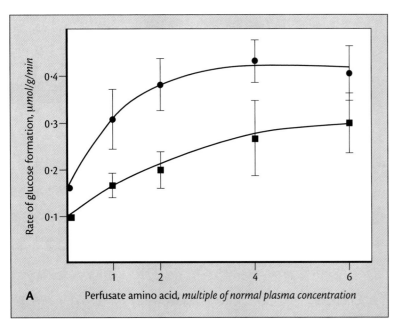

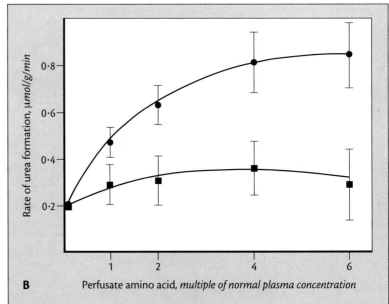

FIGURE 18-7

Protein catabolism in acute renal failure (ARF). Amino acids are redistributed from muscle tissue to the liver. Hepatic extraction of amino acids from the circulation—hepatic gluconeogenesis, **A,** and ureagenesis, **B,** from amino acids all are increased in ARF [12]. The dominant mediator of protein catabolism in ARF is this accelerated hepatic gluconeogenesis, which cannot be suppressed by exogenous substrate infusions (*see* Fig. 18-15). In the liver, protein synthesis and secretion of acute phase proteins are also stimulated. *Circles*—livers from acutely uremic rats; *squares*—livers from sham operated rats. (*From* Fröhlich [12]; with permission.)

CONTRIBUTING FACTORS TO PROTEIN CATABOLISM IN ACUTE RENAL FAILURE

Impairment of metabolic functions by uremia toxins

Endocrine factors

  Insulin resistance

  Increased secretion of catabolic hormones (catecholamines, glucagon, glucocorticoids)

  Hyperparathyroidism

  Suppression of release or resistance to growth factors

Acidosis

Systemic inflammatory response syndrome (activation of cytokine network)

Release of proteases

Inadequate supply of nutritional substrates

Loss of nutritional substrates (renal replacement therapy)

FIGURE 18-8

Protein catabolism in acute renal failure (ARF): contributing factors. The causes of hypercatabolism in ARF are complex and multifold and present a combination of nonspecific mechanisms induced by the acute disease process and underlying illness and associated complications, specific effects induced by the acute loss of renal function, and, finally, the type and intensity of renal replacement therapy.

A major stimulus of muscle protein catabolism in ARF is insulin resistance. In muscle, the maximal rate of insulin-stimulated protein synthesis is depressed by ARF and protein degradation is increased even in the presence of insulin [9].

Acidosis was identified as an important factor in muscle protein breakdown. Metabolic acidosis activates the catabolism of protein and oxidation of amino acids independently of azotemia, and nitrogen balance can be improved by correcting the metabolic acidosis [13]. These findings were not uniformly confirmed for ARF in animal experiments [14].

Several additional catabolic factors are operative in ARF. The secretion of catabolic hormones (catecholamines, glucagon, glucocorticoids), hyperparathyroidism which is also present in ARF (*see* Fig. 18-22), suppression of or decreased sensitivity to growth factors, the release of proteases from activated leukocytes—all can stimulate protein breakdown. Moreover, the release of inflammatory mediators such as tumor necrosis factor and interleukins have been shown to mediate hypercatabolism in acute disease [1, 2].

The type and frequency of renal replacement therapy can also affect protein balance. Aggravation of protein catabolism, certainly, is mediated in part by the loss of nutritional substrates, but some findings suggest that, in addition, both activation of protein breakdown and inhibition of muscular protein synthesis are induced by hemodialysis [15].

Last (but not least), of major relevance for the clinical situation is the fact that inadequate nutrition contributes to the loss of lean body mass in ARF. In experimental animals, starvation potentiates the catabolic response of ARF [7].

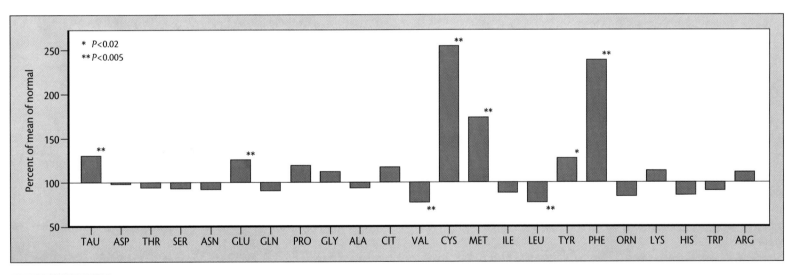

FIGURE 18-9

Amino acid pools and amino acid utilization in acute renal failure (ARF). As a consequence of these metabolic alterations, imbalances in amino acid pools in plasma and in the intracellular compartment occur in ARF. A typical plasma amino acid pattern is seen [16]. Plasma concentrations of cysteine (CYS), taurine (TAU), methionine (MET), and phenylalanine (PHE) are elevated, whereas plasma levels of valine (VAL) and leucine (LEU) are decreased.

Moreover, elimination of amino acids from the intravascular space is altered. As expected from the stimulation of hepatic extraction of amino acids observed in animal experiments, overall amino acid clearance and clearance of most glucoplastic amino acids is enhanced. In contrast, clearances of PHE, proline (PRO), and, remarkably, VAL are decreased [16, 17]. ALA—alanine; ARG—arginine; ASN—asparagine; ASP—aspartate; CIT—citrulline; GLN—glutamine; GLU—glutamate; GLY—glycine; HIS—histidine; ORN—ornithine; PRO—proline; SER—serine; THR—threonine; TRP—tryptophan; TYR—tyrosine. (*From* Druml *et al.* [16]; with permission.)

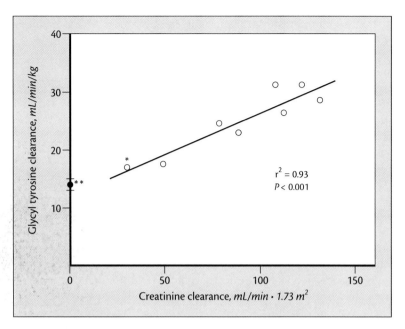

FIGURE 18-10

Metabolic functions of the kidney and protein and amino acid metabolism in acute renal failure (ARF). Protein and amino acid metabolism in ARF are also affected by impairment of the metabolic functions of the kidney itself. Various amino acids are synthe-

sized or converted by the kidneys and released into the circulation: cysteine, methionine (from homocysteine), tyrosine, arginine, and serine [18]. Thus, loss of renal function can contribute to the altered amino acid pools in ARF and to the fact that several amino acids, such as arginine or tyrosine, which conventionally are termed nonessential, might become conditionally indispensable in ARF (*see* Fig. 18-11) [19].

In addition, the kidney is an important organ of protein degradation. Multiple peptides are filtered and catabolized at the tubular brush border, with the constituent amino acids being reabsorbed and recycled into the metabolic pool. In renal failure, catabolism of peptides such as peptide hormones is retarded. This is also true for acute uremia: insulin requirements decrease in diabetic patients who develop of ARF [20].

With the increased use of dipeptides in artificial nutrition as a source of amino acids (such as tyrosine and glutamine) which are not soluble or stable in aqueous solutions, this metabolic function of the kidney may also gain importance for utilization of these novel nutritional substrates. In the case of glycyl-tyrosine, metabolic clearance progressively decreases with falling creatinine clearance (*open circles*, 7 healthy subjects and a patient with unilateral nephrectomy*) but extrarenal clearance in the absence of renal function (*black circles*) is sufficient for rapid utilization of the dipeptide and release of tyrosine [21]. (*From* Druml *et al.* [21]; with permission.)

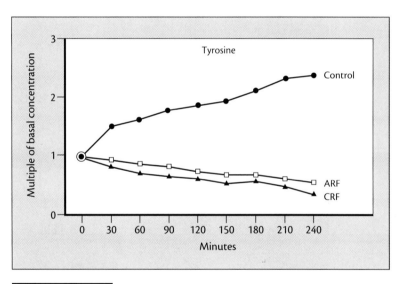

FIGURE 18-11

Amino acids in nutrition of acute renal failure (ARF): Conditionally essential amino acids. Because of the altered metabolic environment of uremic patients certain amino acids designated as nonessential for healthy subjects may become conditionally indispensable to ARF

patients: histidine, arginine, tyrosine, serine, cysteine [19]. Infusion of arginine-free amino acid solutions can cause life-threatening complications such as hyperammonemia, coma, and acidosis.

Healthy subjects readily form tyrosine from phenylalanine in the liver: During infusion of amino acid solutions containing phenylalanine, plasma tyrosine concentration rises (*circles*) [22]. In contrast, in patients with ARF (*triangles*) and chronic renal failure (CRF, *squares*) phenylalanine infusion does not increase plasma tyrosine, indicating inadequate interconversion.

Recently, it was suggested that glutamine, an amino acid that traditionally was designated non-essential exerts important metabolic functions in regulating nitrogen metabolism, supporting immune functions, and preserving the gastrointestinal barrier. Thus, it can become conditionally indispensable in catabolic illness [23]. Because free glutamine is not stable in aqueous solutions, dipeptides containing glutamine are used as a glutamine source in parenteral nutrition. The utilization of dipeptides in part depends on intact renal function, and renal failure can impair hydrolysis (*see* Fig. 18-10) [24]. No systematic studies have been published on the use of glutamine in patients with ARF, and it must be noted that glutamine supplementation increases nitrogen intake considerably.

Protein requirements

ESTIMATING THE EXTENT OF PROTEIN CATABOLISM

Urea nitrogen appearance (UNA) (g/d)

= Urinary urea nitrogen (UUN) excretion

+ Change in urea nitrogen pool

= $(UUN \times V) + (BUN_2 - BUN_1) \, 0.006 \times BW$

+ $(BW_2 - BW_1) \times BUN_2/100$

If there are substantial gastrointestinal losses, add urea nitrogen in secretions:

= volume of secretions $\times BUN_2$

Net protein breakdown (g/d) = UNA $\times$ 6.25

Muscle loss (g/d) = UNA $\times$ 6.25 $\times$ 5

V is urine volume; BUN_1 and BUN_2 are BUN in mg/dL on days 1 and 2

BW_1 and BW_2 are body weights in kg on days 1 and 2

FIGURE 18-12

Estimation of protein catabolism and nitrogen balance. The extent of protein catabolism can be assessed by calculating the urea nitrogen appearance rate (UNA), because virtually all nitrogen arising from amino acids liberated during protein degradation is converted to urea. Besides urea in urine (UUN), nitrogen losses in other body fluids (*eg*, gastrointestinal, choledochal) must be added to any change in the urea pool. When the UNA rate is multiplied by 6.25, it can be converted to protein equivalents. With known nitrogen intake from the parenteral or enteral nutrition, nitrogen balance can be estimated from the UNA calculation.

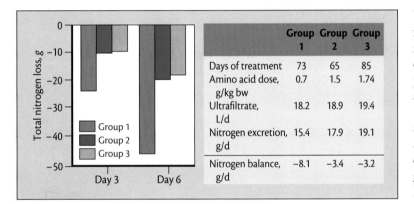

	Group 1	Group 2	Group 3
Days of treatment	73	65	85
Amino acid dose, g/kg bw	0.7	1.5	1.74
Ultrafiltrate, L/d	18.2	18.9	19.4
Nitrogen excretion, g/d	15.4	17.9	19.1
Nitrogen balance, g/d	−8.1	−3.4	−3.2

FIGURE 18-13

Amino acid and protein requirements of patients with acute renal failure (ARF). The optimal intake of protein or amino acids is affected more by the nature of the underlying cause of ARF and the extent of protein catabolism and type and frequency of dialysis than by kidney dysfunction per se. Unfortunately, only a few studies have attempted to define the optimal requirements for protein or amino acids in ARF:

In nonhypercatabolic patients, during the polyuric phase of ARF protein intake of 0.97 g/kg body weight per day was required to achieve a positive nitrogen balance [25]. A similar number (1.03g/kg body weight per day) was derived from a study in which, unfortunately, energy intake was not kept constant [6]. In the polyuric recovery phase in patients with sepsis-induced ARF, a nitrogen intake of 15 g/day (averaging an amino acid intake of 1.3 g/kg body weight per day) as compared to 4.4 g/kg per day (about 0.3 g/kg amino acids) was superior in ameliorating nitrogen balance [26].

Several recent studies have tried to evaluate protein and amino acid requirements of critically ill patients with ARF. Kierdorf and associates found that, in these hypercatabolic patients receiving continuous hemofiltration therapy, the provision of amino acids 1.5 g /kg body weight per day was more effective in reducing nitrogen loss than infusion of 0.7 g (−3.4 versus −8.1 g nitrogen per day) [27]. An increase of amino acid intake to 1. 74 g/kg per day did not further ameliorate nitrogen balance.

Chima and coworkers measured a mean PCR of 1.7 g kg body weight per day in 19 critically ill ARF patients and concluded that protein needs in these patients range between 1.4 and 1.7 g/kg per day [28]. Similarly, Marcias and coworkers have obtained a protein catabolic rate (PCR) of 1.4 g/kg per day and found an inverse relationship between protein and energy provision and PCR and again recommended protein intake of 1.5 to 1.8 g/kg per day [29]. Similar conclusions were drawn by Ikitzler in evaluating ARF patients on intermittent hemodialysis therapy [30]. (*From* Kierdorf *et al.* [27]; with permission.)

Glucose metabolism

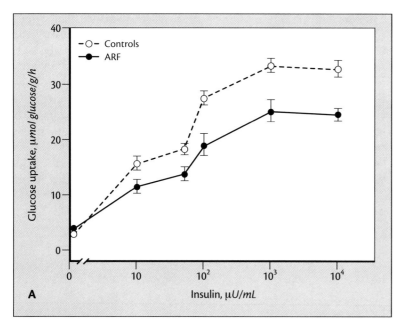

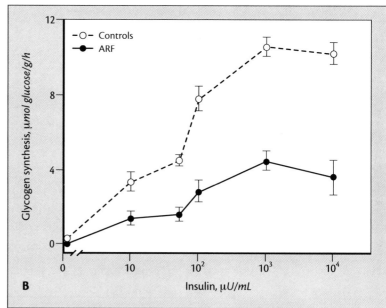

FIGURE 18-14

Glucose metabolism in acute renal failure (ARF): Peripheral insulin resistance. ARF is commonly associated with hyperglycemia. The major cause of elevated blood glucose concentrations is insulin resistance [31]. Plasma insulin concentration is elevated. Maximal insulin-stimulated glucose uptake by skeletal muscle is decreased by 50 %, **A**, and muscular glycogen synthesis is impaired, **B**. However, insulin concentrations that cause half-maximal stimulation of glucose uptake are normal, pointing to a postreceptor defect rather

than impaired insulin sensitivity as the cause of defective glucose metabolism. The factors contributing to insulin resistance are more or less identical to those involved in the stimulation of protein breakdown (*see* Fig. 18-8). Results from experimental animals suggest a common defect in protein and glucose metabolism: tyrosine release from muscle (as a measure of protein catabolism) is closely correlated with the ratio of lactate release to glucose uptake [9]. (*From* May *et al.* [31]; with permission.)

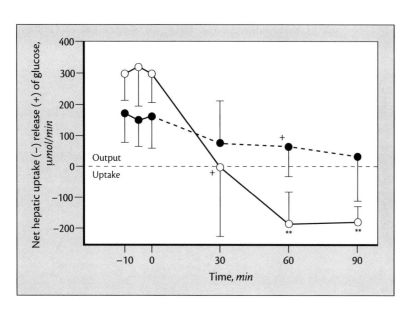

FIGURE 18-15

Glucose metabolism in acute renal failure (ARF): Stimulation of hepatic gluconeogenesis. A second feature of glucose metabolism (and at the same time the dominating mechanism of accelerated protein breakdown) in ARF is accelerated hepatic gluconeogenesis, mainly from conversion of amino acids released during protein catabolism. Hepatic extraction of amino acids, their conversion to glucose, and urea production are all increased in ARF (*see* Fig. 18-7) [12].

In healthy subjects, but also in patients with chronic renal failure, hepatic gluconeogenesis from amino acids is readily and completely suppressed by exogenous glucose infusion. In contrast, in ARF hepatic glucose formation can only be decreased, but not halted, by substrate supply. As can be seen from this experimental study, even during glucose infusion there is persistent gluconeogenesis from amino acids in acutely uremic dogs (•) as compared with controls dogs (o) whose livers switch from glucose release to glucose uptake [32].

These findings have important implications for nutrition support for patients with ARF: 1) It is impossible to achieve positive nitrogen balance; 2) Protein catabolism cannot be suppressed by providing conventional nutritional substrates alone. Thus, for future advances alternative means must be found to effectively suppress protein catabolism and preserve lean body mass. (*From* Cianciaruso *et al.* [32]; with permission.)

Lipid metabolism

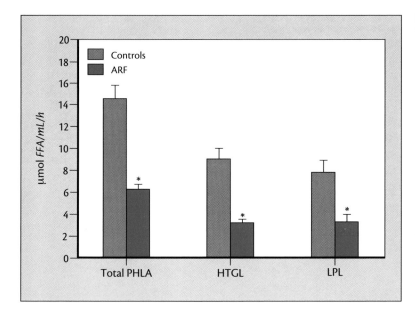

FIGURE 18-16

Lipid metabolism in acute renal failure (ARF). Profound alterations of lipid metabolism occur in patients with ARF. The triglyceride content of plasma lipoproteins, especially very low-density (VLDL) and low-density ones (LDL) is increased, while total cholesterol and in particular high-density lipoprotein (HDL) cholesterol are decreased [33,34]. The major cause of lipid abnormalities in ARF is impairment of lipolysis. The activities of both lipolytic systems, peripheral lipoprotein lipase and hepatic triglyceride lipase are decreased in patients with ARF to less than 50% of normal [35].

Maximal postheparin lipolytic activity (PHLA), hepatic triglyceride lipase (HTGL), and peripheral lipoprotein lipase (LPL) in 10 controls (*open bars*) and eight subjects with ARF (*black bars*). However, in contrast to this impairment of lipolysis, oxidation of fatty acids is not affected by ARF. During infusion of labeled long-chain fatty acids, carbon dioxide production from lipid was comparable between healthy subjects and patients with ARF [36]. FFA—free fatty acids. (*Adapted from* Druml *et al.* [35]; with permission.)

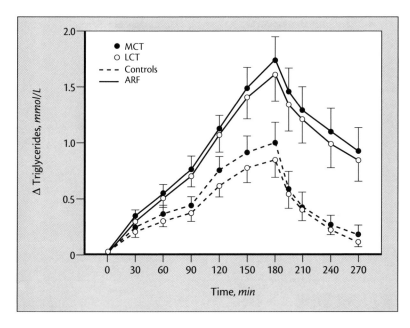

FIGURE 18-17

Impairment of lipolysis and elimination of artificial lipid emulsions in acute renal failure (ARF). Fat particles of artificial fat emulsions for parenteral nutrition are degraded as endogenous very low-density lipoprotein is. Thus, the nutritional consequence of the impaired lipolysis in ARF is delayed elimination of intravenously infused lipid emulsions [33, 34]. The increase in plasma triglycerides during infusion of a lipid emulsion is doubled in patients with ARF (N=7) as compared with healthy subjects (N=6). The clearance of fat emulsions is reduced by more than 50% in ARF. The impairment of lipolysis in ARF cannot be bypassed by using medium-chain triglycerides (MCT); the elimination of fat emulsions containing long chain triglycerides (LCT) or MCT is equally retarded in ARF [34]. Nevertheless, the oxydation of free fatty acid released from triglycerides is not inpaired in patients with ARF [36]. (*From* Druml *et al.* [34]; with permission.)

Electrolytes and micronutrients

CAUSES OF ELECTROLYTE DERANGEMENTS IN ACUTE RENAL FAILURE

Hyperkalemia	Hyperphosphatemia
Decreased renal elimination	Decreased renal elimination
Increased release during catabolism	Increased release from bone
2.38 mEq/g nitrogen	Increased release during catabolism:
0.36 mEq/g glycogen	2 mmol/g nitrogen
Decreased cellular uptake/	Decreased cellular uptake/utilization
increased release	and/or increased release from cells
Metabolic acidosis: 0.6 mmol/L rise/0.1	
decrease in pH	

FIGURE 18-18

Electrolytes in acute renal failure (ARF): causes of hyperkalemia and hyperphosphatemia. ARF frequently is associated with hyperkalemia and hyperphosphatemia. Causes are not only impaired renal excretion of electrolytes but release during catabolism, altered distribution in intracellular and extracellular spaces, impaired cellular uptake, and acidosis. Thus, the type of underlying disease and degree of hypercatabolism also determine the occurrence and severity of electrolyte abnormalities. Either hypophosphatemia or hyperphosphatemia can predispose to the development and maintenance of ARF [37].

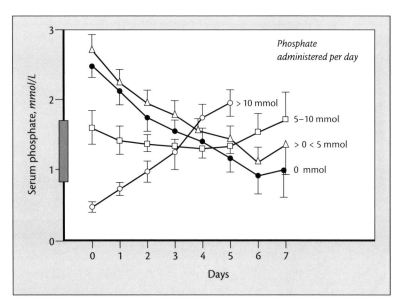

FIGURE 18-19

Electrolytes in acute renal failure (ARF): hypophosphatemia and hypokalemia. It must be noted that a considerable number of patients with ARF do not present with hyperkalemia or hyperphosphatemia, but at least 5% have low serum potassium and more than 12% have decreased plasma phosphate on admission [38]. Nutritional support, especially parenteral nutrition with low electrolyte content, can cause hypophosphatemia and hypokalemia in as many as 50% and 19% of patients respectively [39,40].

In the case of phosphate, phosphate-free artificial nutrition causes hypophosphatemia within a few days, even if the patient was hyperphosphatemic on admission (*black circles*) [41]. Supplementation of 5 mmol per day was effective in maintaining normal plasma phosphate concentrations (*open squares*), whereas infusion of more than 10 mmol per day resulted in hyperphosphatemia, even if the patients had decreased phosphate levels on admission (*open circles*).

Potassium or phosphate depletion increases the risk of developing ARF and retards recovery of renal function. With modern nutritional support, hyperkalemia is the leading indication for initiation of extracorporeal therapy in fewer than 5% of patients [38]. (*Adapted from* Kleinberger *et al.* [41]; with permission.)

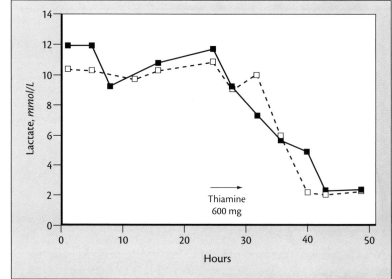

FIGURE 18-20

Micronutrients in acute renal failure (ARF): water-soluble vitamins. Balance studies on micronutrients (vitamins, trace elements) are not available for ARF. Because of losses associated with renal replacement therapy, requirements for water-soluble vitamins are expected to be increased also in patients with ARF. Malnutrition with depletion of vitamin body stores and associated hypercatabolic underlying disease in ARF can further increase the need for vitamins. Depletion of thiamine (vitamin B_1) during continuous hemofiltration and inadequate intake can result in lactic acidosis and heart failure [42]. This figure depicts the evolution of plasma lactate concentration before and after administration of 600 mg thiamine in two patients. Infusion of 600 mg of thiamine reversed the metabolic abnormality within a few hours. An exception to this approach to treatment is ascorbic acid (vitamin C); as a precursor of oxalic acid the intake should be kept below 200 mg per day because any excessive supply may precipitate secondary oxalosis [43]. (*From* Madl *et al.* [42]; with permission.)

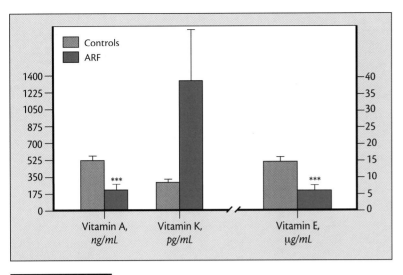

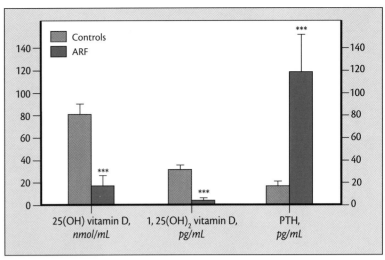

FIGURE 18-21

Micronutrients in acute renal failure (ARF): fat-soluble vitamins (A, E, K). Despite the fact that fat-soluble vitamins are not lost during hemodialysis and hemofiltration, plasma concentrations of vitamins A and E are depressed in patients with ARF and requirements are increased [44]. Plasma concentrations of vitamin K (with broad variations of individual values) are normal in ARF. Most commercial multivitamin preparations for parenteral infusions contain the recommended daily allowances of vitamins and can safely be used in ARF patients. (*From* Druml *et al.* [44]; with permission.)

FIGURE 18-22

Hypocalcemia and the vitamin D–parathyroid hormone (PTH) axis in acute renal failure (ARF). ARF is also frequently associated with hypocalcemia secondary to hypoalbuminemia, elevated serum phosphate, plus skeletal resistance to calcemic effect of PTH and impairment of vitamin-D activation. Plasma concentration of PTH is increased. Plasma concentrations of vitamin D metabolites, 25-OH vitamin D_3 and 1,25-(OH)2 vitamin D_3, are decreased [44]. In ARF caused by rhabdomyolysis rebound hypercalcemia may develop during the diuretic phase. (*Adapted from* Druml *et al.* [44]; with permission.)

FIGURE 18-23

Micronutrients in acute renal failure (ARF): antioxidative factors. Micronutrients are part of the organism's defense mechanisms against oxygen free radical induced injury to cellular components. In experimental ARF, antioxidant deficiency of the organism (decreased vitamin E or selenium status) exacerbates ischemic renal injury, worsens the course, and increases mortality, whereas repletion of antioxidant status exerts the opposite effect [45]. These data argue for a crucial role of reactive oxygen species and peroxidation of lipid membrane components in initiating and mediating ischemia or reperfusion injury.

In patients with multiple organ dysfunction syndrome and associated ARF (*lightly shaded bars*) various factors of the oxygen radical scavenger system are profoundly depressed as compared with healthy subjects (*black bars*): plasma concentrations of vitamin C, of β-carotene, vitamin E, selenium, and glutathione all are profoundly depressed, whereas the end-product of lipid peroxidation, malondialdehyde, is increased (double asterisk, $P < 0.01$; triple asterisk, $P < 0.001$). This underlines the importance of supplementation of antioxidant micronutrients for patients with ARF. (*Adapted from* Druml *et al.* [46]; with permission.)

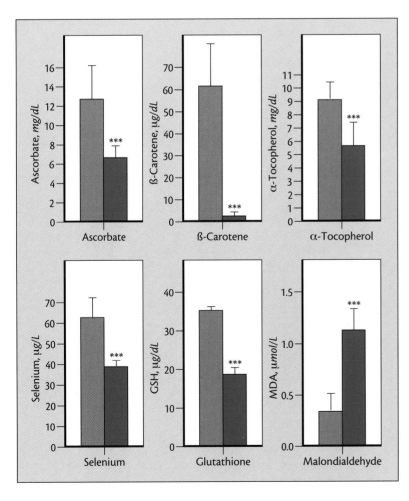

Metabolic Impact of Renal Replacement Therapy

METABOLIC EFFECTS OF CONTINUOUS RENAL REPLACEMENT THERAPY

Amelioration of uremia intoxication (renal replacement)
Plus
  Heat loss
  Excessive load of substrates (eg, lactate, glucose)
  Loss of nutrients (eg, amino acids, vitamins)
  Elimination of short-chain proteins (hormones, mediators?)
  Induction or activation of mediator cascades
  Stimulation of protein catabolism?

FIGURE 18-24

Metabolic impact of extracorporeal therapy. The impact of hemodialysis therapy on metabolism is multifactorial. Amino acid and protein metabolism are altered not only by substrate losses but also by activation of protein breakdown mediated by release of leukocyte-derived proteases, of inflammatory mediators (interleukins and tumor necrosis factor) induced by blood-membrane interactions or endotoxin. Dialysis can also induce inhibition of muscle protein synthesis [15].

In the management of patients with acute renal failure (ARF), continuous renal replacement therapies (CRRT), such as continuous (arteriovenous) hemofiltration (CHF) and continuous hemodialysis have gained wide popularity. CRRTs are associated with multiple metabolic effects in addition to "renal replacement" [47].

By cooling of the extracorporeal circuit and infusion of cooled substitution fluids, CHF may induce considerable heat loss (350 to 700 kcal per day). On the other hand, hemofiltration fluids contain lactate as anions, oxidation of which in part compensates for the heat loss. This lactate load can result in hyperlactemia in the presence of liver dysfunction or increased endogenous lactate formation such as in circulatory shock.

Several nutrients with low protein binding and small molecular weight (sieving coefficient 0.8 to 1.0), such as vitamins or amino acids are eliminated during therapy. Amino acid losses can be estimated from the volume of the filtrate and average plasma concentration, and usually this accounts for a loss of approximately 0.2 g/L of filtrate and, depending on the filtered volume, 5 to 10 g of amino acid per day, respectively, representing about 10 % of amino acid input, but it can be even higher during continuous hemodiafiltration [48].

With the large molecular size cut-off of membranes used in hemofiltration, small proteins such as peptide hormones are filtered. In view of their short plasma half-life hormone losses are minimal and probably not of pathophysiologic importance. Quantitatively relevant elimination of mediators by CRRT has not yet been proven. On the other hand, prolonged blood-membrane interactions can induce consequences of bioincompatibility and activation of various endogenous cascade systems.

Nutrition, Renal Function, and Recovery

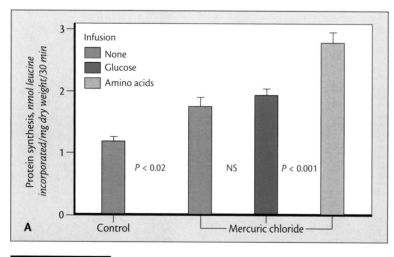

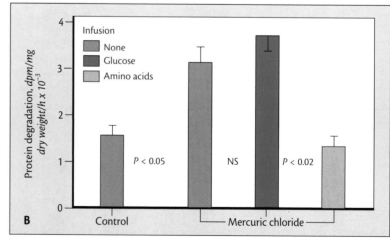

FIGURE 18-25

A, B, Impact of nutritional interventions on renal function and course of acute renal failure (ARF). Starvation accelerates protein breakdown and impairs protein synthesis in the kidney, whereas refeeding exerts the opposite effects [49]. In experimental animals, provision of amino acids or total parenteral nutrition accelerates tissue repair and recovery of renal function [50]. In patients, however, this has been much more difficult to prove, and only one study has reported on a positive effect of TPN on the resolution of ARF [51].

Infusion of amino acids raised renal cortical protein synthesis as evaluated by ^{14}C-leucine incorporation and depressed protein breakdown in rats with mercuric chloride–induced ARF [49]. On the other hand, in a similar model of ARF, infusions of varying quantities of essential amino acids (EAA) and nonessential amino acids (NEAA) did not provide any protection of renal function and in fact increased mortality [52]. However, in balance available evidence suggests that provision of substrates may enhance tissue regeneration and wound healing, and potentially, also renal tubular repair [49]. (*From* Toback *et al.* [50]; with permission.)

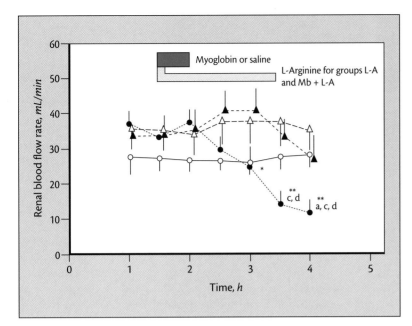

FIGURE 18-26

Impact of nutritional interventions on renal function in acute renal failure (ARF). Amino acid infused before or during ischemia or nephrotoxicity may enhance tubule damage and accelerate loss of renal function in rat models of ARF. In part, this therapeutic paradox [53] from amino acid alimentation in ARF is related to the increase in metabolic work for transport processes when oxygen supply is limited, which may aggravate ischemic injury [54]. Similar observations have been made with excess glucose infusion during renal ischemia. Amino acids may as well exert a protective effect on renal function. Glycine, and to a lesser degree alanine, limit tubular injury in ischemic and nephrotoxic models of ARF [55]. Arginine (possibly by producing nitric oxide) reportedly acts to preserve renal perfusion and tubular function in both nephrotoxic and ischemic models of ARF, whereas inhibitors of nitric oxide synthase exert an opposite effect [56,57]. In myoglobin-induced ARF the drop in renal blood flow (*black circles*, ARF controls) is prevented by L-arginine infusion (*black triangles*) [57]. (*From* Wakabayashi *et al.* [57]; with permission.)

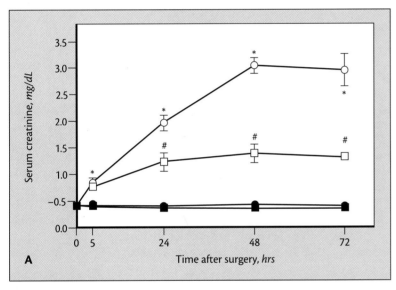

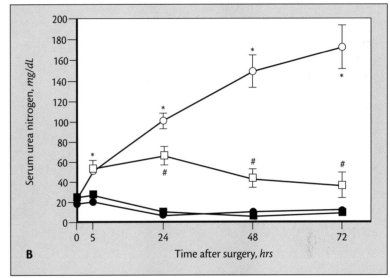

FIGURE 18-27

Impact of endocrine-metabolic interventions on renal function and course of acute renal failure (ARF). Various other endocrine-metabolic interventions (*eg*, thyroxine, human growth hormone [HGH], epidermal growth factor, insulin-like growth factor 1 [IGF-1]) have been shown to accelerate regeneration after experimental ARF [51]. In a rat model of postischemic ARF, treatment with IGF-1 starting 5 hours after induction of ARF accelerates recovery from ischemic ARF, **A**, but also reduces the increase in BUN and improves nitrogen balance, **B**, [58]. (*open circles*) ARF plus vehicle; (*black circles*, sham-operated rats plus vehicle; *open squares*, ARF plus rhIGF-I; *black squares*, sham operated rats plus rhIGF-I.) Unfortunately, efficacy of these interventions was not uniformly confirmed in clinical studies [59, 60]. (*From* Ding *et al.* [58]; with permission.)

Decision Making, Patient Classification, and Nutritional Requirements

DECISIONS FOR NUTRITION IN PATIENTS WITH ACUTE RENAL FAILURE

Decisions dependent on

Patients ability to resume oral diet (within 5 days?)

Nutritional status

Underlying illness/degree of associated hypercatabolism

1. What patient with acute renal failure needs nutritional support?

2. When should nutritional support be initiated?

3. At what degree of impairment in renal function should the nutritional regimen be adapted for renal failure?

4. In a patient with multiple organ dysfunction, which organ determines the type of nutritional support?

5. Is enteral or parenteral nutrition the most appropriate method for providing nutritional support?

FIGURE 18-28

Nutrition in patients with acute renal failure (ARF): decision making. Not every patient with ARF requires nutritional support. It is important to identify those who will benefit and to define the optimal time to initiate therapy [1].

The decision to initiate nutritional support is influenced by the patient's ability to cover nutritional requirements by eating, in addition to the nutritional status of the patient as well as the type of underlying illness involved. In any patient with evidence of malnourishment, nutritional therapy should be instituted regardless of whether the patient will be likely to eat. If a well-nourished patient can resume a normal diet within 5 days, no specific nutritional support is necessary. The degree of accompanying catabolism is also a factor. For patients with underlying diseases associated with excess protein catabolism, nutritional support should be initiated early.

If there is evidence of malnourishment or hypercatabolism, nutritional therapy should be initiated early, even if the patient is likely to eat before 5 days. Modern nutritional strategies should be aimed at avoiding the development of deficiency states and of "hospital-acquired malnutrition." During the acute phase of ARF (the first 24 hours after trauma or surgery) nutritional support should be withheld because nutrients infused during this "ebb phase" are not utilized, could increase oxygen requirements, and aggravate tissue injury and renal dysfunction.

The nutritional regimen should be adapted for renal failure when renal function is impaired. The multiple metabolic alterations characteristic of ARF occur when kidney function is below 30% of normal. Thus, when creatinine clearance falls below 50 to 30 mL per minute/1.73 m^2 (or serum creatinine rises above 2.5 to 3.0 mg/dL) the nutritional regimen should be adapted to ARF. With the exception of severe hepatic failure and massively deranged amino acid metabolism (hyperammonemia) or protein synthesis (depletion of coagulation factors) renal failure is the major determinant of the nutritional regimen in patients with multiple organ dysfunction.

Enteral feeding is preferred for all patients, including those with ARF. Nevertheless, for a large portion of patients, parenteral nutrition—total or partial—will be necessary to meet nutritional requirements.

PATIENT CLASSIFICATION AND SUBSTRATE REQUIREMENTS IN PATIENTS WITH ACUTE RENAL FAILURE

	Extent of Catabolism		
	Mild	Moderate	Severe
Excess urea appearance (above nitrogen intake)	>6 g	6–12 g	>12 g
Clinical setting (examples)	Drug toxicity	Elective surgery ± infection	Severe injury or sepsis
Mortality	20 %	60%	>80%
Dialysis or hemofiltration frequency	Rare	As needed	Frequent
Route of nutrient administration	Oral	Enteral or parenteral	Enteral or parenteral
Energy recommendations (kcal/kg BW/d)	25	25–30	25–35
Energy substrates	Glucose	Glucose + fat	Glucose + fat
Glucose (g/kg BW/d)	3.0–5.0	3.0–5.0	3.0–5.0 (max. 7.0)
Fat (g/kg BW/d)		0.5–1.0	0.8–1.5
Amino acids/protein (g/kg/d)	0.6–1.0	0.8–1.2	1.0–1.5
	EAA (+NEAA)	EAA + NEAA	EAA + NEAA
Nutrients used	Foods	Enteral formulas	Enteral formulas
		Glucose 50%–70% + fat emulsions 10% or 20%	Glucose 50%–70% + fat emulsions 10% or 20%
	EAA + specific NEAA solutions (general or "nephro")		
	Multivitamin and multitrace element preparations		

BW—body weight; EAA—essential amino acids; NEAA—nonessential amino acids.

FIGURE 18-29

Patient classification: substrate requirements. Ideally, a nutritional program should be designed for each individual acute renal failure (ARF) patient. In clinical practice, it has proved useful to distinguish three groups of patients based on the extent of protein catabolism associated with the underlying disease and resulting levels of dietary requirements.

Group I includes patients without excess catabolism and a UNA of less than 6 g of nitrogen above nitrogen intake per day. ARF is usually caused by nephrotoxins (aminoglycosides, contrast media, mismatched blood transfusion). In most cases, these patients are fed orally and the prognosis for recovery of renal function and survival is excellent.

Group II consists of patients with moderate hypercatabolism and a UNA exceeding nitrogen intake 6 to 12 g of nitrogen per day. Affected patients frequently suffer from complicating infections, peritonitis, or moderate injury in association with ARF. Tube feeding or intravenous nutritional support is generally required, and dialysis or hemofiltration often becomes necessary to limit waste product accumulation.

Group III are patients who develop ARF in association with severe trauma, burns, or overwhelming infection. UNA is markedly elevated (more than 12 g of nitrogen above nitrogen intake). Treatment strategies are usually complex and include parenteral nutrition, hemodialysis or continuous hemofiltration plus blood pressure and ventilatory support. To reduce catabolism and avoid protein depletion nutrient requirements are high and dialysis is used to maintain fluid balance and blood urea nitrogen below 100 mg/dL. Mortality in this group of patients exceeds 60% to 80%, but it is not the loss of renal function that accounts for the poor prognosis. It is superimposed hypercatabolism and the severity of the underlying illness. (*Adapted from* Druml [1]; with permission.)

Enteral Nutrition

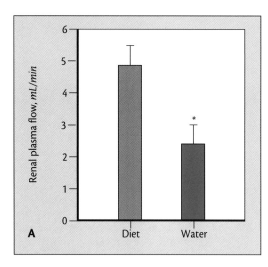

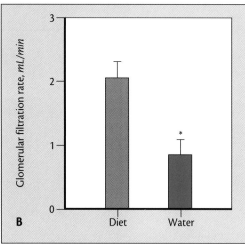

FIGURE 18-30

Enteral nutrition (tube feeding). The gastrointestinal tract should be used whenever possible because enteral nutrients may help to maintain gastrointestinal function and the mucosal barrier and thus prevent translocation of bacteria and systemic infection [61]. Even small amounts of enteral diets exert a protective effect on the intestinal mucosa. Recent animal experiments suggest that enteral feeds may exert additional advantages in acute renal failure (ARF) patients [63]: in glycerol-induced ARF in rats enteral feeding improved renal perfusion, **A**, and preserved renal function, **B**. For patients with ARF who are unable to eat because of cerebral impairment, anorexia, or nausea, enteral nutrition should be provided through small, soft feeding tubes with the tip positioned in the stomach or jejunum [61]. Feeding solutions can be administered by pump intermittently or continuously. If given continuously, the stomach should be aspirated every 2 to 4 hours until adequate gastric emptying and intestinal peristalsis are established. To avoid diarrhea, the amount and concentration of the solution should be increased gradually over several days until nutritional requirements are met. Undesired, but potentially treatable side effects include nausea, vomiting, abdominal distension and cramping and diarrhea. (*From* Roberts *et al.* [62]; with permission.)

SPECIFIC ENTERAL FORMULAS FOR NUTRITIONAL SUPPORT OF PATIENTS WITH RENAL FAILURE

	Amin-Aid	Travasorb renal*	Salvipeptide nephro†	Survimed renal‡	Suplena§	Nepro§
Volume (mL)	750	1050	500	1000	500	500
Calories (kcal)	1467	1400	1000	1320	1000	1000
(cal/mL)	1.96	1.35	2.00	1.32	2.00	2.00
Energy distribution						
Protein:fat:carbohydrates (%)	4:21:75	7:12:81	8:22:70	6:10:84	6:43:51	14:43:43
kcal/g N	832:1	389:1	313:1	398:1	418:1	179:1
Proteins (g)	14.6	24.0	20.0	20.8	15.0	35
EAA (%)	100	60	23			
NEAA (%)	—	30	20			
Hydrolysate (%)	—	—	23	100		
Full protein (%)	—	—	34	—	100	100
Nitrogen (g)	1.76	3.6	3.2	3.32	2.4	5.6
Carbohydrates (g)	274	284	175	276	128	108
Monodisaccharides (%)	100	100	3		10	12
Oligosaccharides (%)	—	—	28			
Polysaccharides (%)	—	—	69	88		90
Fat (g)	34.6	18.6	24	15.2	48	47.8
LCT (%)		30	50		100	100
Essential GA (%)		18	31	52	22	
MCT (%)		70	50	30	0	0
Nonprotein (cal/g N)	502	363	288	374	393	154
Osmol (mOsm/kg)	1095	590	507	600	635	615
Sodium (mmol/L)	11	—	7.2	15.2	32	34.0
Potassium (mmol/L)	—	—	1.5	8	27.0	28.5
Phosphate (mmol)	—	16.1	6.13	6.4	11.0	11.0
Vitamins	b	a	a	a	a	a
Minerals	b	b	a	a	a	a

* 3 bags + 810 mL = 1050 mL

† component I + component II + 350 mL = 500 mL

‡ 4 bags + 800 mL = 1000 mL

§ Liquid formula, cans 8 fl oz (=237.5 mL), supplemented with carnitine, taurine with a low-protein (Suplena) or moderate-protein content (Nepro)

a 2000 kcal/d meets RDA for most vitamins/trace elements

b Must be added

EAA—essential amino acids; FA—fatty acids; LCT—long-chain triglycerides; MCT—medium-chain triglycerides; N—nitrogen; NEAA—non-essential amino acids.

FIGURE 18-31

Enteral feeding formulas. There are standardized tube feeding formulas designed for subjects with normal renal function that can also be given to patients with acute renal failure (ARF). Unfortunately, the fixed composition of nutrients, including proteins and high content of electrolytes (especially potassium and phosphate) often limits their use for ARF.

Alternatively, enteral feeding formulas designed for nutritional therapy of patients with chronic renal failure (CRF) can be used. The preparations listed here may have advantages also for patients with ARF. The protein content is lower and is confined to high-quality proteins (in part as oligopeptides and free amino acids), the electrolyte concentrations are restricted. Most formulations contain recommended allowances of vitamins and minerals.

In part, these enteral formulas are made up of components that increase the flexibility in nutritional prescription and enable adaptation to individual needs. The diets can be supplemented with additional electrolytes, protein, and lipids as required. Recently, ready-to-use liquid diets have also become available for renal failure patients.

Parenteral Nutrition

RENAL FAILURE FLUID—ALL-IN-ONE SOLUTION

Component	Quantity	Remarks
Glucose 40%–70%	500 mL	In the presence of severe insulin resistance switch to D30W
Fat emulsion 10%–20%	500 mL	Start with 10%, switch to 20% if triglycerides are < 350 mg/dL
Amino acids 6.5%–10%	500 mL	General or special "nephro" amino acid solutions, including EAA and NEAA
Water-soluble vitamins	Daily	Limit vitamin C intake < 200 mg/d
Fat-soluble vitamins*	Daily	
Trace elements*	Twice weekly	Caveats: toxic effects
Electrolytes	As required	Caveats: hypophosphatemia or hypokalemia after initiation of TPN
Insulin	As required	Added directly to the solution or given separately

* Combination products containing the recommended daily allowances.

FIGURE 18-32

Parenteral solutions. Standard solutions are available with amino acids, glucose, and lipids plus added vitamins, trace elements, and electrolytes contained in a single bag ("total admixture" solutions, "all-in-one" solutions). The stability of fat emulsions in such mixtures should be tested. If hyperglycemia is present, insulin can be added to the solution or administered separately.

To ensure maximal nutrient utilization and avoid metabolic derangements as mineral imbalance, hyperglycemia or blood urea nitrogen rise, the infusion should be started at a slow rate (providing about 50% of requirements) and gradually increased over several days. Optimally, the solution should be infused continuously over 24 hours to avoid marked derangements in substrate concentrations in the presence of impaired utilization for several nutritional substrates in patients with acute renal failure. EAA, NEAA—essential and nonessential amino acids; TPN—total parenteral nutrition.

AMINO ACID SOLUTIONS FOR THE TREATMENT OF ACUTE RENAL FAILURE ("NEPHRO" SOLUTIONS)

	Rose-Requirements	RenAmin (Clintec)	Aminess (Clintec)	Aminosyn RF (Abbott)	NephrAmine (McGaw)	Nephrotect (Fresenius)
Amino acids (g/L)		65	52	52	54	100
(= g/%)		6.5	5.2	5.2	5.4	10
Volume (mL)		500	400	1000	1000	500
(mOsm/L)		600	416	475	435	908
Nitrogen (g/L)		10	8.3	8.3	6.5	16.3
Essential amino acids (g/L)						
Isoleucine	1.40	5.00	5.25	4.62	5.60	5.80
Leucine	2.20	6.00	8.25	7.26	8.80	12.80
Lysine acetate/HCl	1.60	4.50	6.00	5.35	6.40	12.00
Methionine	2.20	5.00	8.25	7.26	8.80	2.00
Phenylalanine	2.20	4.90	8.25	7.26	8.80	3.50
Threonine	1.00	3.80	3.75	3.30	4.00	8.20
Tryptophan	0.50	1.60	1.88	1.60	2.00	3.00
Valine	1.60	8.20		5.20	6.40	8.70
Nonessential amino acids (g/L)						
Alanine		5.60				6.20
Arginine		6.30	6.00	6.00		8.20
Glycine		3.00				6.30*
Histidine		4.20	4.12	4.29	2.50	9.80
Proline		3.50				3.00
Serine		3.00				7.60
Tyrosine		0.40				3.00†
Cysteine					0.20	0.40

* Glycine is a componenet of the dipeptide.

† Tyrosine is included as dipeptide (glycyl-L-tyrosine).

FIGURE 18-33

Amino acid (AA) solutions for parenteral nutrition in acute renal failure (ARF). The most controversial choice regards the type of amino acid solution to be used: either essential amino acids (EAAs) exclusively, solutions of EAA plus nonessential amino acids (NEAAs), or specially designed "nephro" solutions of different proportions of EAA and specific NEAA that might become "conditionally essential" for ARF (see Fig. 18-11).

Use of solutions of EAA alone is based on principles established for treating chronic renal failure (CRF) with a low-protein diet and an EAA supplement. This may be inappropriate as the metabolic adaptations to low-protein diets in response to CRF may not have occurred in patients with ARF. Plus, there are fundamental differences in the goals of nutritional therapy in the two groups of patients, and consequently, infusion solutions of EAA may be sub-optimal.

Thus, a solution should be chosen that includes both essential and nonessential amino acids (EAA, NEAA) in standard proportions or in special proportions designed to counteract the metabolic changes of renal failure ("nephro" solutions), including the amino acids that might become conditionally essential in ARF.

Because of the relative insolubility of tyrosine in water, dipeptides containing tyrosine (such as glycyl-tyrosine) are contained in modern nephro solutions as the tyrosine source [22, 23]. One should be aware of the fact that the amino acid analogue N-acetyl tyrosine, which previously was used frequently as a tyrosine source, cannot be converted into tyrosine in humans and might even stimulate protein catabolism [21].

Despite considerable investigation, there is no persuasive evidence that amino acid solutions enriched in branched-chain amino acids exert a clinically significant anticatabolic effect. Systematic studies using glutamine supplementation for patients with ARF are lacking (see Fig. 18-11).

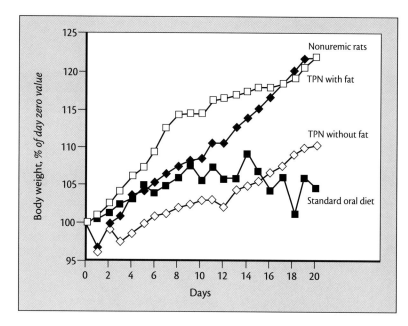

FIGURE 18-34

Energy substrates in total parenteral nutrition (TPN) in acute renal failure (ARF): glucose and lipids. Because of the well-documented effects of overfeeding, energy intake of patients with ARF must not exceed their actual energy expenditure (*ie*, in most cases 100% to 130% of resting energy expenditure [REE]; *see* Figs. 18-3 and 18-4) [2].

Glucose should be the principal energy substrate because it can be utilized by all organs, even under hypoxic conditions, and has the potential for nitrogen sparing. Since ARF impairs glucose tolerance, insulin is frequently necessary to maintain normoglycemia. Any hyperglycemia must be avoided because of the untoward associated side effects—such as aggravation of tissue injury, glycation of proteins, activation of protein catabolism, among others [2]. When intake is increased above 5 g/kg of body weight per day infused glucose will not be oxidized but will promote lipogenesis with fatty infiltration of the liver and excessive carbon dioxide production and hypercarbia. Often, energy requirements cannot be met by glucose infusion without adding large amounts of insulin, so a portion of the energy should be supplied by lipid emulsions [2].

The most suitable means of providing the energy substrates for parenteral nutrition for patients with ARF is not glucose or lipids, but glucose *and* lipids [2]. In experimental uremia in rats, TPN with 30% of nonprotein energy as fat promoted weight gain and ameliorated the uremic state and survival [63]. (*From* Wennberg *et al.* [63]; with permission.)

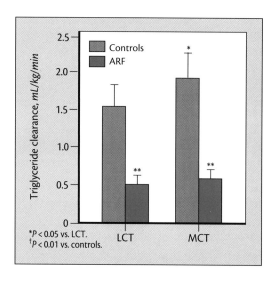

FIGURE 18-35

Energy substrates in parenteral nutrition: lipid emulsions. Advantages of intravenous lipids include high specific energy content, low osmolality, provision of essential fatty acids and phospholipids to prevent deficiency syndromes, fewer hepatic side effects (such as steatosis, hyperbilirubinemia), and reduced carbon dioxide production, especially relevant for patients with respiratory failure.

Changes in lipid metabolism associated with acute renal failure (ARF) should not prevent the use of lipid emulsions. Instead, the amount infused should be adjusted to meet the patient's capacity to utilize lipids. Usually, 1 g/kg of body weight per day of fat will not increase plasma triglycerides substantially, so about 20% to 25% of energy requirements can be met [1]. Lipids should not be administered to patients with hyperlipidemia (*ie*, plasma triglycerides above 350 mg/dL) activated intravascular coagulation, acidosis (pH below 7.25), impaired circulation or hypoxemia.

Parenteral lipid emulsions usually contain long-chain triglycerides (LCT), most derived from soybean oil. Recently, fat emulsions containing a mixture of LCT and medium-chain triglycerides (MCT) have been introduced for intravenous use. Proposed advantages include faster elimination from the plasma owing to higher affinity to the lipoprotein lipase enzyme, complete, rapid, and carnitine-independent metabolism, and a triglyceride-lowering effect; however, use of MCT does not promote lipolysis, and elimination of triglycerides of both types of fat emulsions is equally retarded in ARF [34]. (*Adapted from* [34]; with permission.)

SUGGESTED SCHEDULE FOR MINIMAL MONITORING OF PARENTERAL NUTRITION

Variables	Metabolic Status	
	Unstable	Stable
Blood glucose	1–6 × daily	Daily
Osmolality	Daily	2× weekly
Electrolytes (Na+, K+, Cl+)	Daily	Daily
Calcium, phosphate, magnesium	Daily	3× weekly
Daily BUN increment	Daily	Daily
Urea nitrogen appearance rate	Daily	2 × weekly
Triglycerides	Daily	2 × weekly
Blood gas analysis, pH	Daily	1× weekly
Ammonia	2 × weekly	1 × weekly
Transaminases + bilirubin	2 × weekly	1 × weekly

FIGURE 18-36

Complications and monitoring of nutritional support in acute renal failure (ARF).

Complications: Technical problems and infectious complications originating from the central venous catheter, chemical incompatibilities, and metabolic complications of parenteral nutrition are similar in ARF patients and in nonuremic subjects. However, tolerance to volume load is limited, electrolyte derangements can develop rapidly, exaggerated protein or amino acid intake stimulates excessive blood urea nitrogen (BUN) and waste product accumulation and glucose intolerance, and decreased fat clearance can cause hyperglycemia and hypertriglyceridemia. Thus, nutritional therapy for ARF patients requires more frequent monitoring than it does for other patient groups, to avoid metabolic complications.

Monitoring: This table summarizes laboratory tests that monitor parenteral nutrition and avoid metabolic complications. The frequency of testing depends on the metabolic stability of the patient. In particular, plasma glucose, potassium, and phosphate should be monitored repeatedly after the start of parenteral nutrition.

References

1. Druml W: Nutritional support in acute renal failure. In *Nutrition and the Kidney*. Edited by Mitch WE, Klahr S. Philadelphia: Lippincott-Raven, 1998.
2. Druml W, Mitch WE: Metabolism in acute renal failure. *Sem Dial* 1996, 9:484–490.
3. Om P, Hohenegger M: Energy metabolism in acute uremic rats. *Nephron* 1980, 25:249–253.
4. Schneeweiss B, Graninger W, Stockenhuber F, *et al.*: Energy metabolism in acute and chronic renal failure. *Am J Clin Nutr* 1990, 52:596–601.
5. Soop M, Forsberg E, Thôrne A, Alvestrand A: Energy expenditure in postoperative multiple organ failure with acute renal failure. *Clin Nephrol* 1989, 31:139–145.
6. Spreiter SC, Myers BD, Swenson RS: Protein-energy requirements in subjects with acute renal failure receiving intermittent hemodialysis. *Am J Clin Nutr* 1980, 33:1433–1437.
7. Mitch WE: Amino acid release from the hindquarter and urea appearance in acute uremia. *Am J Physiol* 1981, 241:E415–E419.
8. Salusky IB, Flügel-Link RM, Jones MR, Kopple JD: Effect of acute uremia on protein degradation and amino acid release in the rat hemicorpus. *Kidney Int* 1983, 24(Suppl. 16):S41–S42.
9. Clark AS, Mitch WE: Muscle protein turnover and glucose uptake in acutely uremic rats. *J Clin Invest* 1983, 72:836–845.
10. Maroni BJ, Karapanos G, Mitch WE: System A amino acid transport in incubated muscle: Effects of insulin and acute uremia. *Am J Physiol* 1986, 251:F74–F80.
11. Druml W, Kelly RA, Mitch WE, May RC: Abnormal cation transport in uremia. *J Clin Invest* 1988, 81:1197–1203.
12. Fröhlich J, Hoppe-Seyler G, Schollmeyer P, *et al.*: Possible sites of interaction of acute renal failure with amino acid utilization for gluconeogenesis in isolated perfused rat liver. *Eur J Clin Invest* 1977, 7:261–268.
13. May RC, Kelly RA, Mitch WE: Mechanisms for defects in muscle protein metabolism in rats with chronic uremia: The influence of metabolic acidosis. *J Clin Invest* 1987; 79:1099–1103.
14. Kuhlmann MK, Shahmir E, Maasarani E, *et al.*: New experimental model of acute renal failure and sepsis in rats. *JPEN* 1994, 18:477–485.
15. Bergström J: Factors causing catabolism in maintenance hemodialysis patients. *Miner Electrolyte Metab* 1992, 18:280–283.
16. Druml W, Bürger U, Kleinberger G, *et al.*: Elimination of amino acids in acute renal failure. *Nephron* 1986, 42:62–67.
17. Druml W, Fischer M, Liebisch B, *et al.*: Elimination of amino acids in renal failure. *Am J Clin Nutr* 1994, 60:418–423.
18. Mitch WE, Chesney RW: Amino acid metabolism by the kidney. *Miner Electrolyte Metab* 1983, 9:190–202.
19. Laidlaw SA, Kopple JD: Newer concepts of indispensable amino acids. *Am J Clin Nutr* 1987, 46:593–605.
20. Naschitz JE, Barak C, Yeshurun D: Reversible diminished insulin requirement in acute renal failure. *Postgrad Med J* 1983, 59:269–271.
21. Druml W, Lochs H, Roth E, *et al.*: Utilisation of tyrosine dipeptides and acetyl-tyrosine in normal and uremic humans. *Am J Physiol* 1991, 260:E280–E285.
22. Druml W, Roth E, Lenz K, *et al.*: Phenylalanine and tyrosine metabolism in renal failure. *Kidney Int* 1989, 36(Suppl 27):S282–S286.
23. Fürst P. Stehle P: The potential use of dipeptides in clinical nutrition. *Nutr Clin Pract* 1993, 8:106–114.
24. Hübl W, Druml W, Roth E, Lochs H: Importance of liver and kidney for the utilization of glutamine-containing dipeptides in man. *Metabolism* 1994, 43:1104–1107.
25. Hasik J, Hryniewiecki L, Baczyk K, Grala T: An attempt to evaluate minimum requirements for protein in patients with acute renal failure. *Pol Arch Med Wewn* 1979, 61:29–36.
26. Lopez-Martinez J, Caparros T, Perez-Picouto F: Nutrition parenteral en enfermos septicos con fracaso renal agudo en fase poliurica. *Rev Clin Esp* 1980, 157:171–178.
27. Kierdorf H: Continuous versus intermittent treatment: Clinical results in acute renal failure. *Contrib Nephrol* 1991, 93:1–12.

28. Chima CS, Meyer L, Hummell AC, *et al.*: Protein catabolic rate in patients with acute renal failure on continuous arteriovenous hemofiltration and total parenteral nutrition. *J Am Soc Nephrol* 1993, 3:1516–1521.

29. Macias WL, Alaka KJ, Murphy MH, *et al.*: Impact of nutritional regimen on protein catabolism and nitrogen balance in patients with acute renal failure. *JPEN* 1996, 20:56–62.

30. Ikizler TA, Greene JH, Wingard RL, Hakim RM: Nitrogen balance in acute renal failure patients. *J Am Soc Nephrol* 1995, 6:466A.

31. May RC, Clark AS, Goheer MA, Mitch WE: Specific defects in insulin-mediated muscle metabolism in acute uremia. *Kidney Int* 1985, 28:490–497.

32. Cianciaruso B, Bellizzi V, Napoli R, *et al.*: Hepatic uptake and release of glucose, lactate and amino acids in acutely uremic dogs. *Metabolism* 1991, 40:261–290.

33. Druml W, Laggner A, Widhalm K, *et al.*: Lipid metabolism in acute renal failure. *Kidney Int* 1983, 24(Suppl 16):S139–S142.

34. Druml W, Fischer M, Sertl S, *et al.*: Fat elimination in acute renal failure: Long-chain versus medium-chain triglycerides. *Am J Clin Nutr* 1992, 55:468–472.

35. Druml W, Zechner R, Magometschnigg D, *et al.*: Post-heparin lipolytic activity in acute renal failure. *Clin Nephrol* 1985, 23:289–293.

36. Adolph M, Eckart J, Metges C, *et al.*: Oxidative utilization of lipid emulsions in septic patients with and without acute renal failure. *Clin Nutr* 1995, 14(Suppl 2):35A.

37. Dobyan DC, Bulger RE, Eknoyan G: The role of phosphate in the potentiation and amelioration of acute renal failure. *Miner Electrolyte Metab* 1991, 17:112–115.

38. Druml W, Lax F, Grimm G, *et al.*: Acute renal failure in the elderly—1975–1990. *Clin Nephrol* 1994, 41:342–349.

39. Kurtin P, Kouba J: Profound hypophosphatemia in the course of acute renal failure. *Am J Kidney Dis* 1987, 10:346–349.

40. Marik PE, Bedigian MK: Refeeding hypophosphatemia in critically ill patients in an intensive care unit. *Arch Surg* 1996, 131:1043–1047.

41. Kleinberger G, Gabl F, Gassner A, *et al.*: Hypophosphatemia during parenteral nutrition in patients with renal failure. *Wien Klin Wochenschr* 1978, 90:169–172.

42. Madl Ch, Kranz A, Liebisch B, *et al.*: Lactic acidosis in thiamine deficiency. *Clin Nutr* 1993, 12:108–111.

43. Friedman AL, Chesney RW, Gilbert EF, *et al.*: Secondary oxalosis as a complication of parenteral alimentation in acute renal failure. *Am J Nephrol* 1983, 3:248–252.

44. Druml W, Schwarzenhofer M, Apsner R, Hörl WH: Fat soluble vitamins in acute renal failure. *Miner Electrolyte Metab* 1998, 24:220–226.

45. Zurovsky Y, Gispaan I: Antioxidants attenuate endotoxin-induced acute renal failure in rats. *Am J Kidney Dis* 1995, 25:51–57.

46. Druml W, Bartens C, Stelzer H, *et al.*: Impact of acute renal failure on antioxidant status in multiple organ failure syndrome. *JASN* 1993, 4:314A.

47. Druml W: Impact of continuous renal replacement therapies on metabolism. *Int J Artif Organs* 1996, 19:118–120.

48. Frankenfeld DC, Badellino MM, Reynolds HN, *et al.*: Amino acid loss and plasma concentration during continuous hemodiafiltration. *JPEN* 1993, 17:551–561.

49. Toback FG: Regeneration after acute tubular necrosis. *Kidney Int* 1992, 41:226–246.

50. Toback FG, Dodd RC, Maier ER, Havener LJ: Amino acid administration enhances renal protein metabolism after acute tubular necrosis. *Nephron* 1983, 33:238–243.

51. Abel RM, Beck CH, Abbott WM, *et al.*: Improved survival from acute renal failure after treatment with intravenuous essential amino acids and glucose: Results of a prospective double-blind study. *N Engl J Med* 1973, 288:695–699.

52. Oken DE, Sprinkel M, Kirschbaum BB, Landwehr DM: Amino acid therapy in the treatment of experimental acute renal failure in the rat. *Kidney Int* 1980, 17:14–23.

53. Zager RA, Venkatachalam MA: Potentiation of ischemic renal injury by amino acid infusion. *Kidney Int* 1983, 24:620–625.

54. Brezis M, Rosen S, Spokes K, *et al.*: Transport-dependent anoxic cell injury in the isolated perfused rat kidney. *Am J Pathol* 1984, 116:327–341.

55. Heyman SN, Rosen S, Silva P, *et al.*: Protective action of glycine in cisplatin nephrotoxicity. *Kidney Int* 1991, 40:273–279.

56. Schramm L, Heidbreder E, Lopau K, *et al.*: Influence of nitric oxide on renal function in toxic renal failure in the rat. *Miner Electrolyte Metab* 1996, 22:168–177.

57. Wakabayashi Y, Kikawada R: Effect of L-arginine on myoglobin-induced acute renal failure in the rabbit. *Am J Physiol* 1996, 270:F784–F789.

58. Ding H, Kopple JD, Cohen A, Hirschberg R: Recombinant human insulin-like growth factor-1 accelerates recovery and reduces catabolism in rats with ischemic acute renal failure. *J Clin Invest* 1993, 91:2281–2287.

59. Franklin SC, Moulton M, Sicard GA, *et al.*: Insulin-like growth factor 1 preserves renal function postoperatively. *Am J Physiol* 1997, 272:F257–F259.

60. Hirschberg R, Kopple JD, Guler HP, Pike M: Recombinant human insulin-like growth factor-1 does not alter the course of acute renal failure in patients. 8th Int. Congress Nutr Metabol Renal Disease, Naples 1996.

61. Druml W, Mitch WE: Enteral nutrition in renal disease. In *Enteral and Tube Feeding*. Edited by Rombeau JL, Rolandelli RH. Philadelphia: WB Saunders, 1997:439–461.

62. Roberts PR, Black KW, Zaloga GP: Enteral feeding improves outcome and protects against glycerol-induced acute renal failure in the rat. *Am J Respir Crit Care Med* 1997, 156:1265–1269.

63. Wennberg A, Norbeck HE, Sterner G, Lundholm K: Effects of intravenous nutrition on lipoprotein metabolism, body composition, weight gain and uremic state in experimental uremia in rats. *J Nutr* 1991, 121:1439–1446.

Supportive Therapies: Intermittent Hemodialysis, Continuous Renal Replacement Therapies, and Peritoneal Dialysis

Ravindra L. Mehta

O ver the last decade, significant advances have been made in the availability of different dialysis methods for replacement of renal function. Although the majority of these have been developed for patients with end-stage renal disease, more and more they are being applied for the treatment of acute renal failure (ARF). The treatment of ARF, with renal replacement therapy (RRT), has the following goals: 1) to maintain fluid and electrolyte, acid-base, and solute homeostasis; 2) to prevent further insults to the kidney; 3) to promote healing and renal recovery; and 4) to permit other support measures such as nutrition to proceed without limitation. Ideally, therapeutic interventions should be designed to achieve these goals, taking into consideration the clinical course. Some of the issues that need consideration are the choice of dialysis modality, the indications for and timing of dialysis intervention, and the effect of dialysis on outcomes from ARF. This chapter outlines current concepts in the use of dialysis techniques for ARF.

CHAPTER

19

Dialysis Methods

DIALYSIS MODALITIES FOR ACUTE RENAL FAILURE

Intermittent therapies	Continuous therapies
Hemodialysis (HD)	Peritoneal (CAPD, CCPD)
Single-pass	Ultrafiltration (SCUF)
Sorbent-based	Hemofiltration (CAVH, CVVH)
Peritoneal (IPD)	Hemodialysis (CAVHD, CVVHD)
Hemofiltration (IHF)	Hemodiafiltration (CAVHDF, CVVHDF)
Ultrafiltration (UF)	CVVHDF

FIGURE 19-1

Several methods of dialysis are available for renal replacement therapy. While most of these have been adapted from dialysis procedures developed for end-stage renal disease several variations are available specifically for ARF patients [1] .

Of the intermittent procedures, intermittent hemodialysis (IHD) is currently the standard form of therapy worldwide for treatment of ARF in both intensive care unit (ICU) and non-ICU settings. The vast majority of IHD is performed using single-pass systems with moderate blood flow rates (200 to 250 mL/min) and countercurrent dialysate flow rates of 500 mL/min. Although this method is very efficient, it is also associated with hemodynamic instability resulting from the large shifts of solutes and fluid over a short time. Sorbent system IHD that regenerates small volumes of dialysate with an in-line Sorbent cartridge have not been very popular; however, they are a useful adjunct if large amounts of water are not available or in disasters [2]. These systems depend on a sorbent cartridge with multiple layers of different chemicals to regenerate the dialysate. In addition to the advantage of needing a small amount of water (6 L for a typical

run) that does not need to be pretreated, the unique characteristics of the regeneration process allow greater flexibility in custom tailoring the dialysate. In contrast to IHD, intermittent hemodiafiltration (IHF), which uses convective clearance for solute removal, has not been used extensively in the United States, mainly because of the high cost of the sterile replacement fluid [3]. Several modifications have been made in this therapy, including the provision of on-line preparation of sterile replacement solutions. Proponents of this modality claim a greater degree of hemodynamic stability and improved middle molecule clearance, which may have an impact on outcomes.

As a more continuous technique, peritoneal dialysis (PD) is an alternative for some patients. In ARF patients two forms of PD have been used. Most commonly, dialysate is infused and drained from the peritoneal cavity by gravity. More commonly a variation of the procedure for continuous ambulatory PD termed continuous equilibrated PD is utilized [4]. Dialysate is instilled and drained manually and continuously every 3 to six hours, and fluid removal is achieved by varying the concentration of dextrose in the solutions. Alternatively, the process can be automated with a cycling device programmed to deliver a predetermined volume of dialysate and drain the peritoneal cavity at fixed intervals. The cycler makes the process less labor intensive, but the utility of PD in treating ARF in the ICU is limited because of: 1) its impact on respiratory status owing to interference with diaphragmatic excursion; 2) technical difficulty of using it in patients with abdominal sepsis or after abdominal surgery; 3) relative inefficiency in removing waste products in "catabolic" patients; and 4) a high incidence of associated peritonitis. Several continuous renal replacement therapies (CRRT) have evolved that differ only in the access utilized (arteriovenous [nonpumped: SCUF, CAVH, CAVHD, CAVHDF] versus venovenous [pumped: CVVH, CVVHD, CVVHDF]), and, in the principal method of solute clearance (convection alone [UF and H], diffusion alone [hemodialyis (HD)], and combined convection and diffusion [hemodiafiltration (HDF)]).

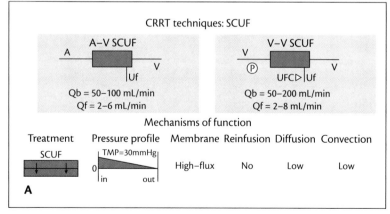

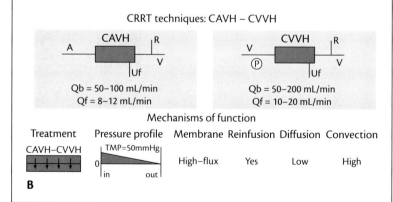

FIGURE 19-2

Schematics of different CRRT techniques. **A**, Schematic representation of SCUF therapy. **B**, Schematic representation of continuous arteriovenous or venovenous hemofiltration (CAVH/CVVH) therapy.

(Continued on next page)

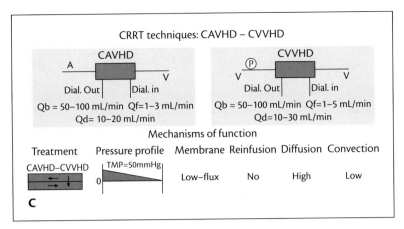

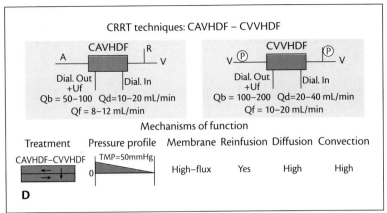

FIGURE 19-2 *(Continued)*

C, Schematic representation of continuous arteriovenous/venovenous hemodialysis (CAVHD-CVVHD) therapy. D, Schematic representation of continuous arteriovenous/venovenous hemodiafiltration (CAVHDF/CVVHDF) therapy. A—artery; V—vein; Uf—ultrafiltrate; R—replacement fluid; P—peristaltic pump; Qb—blood flow; Qf—ultrafiltration rate; TMP—transmembrane pressure; in—dilyzer inlet; out—dialyzer outlet; UFC—ultrafiltration control system; Dial—dialysate; Qd—dialysate flow rate. *(From* Bellomo *et al.* [5]; with permission.)

CONTINUOUS RENAL REPLACEMENT THERAPY: COMPARISON OF TECHNIQUES

	SCUF	CAVH	CVVH	CAVHD	CAVHDF	CVVHD	CVVHDF	PD
Access	AV	AV	VV	AV	AV	VV	VV	Perit. Cath.
Pump	No	No	Yes	No	No	Yes	Yes	No[†]
Filtrate (mL/h)	100	600	1000	300	600	300	800	100
Filtrate (L/d)	2.4	14.4	24	7.2	14.4	7.2	19.2	2.4
Dialysate flow (L/h)	0	0	0	1.0	1.0	1.0	1.0	0.4
Replacement fluid (L/d)	0	12	21.6	4.8	12	4.8	16.8	0
Urea clearance (mL/min)	1.7	10	16.7	21.7	26.7	21.7	30	8.5
Simplicity*	1	2	3	2	2	3	3	2
Cost*	1	2	4	3	3	4	4	3

* 1 = most simple and least expensive; 4 = most difficult and expensive

† cycler can be used to automate exchanges, but they add to the cost and complexity

FIGURE 19-3

In contrast to intermittent techniques, until recently, the terminology for continuous renal replacement therapy (CRRT) techniques has been subject to individual interpretation. Recognizing this lack of standardization an international group of experts have proposed standardized terms for these therapies [5]. The basic premise in the development of these terms is to link the nomenclature to the operational characteristics of the different techniques. In general all these techniques use highly permeable synthetic membranes and differ in the driving force for solute removal. When arteriovenous (AV) circuits are used, the mean arterial pressure provides the pumping mechanism. Alternatively, external pumps generally utilize a venovenous (VV) circuit and permit better control of blood flow rates. The letters AV or VV in the terminology serve to identify the driving force in the technique. Solute removal in these techniques is achieved by convection, diffusion, or a combination of these two. Convective techniques include ultrafiltration (UF) and hemofiltration (H) and depend on solute removal by solvent drag [6].

Diffusion-based techniques similar to intermittent hemodialysis (HD) are based on the principle of a solute gradient between the blood and the dialysate. If both diffusion and convection are used in the same technique the process is termed hemodiafiltration (HDF). In this instance, both dialysate and a replacement solution are used, and small and middle molecules can both be removed easily. The letters UF, H, HD, and HDF identify the operational characteristics in the terminology. Based on these principles, the terminology for these techniques is easier to understand. As shown in Figure 19-1 the letter C in all the terms describes the continuous nature of the methods, the next two letters [AV or VV] depict the driving force and the remaining letters [UF, H, HD, HDF] represent the operational characteristics. The only exception to this is the acronym SCUF (slow continuous ultrafiltration), which remains as a reminder of the initiation of these therapies as simple techniques harnessing the power of AV circuits. *(Modified from* Mehta [7]; with permission.)

Operational Characteristics

Anticoagulation

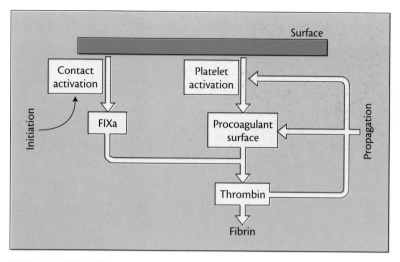

FIGURE 19-4

Pathways of thrombogenesis in extracorporeal circuits. (*Modified from* Lindhout [8]; with permission.)

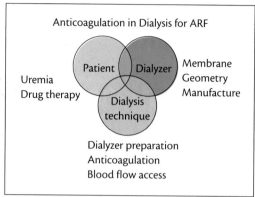

FIGURE 19-5

Factors influencing dialysis-related thrombogenicity. One of the major determinants of the efficacy of any dialysis procedure in acute renal failure (ARF) is the ability to maintain a functioning extracorporeal circuit. Anticoagulation becomes a key component in this regard and requires a balance between an appropriate level of anticoagulation to maintain patency of the circuit and prevention of complications. Figures 19-4 and 19-5 show the mechanisms of thrombus formation in an extracorporeal circuit and the interaction of various factors in this process. (*From* Ward [9]; with permission.)

FIGURE 19-6

Modalities for anticoagulation for continuous renal replacement therapy. While systemic heparin is the anticoagulant most commonly used for dialysis, other modalities are available. The utilization of these modalities is largely influenced by prevailing local experience. Schematic diagrams for heparin, **A**, and citrate, **B**, anticoagulation techniques for continuous renal replacement therapy (CRRT). A schematic of heparin and regional citrate anticoagulation for CRRT techniques. Regional citrate anticoagulation minimizes the major complication of bleeding associated with heparin, but it requires monitoring of ionized calcium. It is now well-recognized that the longevity of pumped or nonpumped CRRT circuits is influenced by maintaining the filtration fraction at less than 20%. Nonpumped circuits (CAVH/HD/HDF) have a decrease in efficacy over time related to a decrease in blood flow (BFR), whereas in pumped circuits (CVVH/HD/HDF) blood flow is maintained; however, the constant pressure across the membrane results in a layer of protein forming over the membrane reducing its efficacy. This process is termed concentration repolarization [10]. CAVH/CVVH—continuous arteriovenous/venovenous hemofiltration. (*From* Mehta RL, *et al.* [11]; with permission.)

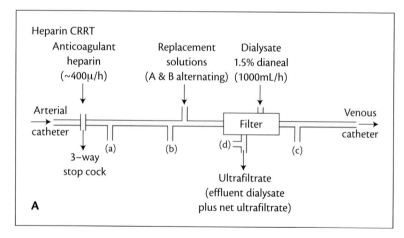

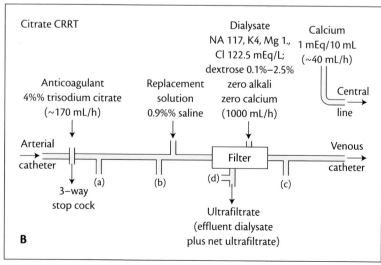

Solute Removal

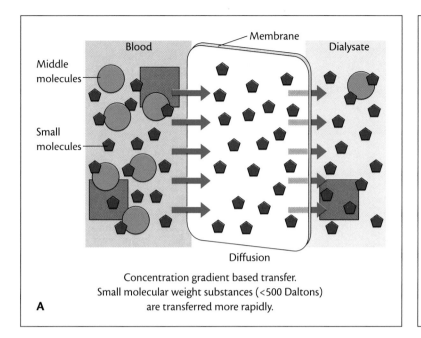

Diffusion

Concentration gradient based transfer.
Small molecular weight substances (<500 Daltons)
are transferred more rapidly.

A

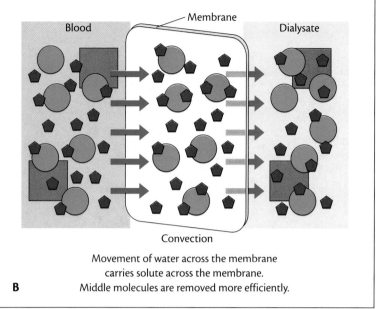

Convection

Movement of water across the membrane
carries solute across the membrane.
Middle molecules are removed more efficiently.

B

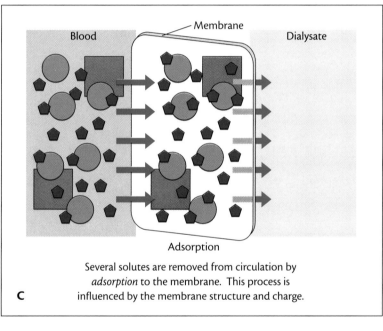

Adsorption

Several solutes are removed from circulation by
adsorption to the membrane. This process is
influenced by the membrane structure and charge.

C

FIGURE 19-7

Mechanisms of solute removal in dialysis. The success of any dialysis procedure depends on an understanding of the operational characteristics that are unique to these techniques and on appropriate use of specific components to deliver the therapy. Solute removal is achieved by diffusion (hemodialysis), **A**, convection (hemofiltration), **B**, or a combination of diffusion and convection (hemodiafiltration), **C**.

DETERMINANTS OF SOLUTE REMOVAL IN DIALYSIS TECHNIQUES FOR ACUTE RENAL FAILURE

	IHD	CRRT	PD
Small solutes (MW <300)	Diffusion:	Diffusion:	Diffusion:
	Q_b	Q_d	Q_d
	Membrane width	Convection:	Convection:
	Qd	Q_f	Q_f
Middle molecules (MW 500–5000)	Diffusion		
	Convection:	Convection:	Convection:
	Q_f	Q_f	Q_f
	SC	SC	SC
LMW proteins (MW 5000–50,000)	Convection	Convection	Convection
	Diffusion	Adsorption	
	Adsorption		
Large proteins (MW >50,000)	Convection	Convection	Convection

FIGURE 19-8

Determinants of solute removal in dialysis techniques for acute renal failure. Solute removal in these techniques is achieved by convection, diffusion, or a combination of these two. Convective techniques include ultrafiltration (UF) and hemofiltration (H) and they depend on solute removal by solvent drag [6]. As solute removal is solely dependent on convective clearance it can be enhanced only by increasing the volume of ultrafiltrate produced. While ultrafiltration requires fluid removal only, to prevent significant volume loss and resulting hemodynamic compromise, hemofiltration necessitates partial or total replacement of the fluid removed. Larger molecules are removed more efficiently by this process and, thus, middle molecular clearances are superior. In intermittent hemodialysis (IHD) ultrafiltration is achieved by modifying the transmembrane pressure and generally does not contribute significantly to solute removal. In peritoneal dialysis (PD) the UF depends on the osmotic gradient achieved by the concentration of dextrose solution (1.55% to 4.25%) utilized the number of exchanges and the dwell time of each exchange. In continuous arteriovenous and venovenous hemodialysis in most situations ulrafiltration rates of 1 to 3 L/hour are utilized; however recently high-volume hemofiltration with 6 L of ultrafiltrate produced every hour has been utilized to remove middle– and large–molecular weight cytokines in sepsis [12]. Fluid balance is achieved by replacing the ultrafiltrate removed by a replacement solution. The composition of the replacement fluid can be varied and the solution can be infused before or after the filter.

Diffusion-based techniques (hemodialysis) are based on the principle of a solute gradient between the blood and the dialysate. In IHD, typically dialysate flow rates far exceed blood flow rates (200 to 400 mL/min, dialysate flow rates 500 to 800 mL/min) and dialysate flow is single pass. However, unlike IHD, the dialysate flow rates are significantly slower than the blood flow rates (typically, rates are 100 to 200 mL/min, dialysate flow rates are 1 to 2 L/hr [17 to 34mL/min]), resulting in complete saturation of the dialysate. As a consequence, dialysate flow rates become the limiting factor for solute removal and provide an opportunity for clearance enhancement. Small molecules are preferentially removed by these methods. If both diffusion and convection are used in the same technique (hemodiafiltration, HDF) both dialysate and a replacement solution are used and small and middle molecules can both be easily removed.

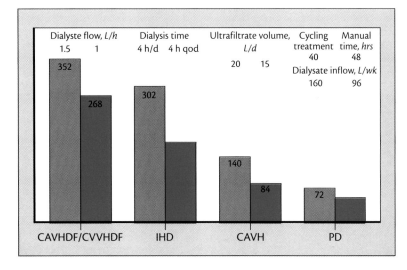

FIGURE 19-9

Comparison of weekly urea clearances with different dialysis techniques. Although continuous therapies are less efficient than intermittent techniques, overall clearances are higher as they are utilized continuously. It is also possible to increase clearances in continuous techniques by adjustment of the ultrafiltration rate and dialysate flow rate. In contrast, as intermittent dialysis techniques are operational at maximum capability, it is difficult to enhance clearances except by increasing the size of the membrane or the duration of therapy. CAV/CVVHDF—continuous arteriovenous/venovenous hemodiafiltration; IHD—intermittent hemodialysis; CAVH—continuous arteriovenous hemodialysis; PD—peritoneal dialysis.

COMPARISON OF DIALYSIS PRESCRIPTION AND DOSE DELIVERED IN CRRT AND IHD

Dialysis Prescription

	IHD	CRRT
Membrane characteristics	Variable permeability	High permeability
Anticoagulation	Short duration	Prolonged
Blood flow rate	≥200 mL/min	<200 mL/min
Dialysate flow	≥500 mL/min	17–34 mL/min
Duration	3–4 hrs	Days
Clearance	High	Low

Dialysis Dose Delivered

	IHD	CRRT
Patient factors		
Hemodynamic stability	+++	+
Recirculation	+++	+
Infusions	++	+
Technique factors		
Blood flow	+++	++
Concentration repolarization	+	+++
Membrane clotting	+	+++
Duration	+++	+
Other factors		
Nursing errors	+	+++
Interference	+	++++

FIGURE 19-10

Comparison of dialysis prescription and dose delivered in continuous renal replacement (CRRT) and intermittent hemodialysis (IHD). The ability of each modality to achieve a particular clearance is influenced by the dialysis prescription and the operational characteristics; however, it must be recognized that there may be a significant difference between the dialysis dose prescribed and that delivered. In general, IHD techniques are limited by available time, and in catabolic patients it may not be possible to achieve a desired level of solute control even by maximizing the operational characteristics.

DRUG DOSING IN CRRT*

Drug	Normal Dose (mg/d)	Dose in CRRT (mg)
Amikacin	1050	250 qd–bid
Netilmycin	420	100–150 qd
Tobramycin	350	100 qd
Vancomycin	2000	500 qd–bid
Ceftazidime	6000	1000 bid
Cefotaxime	12,000	2000 bid
Ceftriaxone	4000	2000 qd
Ciprofloxacin	400	200 qd
Imipenem	4000	500 tid–qid
Metronidazole	2100	500 tid–qid
Piperacillin	24,000	4000 tid
Digoxin	0.29	0.10 qd
Phenobarbital	233	100 bid–qid
Phenytoin	524	250 qd–bid
Theophylline	720	600–900 qd

* Reflects doses for continuous venovenous hemofiltration with ultrafiltration rate of 20 to 30 mL/min.

FIGURE 19-11

Drug dosing in continuous renal replacement (CRRT) techniques. Drug removal in CRRT techniques is dependent upon the molecular weight of the drug and the degree of protein binding. Drugs with significant protein binding are removed minimally. Aditionally, some drugs may be removed by adsorption to the membrane. Most of the commonly used drugs require adjustments in dose to reflect the continuous removal in CRRT. (*Modified from* Kroh *et al.* [13]; with permission.)

NUTRITIONAL ASSESSMENT AND SUPPORT WITH RENAL REPLACEMENT TECHNIQUES

Parameters: Initial Assessment	IHD	CAVH/CVVH	CAVHD/CVVHDF
Energy assessment	HBE x AF x SF, or indirect calorimetry	Same	Same
Dialysate dextrose absorption	Negligible	Not applicable	43% uptake 1.5% dextrose dialysate (525 calories/D)
			45% uptake 2.5% dextrose dialysate (920 calories/D)
			Negligible absorption with dextrose free or dialysate 0.1–0.15% dextrose
Protein assessment			
Visceral proteins	Serum prealbumin	Same	Same
Nitrogen balance: N_2 in–N_2 out	Nitrogen in: protein in TPN +/enteral solutions/6.25	Nitrogen in: same	Nitrogen in: same
	Nitrogen out: urea nitrogen appearance	Nitrogen out: ultrafiltrate urea nitrogen losses	Nitrogen out: ultrafiltrate/dialysate urea nitrogen losses
	UUN[†]	UUN[†]	UUN[†]
	Insensible losses	Insensible losses	Insensible losses
	Dialysis amino acid losses (1.0–1.5 N_2/dialysis therapy)	Ultrafiltrate amino acid losses (1.5–2.0 N_2/D)	Ultrafiltrate/dialysate amino acid losses (1.5–2.0 N_2/D)
Nutrition support prescription: TPN/enteral nutrition	Renal formulas with limited fluid, potassium, phosphorus, and magnesium	Standard TPN/enteral formulations. No fluid or electrolyte restrictions.	Standard TPN/enteral formulations when 0.1–0.15% dextrose dialysate used
			Modified formulations when 1.5–2.5% dextrose dialysate used
			TPN: Low-dextrose solutions to prevent carbohydrate overfeeding; amino acid concentration may be increased to meet protein requirements.
			Enteral: Standard formulas. May require modular protein to meet protein requirements without carbohydrate overfeeding.
Reassessment of requirements and efficacy of nutrition support			
Energy assessment	Weekly HBE x AF x SF*, or indirect calorimetry	Same	Same
Serum prealbumin	Weekly	Same	Same
Nitrogen balance	Weekly	Same	Same

* Harris Benedict equation multiplied by acimity and stress factors
† Collect 24-hour urine for UUN if UOP ≥ 400 ml/d

FIGURE 19-12

Nutritional assessment and support with renal replacement techniques. A key feature of dialysis support in acute renal failure is to permit an adequate amount of nutrition to be delivered to the patient. The modality of dialysis and operational characteristics affect the nutritional support that can be provided. Dextrose absorption occurs form the dialysate in hemodialysis and hemodiafiltration modalities and can result in hyperglycemia. Intermittent dialysis techniques are limited by time in their ability to allow unlimited nutritional support. (*From* Monson and Mehta [14]; with permission.)

Fluid Control

OPERATING CHARACTERISTICS OF CRRT: FLUID REMOVAL VERSUS FLUID REGULATION

	Fluid Removal	Fluid Regulation
Ultrafiltration rate (UFR)	To meet anticipated needs	Greater than anticipated needs
Fluid management	Adjust UFR	Adjust amount of replacement fluid
Fluid balance	Zero or negative balance	Positive, negative, or zero balance
Volume removed	Based on physician estimate	Driven by patient characteristics
Application	Easy, similar to intermittent hemodialysis	Requires specific tools and training

FIGURE 19-13

Operating characteristics of continuous renal replacement (CRRT): fluid removal versus fluid regulation. Fluid management is an integral component in the management of

patients with acute renal failure in the intensive care setting. In the presence of a failing kidney, fluid removal is often a challenge that requires large doses of diuretics with a variable response. It is often necessary in this setting to institute dialysis for volume control rather than metabolic control. CRRT techniques offer a significant advantage over intermittent dialysis for fluid control [14,15]; however, if not carried out appropriately they can result in major complications. To utilize these therapies for their maximum potential it is necessary to recognize the factors that influence fluid balance and have an understanding of the principles of fluid management with these techniques. In general it is helpful to consider dialysis as a method for fluid removal and fluid regulation.

APPROACHES FOR FLUID MANAGEMENT IN CRRT

Approaches	Level 1	Level 2	Level 3
UF volume	Limited	Increase intake	Increase intake
Replacement	Minimal	Adjusted to achieve fluid balance	Adjusted to achieve fluid balance
Fluid balance	8 h	Hourly	Hourly
			Targeted
UF pump	Yes	Yes/No	Yes/No
Examples	SCUF/CAVHD	CAVH/CVVH	CAVHDF/CVVHDF
	CVVHD	CAVHDF/CVVHDF	CVVH
Advantages			
Simplicity	+++	++	+
Achieve fluid balance	+	+++	+++
Regulate volume changes	+	++	+++
CRRT as support	+	++	+++
Disadvantages			
Nursing effort	+	++	+++
Errors in fluid balance	+++	++	+
Hemodynamic instability	++	++	+
Fluid overload	+++	+	+

FIGURE 19-14

Approaches for fluid management in continuous renal replacement therapy (CRRT). CRRT techniques are uniquely situated in providing fluid regulation, as fluid management can be achieved with three levels of intervention [16]. In Level 1, the ultrafiltrate (UF) volume obtained is limited to match the anticipated needs for fluid balance. This calls for an estimate of the amount of fluid to be removed over 8 to 24 hours and subsequent calculation of the ultrafiltration rate. This strategy is similar to that commonly used for intermittent hemodialysis and differs only in that the time to remove fluid is 24 hours instead of 3 to 4 hours. In Level 2 the ultrafiltrate volume every hour is deliberately set to be greater than the hourly intake, and net fluid balance is achieved by hourly replacement fluid administration. In this method a greater degree of control is possible and fluid balance can be set to achieve any desired outcome. The success of this method depends on the ability to achieve ultrafiltration rates that always exceed the anticipated intake. This allows flexibility in manipulation of the fluid balance, so that for any given hour the fluid status could be net negative, positive, or balanced. A key advantage of this technique is that the net fluid balance achieved at the end of every hour is truly a reflection of the desired outcome. Level 3 extends the concept of the Level 2 intervention to target the desired net balance every hour to achieve a specific hemodynamic parameter (eg, central venous pressure, pulmonary artery wedge pressure, or mean arterial pressure). Once a desired value for the hemodynamic parameter is determined, fluid balance can be linked to that value. Each level has advantages and disadvantages; in general greater control calls for more effort and consequently results in improved outcomes. SCUF—ultrafiltration; CAVHD/CVVHD—continuous arteriovenous/venovenous hemodialysis; CAVH/CVVH—continuous arteriovenous/venovenous hemofiltration; CAVHDF/CVVHDF—continuous arteriovenous/venovenous hemodiafiltration.

COMPOSITION OF REPLACEMENT FLUID AND DIALYSATE FOR CRRT

Replacement Fluid

Investigator	Golper [19]	Kierdorf [20]	Lauer [21]	Paganini [22]	Mehta [11]	Mehta [11]
Na^+	147	140	140	140	140.5	154
Cl^-	115	110	—	120	115.5	154
HCO_3^-	36	34	—	6	25	—
K^+	0	0	2	2	0	—
Ca^{2+}	1.2	1.75	3.5	4	4	—
Mg^{2+}	0.7	0.5	1.5	2	—	—
Glucose	6.7	5.6	—	10	—	—
Acetate	—	—	41	40	—	—

Dialysate

Component (mEq/L)	1.5% Dianeal	Hemosol AG 4D	Hemosol LG 4D	Baxter	Citrate
Sodium	132	140	140	140	117
Potassium	—	4	4	2	4
Chloride	96	119	109.5	117	121
Lactate	35	—	40	30	—
Acetate	—	30	—	—	—
Calcium	3.5	3.5	4	3.5	—
Magnesium	1.5	1.5	1.5	1.5	1.5
Dextrose (g/dL)	1.5	0.8	.11	0.1	0.1–2.5

FIGURE 19-15

Composition of dialysate and replacement fluids used for continuous renal replacement therapy (CRRT). One of the key features of any dialysis method is the manipulation of metabolic balance. In general, this is achieved by altering composition of dialysate or replacement fluid . Most commercially available dialysate and replacement solutions have lactate as the base; however, bicarbonate-based solutions are being utilized more and more [17,18].

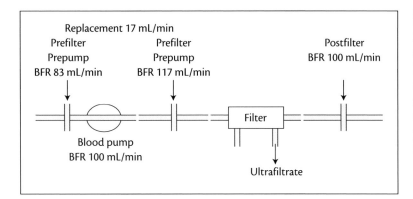

FIGURE 19-16

Effect of site of delivery of replacement fluid: pre- versus postfilter continuous venovenous hemofiltration with ultrafiltration rate of 1 L/hour. Replacement fluids may be administered pre- or postfilter, depending on the circuit involved . It is important to recognize that the site of delivery can influence the overall efficacy of the procedure. There is a significant effect of fluid delivered prepump or postpump, as the amount of blood delivered to the filter is reduced in prepump dilution. BFR—blood flow rate.

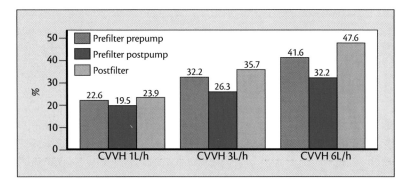

FIGURE 19-17

Pre- versus postfilter replacement fluid: effect on filtration fraction. Prefilter replacement tends to dilute the blood entering the circuit and enhances filter longevity by reducing the filtration fraction; however, in continuous venovenous hemofiltration (CVVH) circuits the overall clearance may be reduced as the amount of solute delivered to the filter is reduced.

Applications and Indications for Dialytic Intervention _____

INDICATIONS AND TIMING OF DIALYSIS FOR ACUTE RENAL FAILURE: RENAL REPLACEMENT VERSUS RENAL SUPPORT

	Renal Replacement	Renal Support
Purpose	Replace renal function	Support other organs
Timing of intervention	Based on level of biochemical markers	Based on individualized need
Indications for dialysis	Narrow	Broad
Dialysis dose	Extrapolated from ESRD	Targeted for overall support

FIGURE 19-18

Dialysis intervention in acute renal failure (ARF): renal replacement versus renal support. An important consideration in the management of ARF is defining the goals of therapy. Several issues must be considered, including the timing of the intervention, the amount and frequency of dialysis, and the duration of therapy. In practice, these issues are based on individual preferences and experience, and no immutable criteria are followed [7,23]. Dialysis intervention in ARF is usually considered when there is clinical evidence of uremia symptoms or biochemical evidence of solute and fluid imbalance. An important consideration in this regard is to recognize that the patient with ARF is somewhat different than the one with end-stage renal disease (ESRD). The rapid decline of renal function associated with multiorgan failure does not permit much of an adaptive response which characterizes the course of the patient with ESRD. As a consequence, the traditional indications for renal replacement may need to be redefined. For instance, excessive volume resuscitation, a common strategy for multiorgan failure, may be an indication for dialysis, even in the absence of significant elevations in blood urea nitrogen. In this respect, it may be more appropriate to consider dialysis intervention in the intensive care patient as a form of renal support rather than renal replacement. This terminology serves to distinguish between the strategy for replacing individual organ function and one to provide support for all organs.

POTENTIAL APPLICATIONS FOR CONTINUOUS RENAL REPLACEMENT THERAPY

Renal Replacement	Renal Support	Extrarenal Applications
Acute renal failure	Fluid management	Cytokine removal ? sepsis
Chronic renal failure	Solute control	Heart failure
	Acid-base adjustments	Cancer chemotherapy
	Nutrition	Liver support
	Burn management	Inherited metabolic disorders

FIGURE 19-19

Potential applications for continuous renal replacement therapy (CRRT). CRRT techniques are increasingly being utilized as support modalities in the intensive care setting and are particularly suited for this function. The freedom to provide continuous fluid management permits the application of unlimited nutrition, adjustments in hemodynamic parameters, and achievement of steady-state solute control, which is difficult with intermittent therapies. It is thus possible to widen the indications for renal intervention and provide a customized approach for the management of each patient.

RELATIVE ADVANTAGES (+) AND DISADVANTAGES (−) OF CRRT, IHD, AND PD

Variable	CRRT	IHD	PD
Continuous renal replacement	+	−	+
Hemodynamic stability	+	−	+
Fluid balance achievement	+	−	−
Unlimited nutrition	+	−	−
Superior metabolic control	+	−	−
Continuous removal of toxins	+	−	+
Simple to perform	±	−	+
Stable intracranial pressure	+	−	+
Rapid removal of poisons	−	+	−
Limited anticoagulation	−	+	+
Need for intensive care nursing support	+	−	+
Need for hemodialysis nursing support	±	+	+
Patient mobility	−	+	−

FIGURE 19-20

Advantages (+) and disadvantages (−) of dialysis techniques. CRRT—continuous renal replacement therapy; IHD—intermittent hemodialysis; PD—peritoneal dialysis.

DETERMINANTS OF THE CHOICE OF TREATMENT MODALITY FOR ACUTE RENAL FAILURE

Patient
  Indication for dialysis
  Presence of multiorgan failure
  Access
  Mobility and location of patient
  Anticipated duration of therapy
Dialysis process
  Components (eg, membrane, anticoagulation)
  Type (intermittent or continuous)
  Efficacy for solute and fluid balance
  Complications
  Outcome
Nursing and other support
  Availability of machines
  Nursing support

FIGURE 19-21

Determinants of the choice of treatment modality for acute renal failure. The primary indication for dialysis intervention can be a major determinant of the therapy chosen because different therapies vary in their efficacy for solute and fluid removal. Each technique has its advantages and limitations, and the choice depends on several factors. Patient selection for each technique ideally should be based on a careful consideration of multiple factors [1]. The general principle is to provide adequate renal support without adversely affecting the patient. The presence of multiple organ failure may limit the choice of therapies; for example, patients who have had abdominal surgery may not be suitable for peritoneal dialysis because it increases the risk of wound dehiscence and infection. Patients who are hemodynamically unstable may not tolerate intermittent hemodialysis (IHD). Additionally, the impact of the chosen therapy on compromised organ systems is an important consideration. Rapid removal of solutes and fluid, as in IHD, can result in a disequilibrium syndrome and worsen neurologic status. Peritoneal dialysis may be attractive in acute renal failure that complicates acute pancreatitis, but it would contribute to additional protein losses in the hypoalbuminemic patient with liver failure.

RECOMMENDATION FOR INITIAL DIALYSIS MODALITY FOR ACUTE RENAL FAILURE (ARF)

Indication	Clinical Condition	Preferred Therapy
Uncomplicated ARF	Antibiotic nephrotoxicity	IHD, PD
Fluid removal	Cardiogenic shock, CP bypass	SCUF, CAVH
Uremia	Complicated ARF in ICU	CVVHDF, CAVHDF, IHD
Increased intracranial pressure	Subarachnoid hemorrhage, hepatorenal syndrome	CVVHD, CAVHD
Shock	Sepsis, ARDS	CVVH, CVVHDF, CAVHDF
Nutrition	Burns	CVVHDF, CAVHDF, CVVH
Poisons	Theophylline, barbiturates	Hemoperfusion, IHD, CVVHDF
Electrolyte abnormalities	Marked hyperkalemia	IHD, CVVHDF
ARF in pregnancy	Uremia in 2nd, 3rd trimester	PD

FIGURE 19-22

Recommendation for initial dialysis modality for acute renal failure (ARF). Patients with multiple organ failure (MOF) and ARF can be treated with various continuous therapies or IHD. Continuous therapies provide better hemodynamic stability; however, if not monitored carefully they can lead to significant volume depletion. In general, hemodynamically unstable, catabolic, and fluid-overloaded patients are best treated with continuous therapies, whereas IHD is better suited for patients who require early mobilization and are more stable. It is likely that the mix of modalities used will change as evidence linking the choice of modality to outcome becomes available. For now, it is probably appropriate to consider all these techniques as viable options that can be used collectively. Ideally, each patient should have an individualized approach for management of ARF.

Outcomes

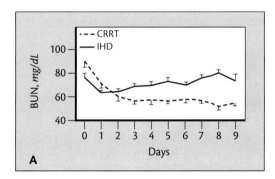

A

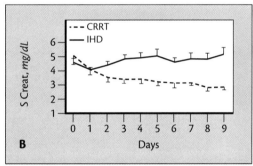

B

FIGURE 19-23

Efficacy of continuous renal replacement therapy (CRRT) versus intermittent hemodialysis (IHD): effect on blood urea nitrogen, **A**, and creatinine levels, **B**, in acute renal failure.

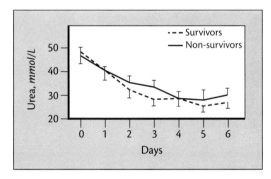

FIGURE 19-24

Blood urea nitrogen (BUN) levels in survivors and non-survivors in acute renal failure treated with continuous renal replacement therapy (CRRT). It is apparent that CRRT techniques offer improved solute control and fluid management with hemodynamic stability, however a relationship to outcome has not been demonstrated. In a recent retrospective analysis van Bommel [24] found no difference in BUN levels among survivors and non-survivors with ARF While it is clear that lower solute concentrations can be achieved with CRRT whether this is an important criteria impacting on various outcomes from ARF still needs to be determined. A recent study form the Cleveland Clinic suggests that the dose of dialysis may be an important determinant of outcome allowing for underlying severity of illness [25]. In this study the authors found that in patients with ARF, 65.4% of all IHD treatments resulted in lower Kt/V than prescribed. There appeared to be an influence of dose of dialysis on outcome in patients with intermediate levels of severity of illness as judged by the Cleveland Clinic Foundation acuity score for ARF (see Fig. 19-25). Patients receiving a higher Kt/V had a lower mortality than predicted. These data illustrate the importance of the underlying severity of illness, which is likely to be a major determinant of outcome and should be considered in the analysis of any studies.

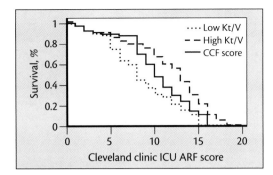

FIGURE 19-25

Effect of dose of dialysis in acute renal failure (ARF) on outcome from ARF.

BIOCOMPATIBLE MEMBRANES IN INTERMITTENT HEMODIALYSIS (IHD) AND ACUTE RENAL FAILURE (ARF): EFFECT ON OUTCOMES

	BCM Group	BICM Group	Probability
Patients, *n*	72	81	
All patients recover of renal function	46 (64%)	35 (43%)	0.001
Survival	41 (57%)	37 (46%)	0.03
Patients nonoliguric before hemodialysis	39	46	
Development of oliguria with dialysis	17 (44%)	32 (70%)	0.03
Recovery of renal function	31 (79%)	21 (46%)	0.0004
Survival	28 (74%)	22 (48%)	0.003
Patients oliguric before hemodialysis	33	35	
Recovery of renal function	15 (45%)	14 (40%)	ns
Survival	12 (36%)	15 (43%)	ns

FIGURE 19-26

Biocompatible membranes in intermittent hemodialysis (IHD) and acute renal failure (ARF): effect outcomes. The choice of dialysis membrane and its influence on survival from ARF has been of major interest to investigators over the last few years. While the evidence tends to support a survival advantage for biocompatible membranes, most of the studies were not well controlled. The most recent multicenter study showed an improvement in mortality and recovery of renal function with biocompatible membranes; however, this effect was not significant in oliguric patients. Further investigations are required in this area. NS—not significant.

MORTALITY IN ACUTE RENAL FAILURE: COMPARISON OF CRRT VERSUS IHD

Investigator	Type of Study	IHD		CRRT		Change, %	P Value
		No	Mortality, %	No	Mortality, %		
Mauritz [32]	Retrospective	31	90	27	70	−20	ns
Alarabi [33]	Retrospective	40	55	40	45	−10	ns
Mehta [34]	Retrospective	24	85	18	72	−13	ns
Kierdorf [20]	Retrospective	73	93	73	77	−16	< 0.05
Bellomo [35]	Retrospective	167	70	84	59	−11	ns
Bellomo [36]	Retrospective	84	70	76	45	−25	< 0.01
Kruczynski [37]	Retrospective	23	82	12	33	−49	< 0.01
Simpson [38]	Prospective	58	82	65	70	−12	ns
Kierdorf [39]	Prospective	47	65	48	60	−4.5	ns
Mehta [40]	Prospective	82	41.5	84	59.5	+18	ns

FIGURE 19-27

Continuous renal replacement therapy (CRRT) versus intermittent hemodialysis (IHD): effect on mortality. Despite significant advances in the management of acute renal failure (ARF) over the last four decades, the perception is that the associated mortality has not changed significantly [26]. Recent publications suggest that there may have been some improvement during the last decade [27]. Both IHD and peritoneal dialysis (PD) were the major therapies until a decade ago, and they improved the outcome from the 100% mortality of ARF to its current level. The effect of continuous renal replacement therapy on overall patient outcome is still unclear [28]. The major studies done in this area do not show a survival advantage for CRRT [29,30]. Although several investigators have not been able to demonstrate an advantage of these therapies in influencing mortality, we believe this may represent the difficulty in changing a global outcome which is impacted by several other factors [31]. It is probably more relevant to focus on other outcomes such as renal functional recovery rather than mortality. We believe that continued research is required in this area; however, there appears to be enough evidence to support the use of CRRT techniques as an alternative that may be preferable to IHD in treating ARF in an intensive care setting.

Future Directions

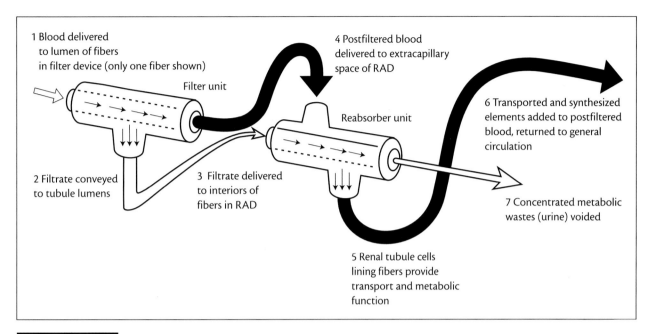

FIGURE 19-28

Schematic for the bioartificial kidney. As experience with these techniques grows, innovations in technology will likely keep pace. Over the last 3 years, most of the major manufacturers of dialysis equipment have developed new pumps dedicated for continuous renal replacement therapy (CRRT). Membrane technology is also evolving, and antithrombogenic membranes are on the horizon [41]. Finally the application of these therapies is likely to expand to other arenas, including the treatment of sepsis, congestive heart failure [42], and multi-organ failure [43]. An exciting area of innovative research is the development of a bioartificial tubule utilizing porcine tubular epithelial cells grown in a hollow fiber to add tubular function to the filtrative function provided by dialysis [44]. These devices are likely to be utilized in combination with CRRT to truly provide complete RRT in the near future. (*From* Humes HD [44]; with permission.)

References

1. Mehta RL: Therapeutic alternatives to renal replacement therapy for critically ill patients in acute renal failure. *Semin Nephro* 1994, 14:64–82.

2. Shapiro WB: The current status of Sorbent hemodialysis. *Semin Dial* 1990, 3:40–45.

3. Botella J, Ghezzi P, Sanz-Moreno C, *et al.*: Multicentric study on paired filtration dialysis as a short, highly efficient dialysis technique. *Nephrol Dial Transplant* 1991, 6:715–721.

4. Steiner RW: Continuous equilibration peritoneal dialysis in acute renal failure. *Perit Dial Intensive* 1989, 9:5–7.

5. Bellomo R, Ronco C, Mehta RL: Nomenclature for continuous renal replacement therapies. *Am J Kidney Dis* 1996, 28(5)S3:2–7.

6. Henderson LW: Hemofiltration: From the origin to the new wave. *Am J Kidney Dis* 1996, 28(5)S3:100–104.

7. Mehta RL: Renal replacement therapy for acute renal failure: Matching the method to the patient. *Semin Dial* 1993, 6:253–259.

8. Lindhout T: Biocompatability of extracorporeal blood treatment. Selection of hemostatic parameters. *Nephrol Dial Transplant* 1994, 9(Suppl. 2):83–89.

9. Ward RA: Effects of hemodialysis on corpulation and platelets: Are we measureing membrane biocompatability? *Nephrol Dial Transplant* 1995, 10(Suppl. 10):12–17.

10. Ronco C, Brendolan A, Crepaldi C, *et al.*: Importance of hollow fiber geometry in CAVH. *Contrib Nephrol* 1991, 15:175–178.

11. Mehta RL, McDonald BR, Aguilar MM, Ward DM: Regional citrate anticoagulation for continuous arteriovenous hemodialysis in critically ill patients. *Kidney Int* 1990, 38:976–981.

12. Grootendorst AF, Bouman C, Hoeben K, *et al.*: The role of continuous renal replacement therapy in sepsis multiorgan failure. *Am J Kidney Dis* 1996, 28(5) S3:S50–S57.

13. Kroh UF, Holl TJ, Steinhausser W: Management of drug dosing in continuous renal replacement therapy. *Semin Dial* 1996, 9:161–165.

14. Monson P, Mehta RL: Nutritional considerations in continuous renal replacement therapies. *Semin Dial* 1996, 9:152–160.

15. Golper TA: Indications, technical considerations, and strategies for renal replacement therapy in the intensive care unit. *J Intensiv Care Med* 1992, 7:310–317.

16. Mehta RL: Fluid management in continuous renal replacement therapy. *Semin Dial* 1996, 9:140–144.

17. Palevsky PM: Continuous renal replacement therapy component selection: replacement fluid and dialysate. *Semin Dial* 1996, 9:107–111.

18. Thomas AN, Guy JM, Kishen R, *et al.*: Comparison of lactate and bicarbonate buffered haemofiltration fluids: Use in critically ill patients. *Nephrol Dial Transplant* 1997, 12(6):1212–1217.

19. Golper TA: Continuous arteriovenous hemofiltration in acute renal failure. *Am J Kidney Dis* 1985, 6:373–386.

20. Kierdorf H: Continuous versus intermittent treatment: clinical results in acute renal failure. *Contrib Nephrol* 1991, 93:1–12.

21. Lauer

22. Paganini EP: Slow continuous hemofiltration and slow continuous ultrafiltration. *Trans Am Soc Artif Intern Organs* 1988, 34:63–66.

23. Schrier RW, Abraham HJ: Strategies in management of acute renal failure in the intensive therapy unit. In *Current Concepts in Critical Care: Acute Renal Failure in the Intensive Therapy Unit.* Edited by Bihari D, Neild G. Berlin:Springer-Verlag, 1990:193–214.

24. Van Bommel EFH, Bouvy ND, So KL, *et al.*: High risk surgical acute renal failure treated by continuous arterio venous hemodiafiltration: Metabolic control and outcomes in sixty patients. *Nephron* 1995, 70:185–196.

25. Paganini EP, Tapolyai M, Goormastic M, *et al.*: Establishing a dialysis therapy/patient outcome link in intensive care unit acute dialysis for patients with acute renal failure. *Am J Kidney Dis* 1996, 28(5)S3:81–90.

26. Wilkins RG, Faragher EB: Acute renal failure in an intensive care unit: Incidence, prediction and outcome. *Anesthesiology* 1983, 38:638.

27. Firth JD: Renal replacement therapy on the intensive care unit. *Q J Med* 1993, 86:75–77.

28. Bosworth C, Paganini EP, Cosentino F, *et al.*: Long term experience with continuous renal replacement therapy in intensive care unit acute renal failure. *Contrib Nephrol* 1991, 93:13–16.

29. Kierdorf H: Continuous versus intermittent treatment: Clinical results in acute renal failure. *Contrib Nephrol* 1991, 93:1–12.

30. Jakob SM, Frey FJ, Uhlinger DE: Does continuous renal replacement therapy favorably influence the outcome of patients? *Nephrol Dial Transplant* 1996, 11:1250–1235.

31. Mehta RL: Acute renal failure in the intensive care unit: Which outcomes should we measure? *Am J Kidney Dis* 1996, 28(5)S3:74–79.

32. Mauritz W, Sporn P, Schindler I, *et al.*: Acute renal failure in abdominal infection: comparison of hemodialysis and continuous arteriovenous hemofiltration. *Anasth Intensivther Notfallmed* 1986, 21:212–217.

33. Alarabi AA, Danielson BG, Wikstrom B, Wahlberg J: Outcome of continuous arteriovenous hemofiltration (CAVH) in one centre. *Ups J Med Sci* 1989, 94:299–303.

34. McDonald BR, Mehta RL: Decreased mortality in patients with acute renal failure undergoing continuous arteriovenous hemodialysis. *Contrib Nephrol* 1991, 93:51–56.

35. Bellomo R, Mansfield D, Rumble S, *et al.*: Acute renal failure in critical illness. Conventional dialysis versus acute continuous hemodiafiltration. *Am Soc Artif Intern Organs J* 1992, 38:654–657.

36. Bellomo R, Boyce N: Continuous venovenous hemodiafiltration compared with conventional dialysis in critically ill patients with acute renal failure. *Am Soc Artif Intern Organs J* 1993, 39:794–797.

37. Kruczynski K, Irvine-Bird K, Toffelmire EB, Morton AR: A comparison of continuous arteriovenous hemofiltration and intermittent hemodialysis in acute renal failure patients in the intensive care unit. *Am Soc Artif Intern Organs J* 1993, 39:778–781.

38. Simpson K, Allison MEM: Dialysis and acute renal failure: can mortality be improved? *Nephrol Dial Transplant* 1993, 8:946.

39. Kierdorf H: Einfuss der kontinuierlichen Hamofiltration auf Proteinkatabolismus, Mediatorsubstanzen und Prognose des akuten Nierenversagens [Habilitation-Thesis], Medical Faculty Technical University of Aachen, 1994.

40. Mehta RL, McDonald B, Pahl M, *et al.*: Continuous vs. intermittent dialysis for acute renal failure (ARF) in the ICU: Results from a randomized multicenter trial. Abstract A1044. *JASN* 1996, 7(9):1456.

41. Yang VC, Fu Y, Kim JS: A potential thrombogenic hemodialysis membranes with impaired blood compatibility. *ASAIO Trans* 1991, 37:M229–M232.

42. Canaud B, Leray-Moragues H, Garred LJ, *et al.*: Slow isolated ultrafiltration for the treatment of congestive heart failure. *Am J Kidney Dis* 1996, 28(5)S3:67–73.

43. Druml W: Prophylactic use of continuous renal replacement therapies in patients with normal renal function. *Am J Kidney Dis* 1996, 28(5)S3:114–120.

44. Humes HD, Mackay SM, Funke AJ, Buffington DA: The bioartificial renal tuble assist device to enhance CRRT in acute renal failure. *Am J Kidney Dis* 1997, 30(Suppl. 4):S28–S30.

Index

Page numbers followed by *t* indicate tables.

Index

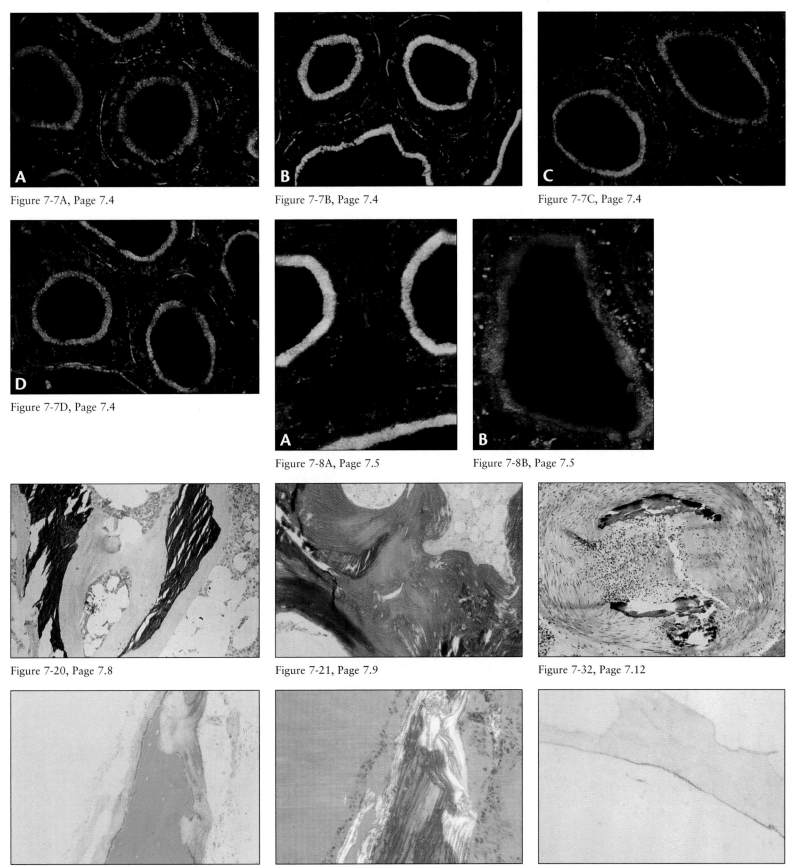

Figure 7-7A, Page 7.4

Figure 7-7B, Page 7.4

Figure 7-7C, Page 7.4

Figure 7-7D, Page 7.4

Figure 7-8A, Page 7.5

Figure 7-8B, Page 7.5

Figure 7-20, Page 7.8

Figure 7-21, Page 7.9

Figure 7-32, Page 7.12

Figure 7-35, Page 7.13

Figure 7-36, Page 7.13

Figure 7-37, Page 7.13

Color Plates

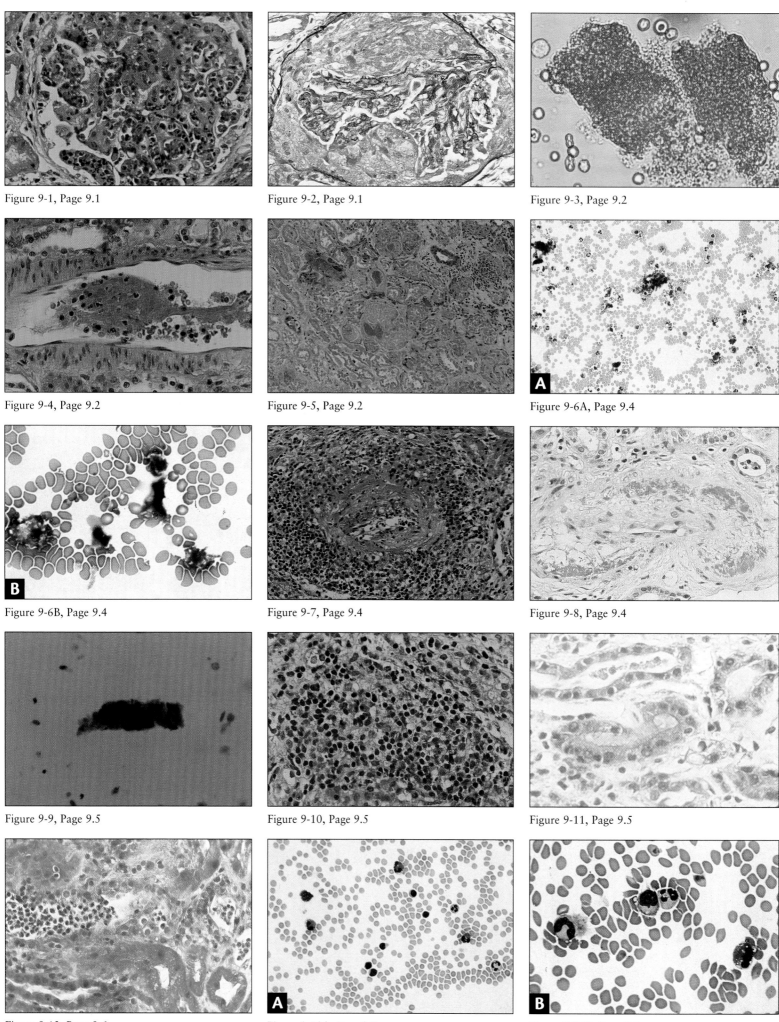

Figure 9-1, Page 9.1

Figure 9-2, Page 9.1

Figure 9-3, Page 9.2

Figure 9-4, Page 9.2

Figure 9-5, Page 9.2

Figure 9-6A, Page 9.4

Figure 9-6B, Page 9.4

Figure 9-7, Page 9.4

Figure 9-8, Page 9.4

Figure 9-9, Page 9.5

Figure 9-10, Page 9.5

Figure 9-11, Page 9.5

Figure 9-12, Page 9.6

Figure 9-13A, Page 9.6

Figure 9-13B, Page 9.6

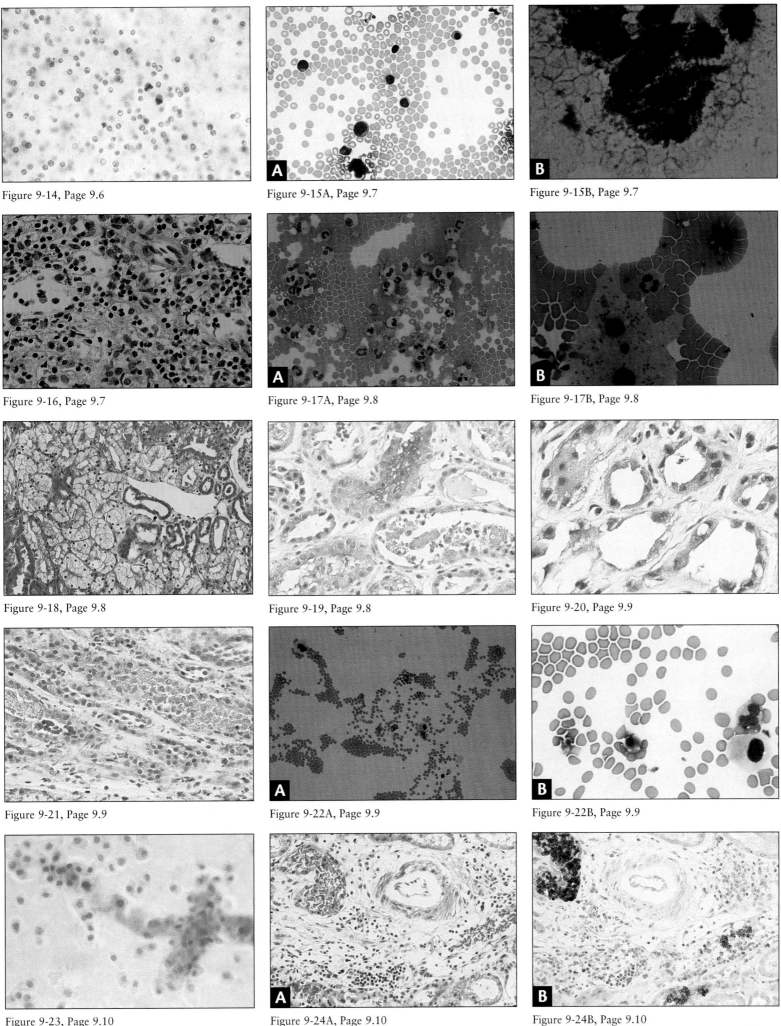

Figure 9-14, Page 9.6

Figure 9-15A, Page 9.7

Figure 9-15B, Page 9.7

Figure 9-16, Page 9.7

Figure 9-17A, Page 9.8

Figure 9-17B, Page 9.8

Figure 9-18, Page 9.8

Figure 9-19, Page 9.8

Figure 9-20, Page 9.9

Figure 9-21, Page 9.9

Figure 9-22A, Page 9.9

Figure 9-22B, Page 9.9

Figure 9-23, Page 9.10

Figure 9-24A, Page 9.10

Figure 9-24B, Page 9.10

Color Plates

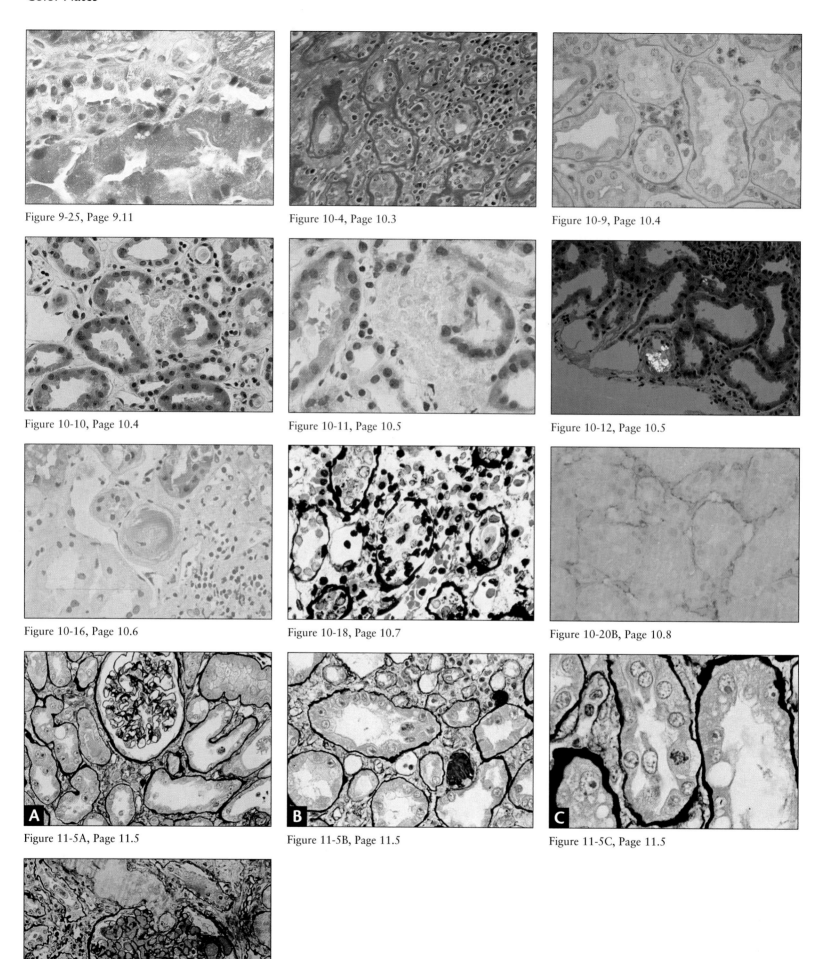

Figure 9-25, Page 9.11

Figure 10-4, Page 10.3

Figure 10-9, Page 10.4

Figure 10-10, Page 10.4

Figure 10-11, Page 10.5

Figure 10-12, Page 10.5

Figure 10-16, Page 10.6

Figure 10-18, Page 10.7

Figure 10-20B, Page 10.8

Figure 11-5A, Page 11.5

Figure 11-5B, Page 11.5

Figure 11-5C, Page 11.5

Figure 11-13, Page 11.10